Ordinary Lives, Death, and Social Class

Ordinary Lives, Death, and Social Class

Dublin City Coroner's Court, 1876–1902

CIARA BREATHNACH

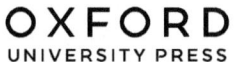

OXFORD
UNIVERSITY PRESS

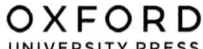

Great Clarendon Street, Oxford, OX2 6DP,
United Kingdom

Oxford University Press is a department of the University of Oxford.
It furthers the University's objective of excellence in research, scholarship,
and education by publishing worldwide. Oxford is a registered trade mark of
Oxford University Press in the UK and in certain other countries

First Edition published in 2022

Impression: 1

Published in the United States of America by Oxford University Press
198 Madison Avenue, New York, NY 10016, United States of America

British Library Cataloguing in Publication Data

Data available

Library of Congress Control Number: 2022932393

ISBN 978–0–19–886578–0

DOI: 10.1093/oso/9780198865780.001.0001

Printed and bound by
CPI Group (UK) Ltd, Croydon, CR0 4YY

I ndíl chuimhne Kathleen Walsh

Acknowledgements

I began gathering data for this book in 2016; initially I used it to formulate my thoughts for a funding application and I was fortunate to have been the recipient of an Irish Research Council Laureate Award 2018–22 for a project entitled Death and Burial Data Ireland, 1864–1922. I acknowledge this generous support. On returning to the research in autumn 2018, I met Cathryn Steele who encouraged me to put a proposal together. It has been a pleasure to work with her since.

Over the past five years I have amassed a debt of gratitude in a number of quarters. First I would like to thank the very wonderful and sadly, late, Gregory O'Connor; both he and Brian Donnelly have encouraged me greatly over the years and provided sage advice and fascinating insights into the records held at the National Archives of Ireland (NAI). Other NAI stalwarts Zoë Reid, Tom Quinlan, Elizabeth McAvoy, Natalie Milne, Suzanne Bedell, Paddy Sarsfield, Ken Robinson, Ken Martin, Brian Birmingham, Darren Kelly, and Jennifer Nolan deserve special mention for their assistance and problem-solving skills during the global pandemic. Similarly, Katherine McSharry, Justin Furlong, Berni Metcalfe, James Harte, and Glenn Dunne at the National Library of Ireland did likewise. I am also very grateful to Eibhlin Colgan, Archive Manager, Guinness Archives, who has been immensely helpful over the past few years. There are many other librarians and archivists who have helped me along my way and I thank them in the footnotes. Maith sibh uilig.

I was fortunate to have Dr Laurence M. Geary as a PhD supervisor; he continues to be an excellent mentor and friend. I have had the benefit of the wisdom of incredible female scholars, Professor Barbara Brookes (who gave me a start in academia in 2002 at the University of Otago); Professors Tiziana Margaria, Orla Muldoon, Lucia Pozzi and Oonagh Walsh have acted as generous mentors, collaborators, and referees when called upon. Several others, Professors Eunan O' Halpin, Anthony McElligott, Mary Kelly, Laura D. Kelley, Thomas Bayer, Erika Hanna, Leanne McCormick, Elaine Farrell, Andrew Sneddon, Peter Hession, Shane Ewan, Rebecca Wynter, Jonathan Reinarz, Sanjoy Bhattacharya, and Niall Bergin have enriched this work and helped in various ways. My students past and present at the University of Limerick are a joy; they have moulded me into the historian that I am. I must mention former and current research students Dr Rose Molloy, Dr Jutta Kruse, Claire McCormick, Maëlle Le Roux, Barbara Watts, Ian Walsh, Stuart Clancy, Helene Haak, Rafflesia Khan, and Mathew Ayodele.

I am very grateful to my fond friends Dr Catherine Lawless, Stephanie Lawless, and Dr Sarah-Anne Buckley who generously read sections of this book, and Dr Rachel Murphy who drew maps and kindly untangled complex genealogical conundrums. Errors are, of course, all mine. Thanks to Ruth Stokes, Sarah Walsh, Catherine Griffin, and Sineád O'Gara for the decades of friendship and laughter. Kevin Maguire, you fill my days with happiness and fun, and have discussed, mapped, and lived this project with me, and much else besides. I cannot thank you enough.

I have to acknowledge my family, especially my sister Deirdre Walsh and nephew Thomas Walsh who took on the task of primary carers for our mother until she passed in September 2021. This book is dedicated to Kathleen Walsh (née Quill of Ballynoe, Causeway), who regularly applied gentle pressure by inquiring when precisely it would be finished, as only a mother can. Much of this book was written and edited as I sat beside her; it is every bit hers as it is mine. Our days are tinged with sadness without you, codladh sámh Mama you 'have done enough in this world'.

Contents

List of Figures, Maps, and Tables

Figures

Maps

Tables

Introduction

Between 3 p.m. and 4 p.m. on 21 April 1900, 26-year-old John Healy rode a brick-laden horse-drawn hackney car down Saint Augustine Street, which linked the busier thoroughfares of Thomas Street and the South Quays of the River Liffey (Figure 0.1 and Map 0.1).[1] As he proceeded down the natural gradient of that street, the horse suddenly bolted. In that moment Healy was thrown forward from his perch; he landed on the uneven cobblestoned street surface and one of the carriage wheels passed over his abdomen. According to the Dublin Metropolitan Police (DMP) preliminary report, three local residents witnessed the accident and all agreed that the impetus for the chain of events was that the horse startled and 'the breeching broke'.[2] Constable Thomas Donohue, registration number 39D,[3] was nearby and Thomas Keogh who was passing in his hackney car (a horse-drawn vehicle colloquially known as an H-car) stopped to give assistance. Together they immediately conveyed Healy to Jervis Street Hospital, located but a short distance away on the north side of the River Liffey.[4] After Healy was admitted to hospital, he was conscious and corroborated the evidence provided in the witness statements to Constable Donohue. His medical prognosis, provided by Resident Physician, Dr Carrol O'Sullivan, was grim as he had suffered serious abdominal trauma and profuse haemorrhaging: Healy, who was described as a labourer living at 1 Malpas Street, died at 7.30 a.m. the following morning.[5] Although a straightforward case of accidental death it proceeded to inquest. It is a significant marker for this study because it was the first case to be

---

[1] In 2020 the collection was assigned a new call reference as follows: National Archives of Ireland/ Crown and Peace/Dublin/Office of Coroner/number of Inquest (NAI/CP/DN/10/1/1). In that configuration no provisions were made for years, so hereafter inquests will be cited by archive/year/number (e.g. NAI/1900/1 for John Healy). Inquests are contained in individual numbered envelopes and can include any number of pages—from two to fifty pages of evidence. Witness statements are not always individually dated, so the date of inquest is used in such instances.

[2] Witnesses were named as follows: Patrick Jordan, 3 Lamb Alley; James Byrne, 13 Walls Lane; and John Cripp, 19 Saint Augustine Street.

[3] For policing purposes, Dublin City centre was arranged into alphabetically named 'divisions' established as A (Castle), B (College), C (Rotunda), and D (Barrack). In 1900, with the redrawing of the city boundary, E (Donnybrook) and F (Kingstown) were added. For a thorough discussion, see Anastasia Dukova, *A History of the Dublin Metropolitan Police and Its Colonial Legacy* (Basingstoke, 2016), p. 57.

[4] In accordance with the Dublin Carriage Act, 1853 (16 &17 Vic.) c.112, Hackney cars were required to be licensed and registered with the local authorities; each received a number. Keogh was from 10 Wood Quay, his hackney car licence number was 1123.

[5] *Dublin Evening Mail*, 21 April 1900; *Freeman's Journal*, 23 April 1900.

Ordinary Lives, Death, and Social Class: Dublin City Coroner's Court, 1876–1902. Ciara Breathnach, Oxford University Press. © Ciara Breathnach 2022. DOI: 10.1093/oso/9780198865780.003.0001

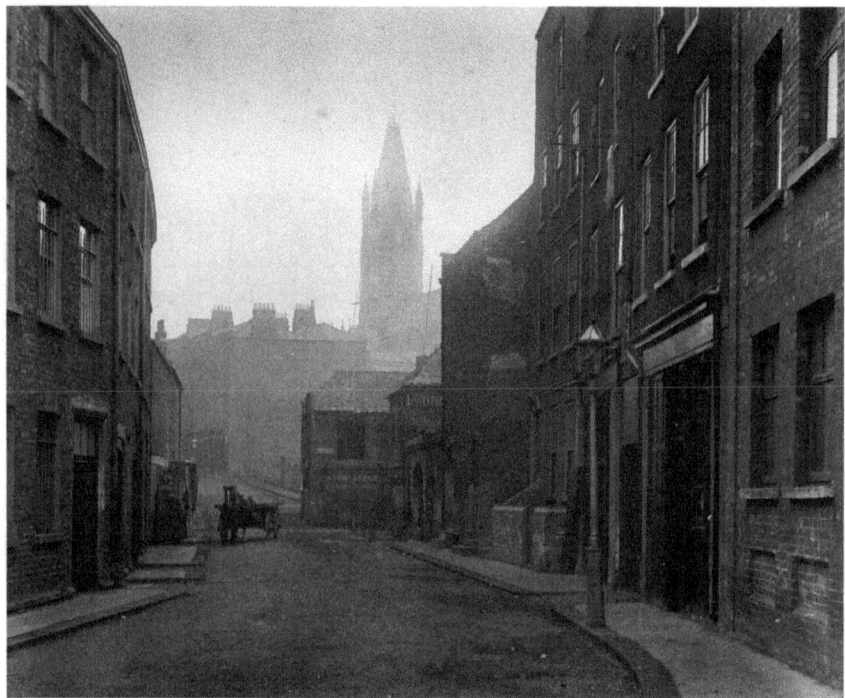

Figure 0.1 Saint Augustine Street from the Quays *c.*1891

Source: National Library of Ireland (NLI) JL15, photographer James Talbot Power. Image reproduction courtesy of the National Library of Ireland.

filed under the tenure of the long-serving Dr Louis Aloysius Byrne, who was elected coroner for the city on 19 April 1900 and served in that post until 1932.[6]

Coroners' inquests are a combination of eyewitness testimony, expert medico-legal language, detailed minutiae of people, places, and occupational identities pinned to a moment in time. Thus they have a simultaneous capacity to reveal histories from both above and below. Rich in geographical, socio-economic, cultural, class, and medical detail, these records collated in a liminal setting about the hour of death bear incredible witness to what has often been termed 'ordinary lives'. Although the term 'ordinary lives' to distinguish between the political elite and the 'masses' is itself contested by social historians, I use it in my title very specifically as it best describes the people coming before the coroners' courts.[7] Ordinariness is an entirely relative concept that hinges on temporal and spatial

[6] *Daily Irish Independent*, 20 April 1900. Dr Louis A. Byrne, Kirkpatrick Index, Royal College of Physicians of Ireland (RCPI) Archive. I am grateful to Harriet Wheelock, archivist RCPI for her assistance. As Vaughan notes, the coroner was the only elected official in local government. W.E. Vaughan, *Murder Trials in Ireland, 1836–1914* (Dublin, 2009), p. 41.

[7] Raphael Samuel, *Theatres of Memory: Past and Present in Contemporary Culture* (London, 1996), pp. 16, 160, 431 uses the term in inverted commas to delineate his concerns.

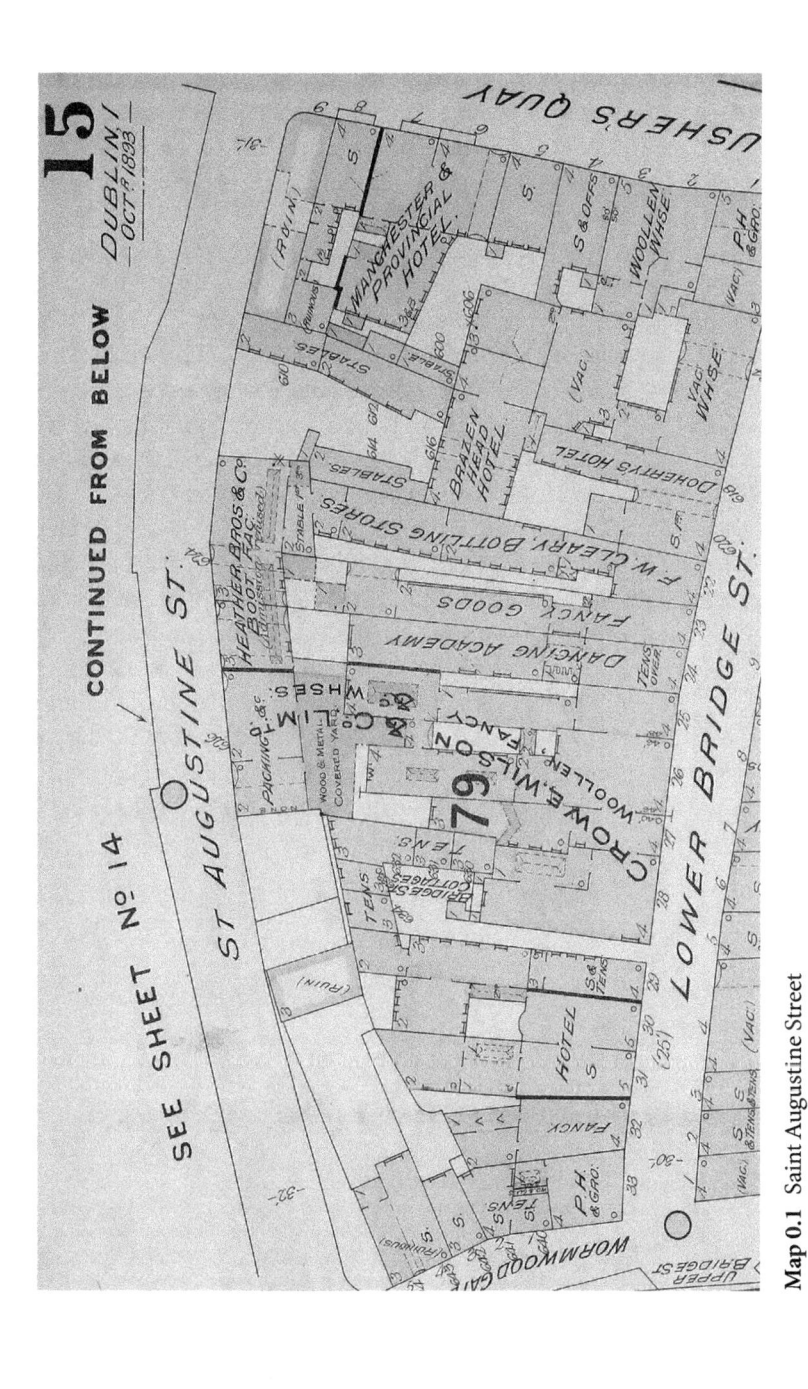

Map 0.1 Saint Augustine Street

Source: British Library 145.b.4. (2). Charles E. Goad, Dublin Map 15.2, 1893. Insurance Plan of the City of Dublin Vol. 1: sheet 15-1 enhanced and modified by author. Available at http://www.bl.uk/onlinegallery/onlineex/firemaps/ireland/largeimage146707.html (accessed 3 February 2019).

parameters to find meaning, and it is often taken for granted. As Claire Langhamer has asserted in her discussion of post-Second World War British identity and local politics, it 'was not necessarily a stable identity. Rather it was bestowed, performed or addressed within specific contexts for particular purposes.'[8] As a conceptual framework, ordinariness operates on a multiplicity of levels and in a highly gendered fashion: the experience of 'ordinary life' for working-class women was subject to far more limitations than that of working-class men in Dublin City.

Bearing all the hallmarks of an emergency medical situation, John Healy's tragic accident brought witnesses into a medico-legal scenario unwittingly and sometimes unwillingly. Despite the statutory requirement being in place since 1864, Healy's birth was unregistered.[9] In fact, the only other civil record to show that he had lived also emanated from the coroner's office when it conveyed the certificate necessary to register his death on 5 June.[10] At that point his age was corrected from 26 to 24 years old.[11] Although circumstances differed from case to case, the scenario was the same and was replicated with extraordinary frequency throughout Dublin City, which averaged about three hundred inquests per year. In this book I present a broad range of the ordinary, the everyday of life and death, as opposed to deaths in years of national mortality crises, for instance in 1881 owing to three successive crop failures or the 1918/19 flu pandemic.[12] For that reason I chose John Healy's case to ground the study; his death is the first in the series of 611 consecutive cases dating from 1900 to 1902 that form the basis of this book (NAI/Dataset 1900–1902). His case represents the normal rhythm of the everyday and the deaths that presented to the Dublin City coroner's court: suspicious deaths, which form the basis of the final section of the book, were the exception.

---

[8] Claire Langhamer, "Who the hell are ordinary people?' Ordinariness as a category of historical analysis', *Transactions of the Royal Historical Society*, 28 (2018), pp. 175–95 at 183. See also 'Introduction', Claire Langhamer, *The English in Love: The Intimate Story of an Emotional Revolution* (Oxford, 2013).

[9] It seems that he was baptised on 9 January 1872, making him 28 years of age when he died: see https://churchrecords.irishgenealogy.ie/churchrecords/display-pdf.jsp?pdfName=st.catherine_baptisms_mf_1811-1880_ba_0695. I am grateful to Dr Rachel Murphy for assistance in tracking this down, via his brother Martin's baptism which gave his mother's maiden name of Eliza Flinter.

[10] *Registration of Deaths in Ireland: A Statistical Nosology, Comprising the Causes of Death, Classified and Alphabetically Arranged* (Dublin, 1864), p. 31: https://civilrecords.irishgenealogy.ie/churchrecords/images/deaths_returns/deaths_1900/05762/4627964.pdf (accessed 3 August 2019).

[11] See https://civilrecords.irishgenealogy.ie/churchrecords/images/birth_returns/births_1877/03024/2108365.pdf (accessed 3 August 2019). On the night of 31 March 1901, his household recorded his widowed mother Elizabeth, brother Martin, and sister Elizabeth, aged 60, 32, and 30, respectively, still sharing a room at 1.2 Malpas Street: http://www.census.nationalarchives.ie/reels/nai003803863/ (accessed 3 August 2019).

[12] Fearghal McGarry, *The Rising: Ireland Easter 1916* (Oxford, 2017); Ida Milne, *Stacking the Coffins: The 1918–19 Flu Pandemic in Ireland* (Manchester, 2018); Patricia Marsh, *The Spanish Flu in Ireland: A Socio-Economic Shock to Ireland, 1918–1919* (London, 2021); Ciara Breathnach and Brian Gurrin, 'Maternal mortality, Dublin 1864–1905', *Social History of Medicine*, 31:1 (2018), pp. 79–105.

The key legislation underpinning the modern court was the 1846 Coroners (Ireland) Act, which divided the country into administrative districts that in turn could administer the appointment and remuneration of personnel.[13] This modern iteration was similar in structure and form to the system in England and Wales, but it was completely separate.[14] The Irish court had in fact a very long lineage, which Michael J. Clark traces to the mid-thirteenth century.[15] An entirely different process, under the auspices of the legal system, was in place in Scotland. Fatal accident inquiries known as precognitions, were undertaken by the Procurator Fiscal, who was a local crown solicitor and the process was overseen by the Lord Advocate.[16]

On the discovery of a body in Ireland, police were supposed to be notified and they were tasked with carrying out preliminary investigations. That inquiry generated a police report, which was sent to the coroner. The coroner had the discretion to decide if an inquest was deemed necessary. If called, the next procedural stage was the issue of a precept to summon a jury. Empanelment of juries was a DMP task. Coronial court juries were composed of no fewer than twelve and up to twenty-three local men from 1881 to 1926, and according to section 22 of the 1846 act they were to be residents and rate-payers of over £4.[17] By these decrees jurors were ordinarily of a higher social standing than the subjects of the Dublin City coroner's court. Irrespective of the property requirement, the good moral standing of jurors was important, as the integrity of subsequent criminal cases could be compromised if inquisitions were quashed.[18] Once assembled jury members were sworn in, usually by the clerk of the court, their first task was to formally view the body; they had to listen to the evidence of medical experts and witnesses, agree a verdict, and sign or put their mark to the inquisition form.[19]

Verdicts, which identified cause of death, were usually established by the facts presented by medical experts arising from a post-mortem examination; they were agreed and returned by the jury. Following the Registration of Births and Deaths Ireland Act 1863 these were submitted by the coroner verbatim and in writing to

---

[13] Coroners (Ireland) Act, 1846 (9 & 10 Vic.) c. 37.

[14] Ian Burney's work has traced the election, powers, and evolution of county and borough coroners in England and Wales. Ian Burney, *Bodies of Evidence: Medicine and the Politics of the English Inquest, 1830–1926* (Baltimore, 2000), pp. 3–5.

[15] Michael J. Clark, 'General practice and coroner's practice: medico-legal work and the Irish medical profession, c.1830–c.1890', in Catherine Cox and Maria Luddy (eds), *Cultures of Care in Irish Medical History, 1750–1970* (Basingstoke, 2010), pp. 37–56.

[16] Fatal Accidents Inquiry (Scotland) Act, 1895 (58 & 59 Vic.) c. 36. Criminal and judicial statistics, 1880, Ireland, Part I, Police—criminal proceedings—prisons; Part II, Civil proceedings in central and larger and smaller district courts [C.3028], p. 13.

[17] Coroners (Ireland) Act 1881 (44 & 45 Vic.) c. 35. The 1846 Act stipulated 'a sufficient number' with respect to jurors but did not state how many.

[18] William G. Huband, *A Practical Treatise on the Law Relating to the Grand Jury in Criminal Cases, the Coroner's Jury and the Petty Jury in Ireland* (London, 1896), p. 239.

[19] Coroners (Ireland) Act, 1846 (9 & 10 Vic.) c. 37. Under section 43, jurors were required to view the body.

the local registrar.[20] The jury was permitted to express opinions in riders, which were sometimes used to praise the heroic deeds of civilians and emergency services alike, but they were used primarily to allocate or exonerate people from blame. There are unmistakeable undertones of morality and religiosity in all cases, but some were overt: one jury rider berated a man named John Lane for acting in 'an unchristian manner.'[21] Those who tried to use the court for legal, sectarian, or political gain received short shrift from the coroner; its purpose was clearly defined under statute and he enforced the law without hesitation. It was a busy court of record that occasionally dealt with three or more inquisitions in one day. On days with multiple cases, invariably the same jury was used for all, but with slight variations in terms of foreman, or juror number 1.

Although separated in legislative terms, work by Elizabeth T. Hurren, Steven King, Ian Burney, Vicky Holmes, Mary Beth Emerlichs, Joe Sim, and Tony Ward on the English coronial courts shows that they were important platforms for the poor and, in terms of social class, the profile of the Irish system in the post-Famine era was no different.[22] Middle-class deaths are largely absent from this study because Dublin City by the turn of the twentieth century was disproportionately populated by the working-class poor who lived in decrepit over-crowded tenements. There are a few exceptions, like Gerald Barry who was 4 years and 6 months old when he died at his home in the opulent surrounds of 50 Merrion Square, in the south side of the city.[23] He had returned from a walk with his nurse Lizzie Rimmer and proceeded to run upstairs. Shortly after that he fell from an open window in the top back room; doctors were called and arrived promptly, but to no avail and the child died from his devastating head injuries.[24] Another unusual case was that of Richard Davies who was found on the landing of his house at 5 Capel Street following 'an overdose of liquor'. A printer and window card writer with no relatives in Ireland but a son in Manchester, he stands apart

---

[20] An Act for the Registration of Births and Deaths in Ireland, 1863 (26 & 27 Vic.) c. 11, section 38.

[21] NAI/1900/207 Inquest on the body of James Moran, 31 December 1900. When James Moran took a fall and sustained a head injury late one evening, his neighbours mistook his groans for that of animals from an adjacent yard on Saint Augustine Street and nobody came to his assistance.

[22] Elizabeth T. Hurren, 'Remaking the medico-legal scene: a social history of the late-Victorian coroner in Oxford', *Journal of the History of Medicine and Allied Sciences*, 65:2 (2010), pp. 207–52; Elizabeth T. Hurren and Steven King, 'Courtship at the coroner's court', *Social History*, 40:2 (2015), pp. 185–207; Burney, *Bodies of Evidence*; Mary Beth Emmerichs, 'Getting away with murder? Homicide and the coroners in 19th century London', *Social Science History*, 25:1 (2001), pp. 93–100; Vicky Holmes, 'Death of an infant', *Home Cultures*, 11:3 (2014), pp. 305–31; V. Holmes, 'Absent fireguards and burnt children: coroners and the development of clause 15 of the Children Act 1908', *Law, Crime, and History*, 2 (2012), pp. 21–58; Joe Sim and Tony Ward, 'The magistrate of the poor? Coroners and deaths in custody in nineteenth-century England', in Michael Clark and Catherine Crawford (eds), *Legal Medicine in History* (Cambridge, 1994), pp. 245–67.

[23] NAI/1901/141 Inquest on the body of Gerald Barry, 18 May 1901, http://www.census.national-archives.ie/reels/nai003818331/. Gerald was the middle of five children. His father Patrick Joseph was a doctor originally from County Clare. Elizabeth 'Lizzie' Rimmer, aged 21, was described as a 'nurse' and domestic servant.

[24] NAI/1901/141 Inquest on the body of Gerald Barry, 18 May 1901; *Munster Express*, 25 May 1901.

from other cases because he had substantial sums of money in the Hibernian & Munster and Leinster banks amounting to £850 and a further deposit of £10 13s. 6d. in Whites Bank.[25]

More typical of the profile of the Dublin City coronial court was the case of John Healy, whose age and circumstances of death ensured that his case progressed from the DMP report to the order of inquest. It was held at Jervis Street Hospital, where a jury of fourteen local men gave its verdict of 'accidental death'. Benevolent societies had a strong presence in early twentieth-century Dublin, but little survives by way of records and we have no way of knowing if Healy was a member. Nuanced by socio-economic sensitivities, the jury added an all-important rider attaching 'no blame to anyone'; instead, the court expressed its 'heartfelt' sympathies to his relatives. In that instance the owner of the H-car was not an affluent employer like, for instance, the nearby Messrs Guinness & Co. Brewery, so no pressure was brought to bear for compensation.[26]

Situating Coronial Court Records: Power, Class, and Agency

Coronial court records, as scholars of the British courts have so ably shown, offer unprecedented access to ordinary lives and have enormous potential to deepen our understanding of medico-legal literacy.[27] I argue and show throughout this book that these records contain clear voices of the poor even if their experiences are mediated through the DMP and the court clerk. This contention raises fundamental textual and contextual problems: where, how, and can we locate coronial court records in terms of agency of the poor and authenticity of voices. With respect to genre, depositions both in witness statements to the DMP and subsequently taken in evidence at the coroner's court bear more of a resemblance to criminal court records than any other classification of document.[28] But unlike the

---

[25] NAI/1901/102 Inquest on the body of Charles Young, 10 April 1901. He had no relatives in Ireland, a son in Manchester.

[26] NAI/1900/1 Inquest on the body of John Healy, 21 April 1900. The hackney car was the property of James Maher, 134 Cork Street; he is not listed in directories as being a substantial service provider. In the 1901 census his occupation is listed as general labourer http://www.census.nationalarchives.ie/reels/nai003713874/ (accessed 2 April 2021). In England, the law of deodands existed from the eleventh century until the Fatal Accidents Act, 1846 (9th & 10th Vict.) c. 62. It permitted the forfeiture of good or animals responsible for death. See William G. Huband, *A Practical Treatise on the Law Relating to the Grand Jury in Criminal Cases, the Coroner's Jury and the Petty Jury in Ireland* (London, 1896), p. 25; Caoimhe Gethings, 'Not so saved by the bell: the deodand in Irish and English law', *Irish law Times*, 38:15 (2020), pp. 223–8. Deaths in the workplace and the compensation of relatives are discussed further in Chapter 4.

[27] Holmes, 'Death of an infant', pp. 305–31; Holmes, 'Absent fireguards and burnt children', pp. 21–58; Hurren, 'Remaking the medico-legal scene', pp. 207–52; Hurren and King 'Courtship at the coroner's court', pp. 185–207; Mary Beth Emmerichs, 'Getting away with murder?', pp. 93–100.

[28] William Reddy, *The Navigation of Feelings: A Framework for the History of Emotions* (Cambridge, 2001).

criminal setting the coronial court inquest occurred usually within hours and not more than a day after the discovery of the body, and apart from age discrepancies, witness statements were usually in step with one another. Dishonesty was not as much of a factor in the coroners' as it would have been in adversarial courts, where witnesses had time to prepare their responses and performativity which, as Katie Barclay argues, was perhaps more of a factor.[29]

Viewed from the perspective of the Dublin City coroner's court, urban streetscapes at the turn of the twentieth century were fraught with the perils of licensed yet inconsistently regulated, fast-moving and powerful draft horses, carts, carriages, trams, and trains, which combined with uneven surfaces and falling debris to pose pervasive threats to life. For the risk-averse poor, the very architecture of the home offered cold comfort; crumbling tenements, poor lighting, limited space, and inadequate cooking facilities led to falls, burns, and scalds, which featured heavily as cause of 'accidental death' in domestic settings, especially in cases concerning children. In both public and domestic spaces, periodic eruptions of violence often precipitated deaths in suspicious circumstances. Dublin City at the turn of the nineteenth century embraced and resisted modernity in equal measures, and it was a very challenging place in which to live and work. Facets of Dublin life contributed greatly to the untimely deaths coming before Dr Byrne.

City life was bounded by the physical thresholds of the River Liffey and the Grand and Royal Canals, but other dynamics like the law, morality, class, and gender expectations were in perpetual silent motion. It is important for this study to consider the overarching implications of the Foucauldian concept of biopower (*biopouvoir*, 'an explosion of numerous and diverse techniques for achieving the subjugation of bodies and the control of populations'[30]) as a framework to outline and examine the power dynamics of late Victorian Dublin.[31] Together with governmentality (the way in which the state exercises control over, or governs, the body of its populace), biopower was simply mentioned and not developed by Michel Foucault during his 1970s lectures at the Collège de France, Paris. Conceptually he was building on his previous theories on power, institutions, medicalisation, and sexuality but it was other scholars who developed the field.[32] With few exceptions, Foucauldian hypotheses have not been applied to Irish historical studies of power, which has focused predominantly on 'hard' political power from empirical perspectives.[33] Both biopower and governmentality had a

[29] Katie Barclay, 'Singing and lower-class masculinity in the Dublin Magistrate's Court, 1800–1845', *Journal of Social History*, 47:3 (2014), pp. 746–68; Katie Barclay, *Men on Trial: Performing Emotion, Embodiment and Identity in Ireland, 1800–45* (Manchester, 2019).

[30] Michel Foucault, *The History of Sexuality. Volume I: An Introduction*, translated from the French by Robert Hurley (New York, 1978), p. 140.

[31] Patrick Joyce, *The Rule of Freedom: Liberalism and the Modern City* (London, 2003).

[32] Paul Rabinow and Nikolas Rose, 'Biopower today', *BioSocieties*, 1 (2006), pp. 195–217.

[33] Tom Inglis, 'Origins and legacies of Irish prudery: sexuality and social control in modern Ireland', *Éire-Ireland*, 30:3–4 (2005), pp. 9–37; Tom Inglis, 'Foucault, Bourdieu and the field of Irish sexuality', *Irish Journal of Sociology*, 7 (1997), pp. 5–28.

strong bearing on the lives of ordinary people; its creeping progress permitted the state an increasing level of knowledge and control over what was previously considered personal and private.

Although a deposed capital, opportunities for social mobility gradually emerged in the late nineteenth century for the Roman Catholic elite but, for the poor, especially the Dublin-born poor, class lines continued to prove impenetrable until educational opportunities and labour rights were more firmly established. Central to the maintenance of these social barriers in Dublin City was its physical and municipal organisation, which when combined with surveillance mechanisms of civil registration and policing ensured conformity with instruments of biopower and governmentality. Nikolas Rose and Carlos Novas have termed these touchpoints with officialdom 'biological citizenship' and with respect to individual inquests the fear of engagement with such instruments, especially for the most disadvantaged, is apparent.[34] In the context of the coroner's court, medical experts, police constables, fire brigade officers, ambulance drivers, and jurors all played their part in the surveillance of the poor and there are glimpses of compassion, and indeed cruelty, in the ways in which regulations were implemented.[35] A cursory example of this compassion is the use of euphemistic language or alternative causes of death in cases of suicide, which could have longer-term ramifications for relatives of the deceased.[36] Empathy was not selflessly motivated; many of these surveillance foot soldiers were only just a rung above the very poor and there was always a sense that in precarious times hard won upward mobility gains could be easily lost.[37]

Notoriously challenging and elusive, the Irish poor had a strong track record of evading the authorities and the instruments of biopower where possible. Modern biopower depends heavily on biopolitics (technologies of power) and has its origins in the late nineteenth century when the clinical gaze in Ireland was gradually vested with political and legal authority. Together biopower, governmentality, and biopolitics unhinged the hegemony of traditional modes of corporeal care and civil, religious, and legal codes in nineteenth-century Ireland.[38] The architecture of modern biopower was introduced in quick succession; unlike England, Scotland and Wales, Ireland did not have an 'old' Poor Law. Roman Catholics

---

[34] Nikolas Rose and Carlos Novas, 'Biological citizenship', in Aihwa Ong and Stephen J. Collier (eds), *Global Assemblages: Technology, Politics, and Ethics as Anthropological Problems* (Oxford, 2004), pp. 439–63.

[35] NSPCC Inspectors were involved to a much lesser extent in the coronial courts: see Chapter 3.

[36] Graham Mooney, *Intrusive Interventions: Public Health, Domestic Space, and Infectious Disease Surveillance in England 1840–1914* (Rochester, 2015).

[37] David Dickson, *Dublin: The Making of a Capital City* (Dublin, 2014), pp. 379–424 adopts an empirical approach to provide an overview of the city's power brokerage and municipal innovations, 1880–1913.

[38] Foucault, *The History of Sexuality. Volume I*, p. 141.

numbered approximately 75 per cent of the entire populace in the post-Famine period; for most, the religious rites of baptism took precedence over birth registration and burial rites over death registration. The poor had much to learn. Several acts were passed to count the people from the introduction of civil registration of births, deaths, and marriages in 1864 to the decennial census conducted from 1821 to 1911.[39] A total of 151 DMP constables were involved in the 1901 enumeration of Dublin City, which was overseen by six district inspectors. Each enumerator was responsible for an average of 2,533 people, of a total population of 332,471, within the newly defined city parameters.[40] This engagement brought DMP constables into tenements and homes. In turn this amplified their visibility, it bolstered their ability to create and maintain relationships, and offered the opportunity to keep watch over communities.

In instances where relatives were compliant with birth and death registration, General Registrar Office (GRO) data can give the parameters of a life course, but compliance was not always a given.[41] With Brian Gurrin, I have described elsewhere how the registrar general used burial records to correct deficient returns in Dublin City from 1878 onwards and raised questions about personal agency, and resistance either passive or active (aware of the laws and deliberately defying) to the agents of biopower.[42] Passive resistance was usually described as 'ignorance of the law', which is problematic. Ignorance places responsibility for medico-legal literacy on individuals and implies that the function of the state and its instruments is simply to police and monitor observance of the law without actively engaging in educating the populace about systems and processes.[43] The Annual Reports of the Registrar General (ARRG) included a section on the number of prosecutions brought before the petty sessions for non-compliance with the civil registration acts. Although rare, there are examples of abuse of the acts, like the case of a man who was prosecuted in 1894 for attempting to register the birth of a fictitious child presumably to commit life insurance policy fraud at a later date. Far more common were cases of underreporting of life events, some of which came before the lower courts.[44] In 1900, only 612 offences against the registration acts were registered nationally, resulting in eighty-nine prosecutions and forty-seven convictions for neglect to register marriages, births, and deaths; neglect of a

---

[39] An Act for the Registration of Births and Deaths in Ireland, 1863 (26 & 27 Vic.) c. 11.

[40] Census of Ireland, 1901, Part II, General report with illustrative maps and diagrams, tables, and appendix [Cd. 1190], p. 4.

[41] I am grateful to the General Registrar Office for permission to access and use these data for research and publication purposes.

[42] Breathnach and Gurrin, 'Maternal mortality, Dublin 1864–1905', pp. 79–105.

[43] Patrick E. Carroll, 'Medical police and the history of public health', *Medical History*, 46 (2002), pp. 461–94.

[44] Thirty-first detailed annual report of the Registrar-General (Ireland), containing a general abstract of the numbers of marriages, births, and deaths registered in Ireland during the year 1894 [C. 7800], p. 196.

coroner to furnish certificates of inquest; and some cases of falsified age of death information.[45] These are relatively low numbers considering that the law was nei- ther fully observed nor properly policed. Absences are just as important as pres- ences in the reconstruction of ordinary lives from official sources, as they provide an invaluable prism on power brokerage albeit predominantly the weak positioning of the poor. Entire cohorts are missing from civil registration data and in as much as a spectrum of poverty existed, so too did a myriad of socio-economic reasons for non-compliance with census and GRO legislation. Some people were simply fearful of engagement with the instruments of biopower, especially those of British Administration in Ireland.

Foucault's musings on biopower have since the 1970s burgeoned into an entire research area and most criticisms of his work point to the fact that he gives indi- vidual agency no quarter. Although subject to several mechanisms, people reacted and found clever ways to negotiate power, and scholars of the poor and institu- tionalised have slowly been uncovering evidence of individual agency over the past few decades. Although E.P. Thompson's *The Making of the English Working Class* is not without its limitations, it is widely regarded as a watershed in the development of history from below.[46] Since its publication in 1963, historians have been working on various sources to draw out the experience of poverty in different countries and thus the study of individual agency and ordinary lives has emerged. The English poor has received careful consideration in pioneering work by, for example, Thomas Sokoll on Essex pauper letters, and more recently Steven King's work on how the poor actively negotiated the system through deft pen- manship to advocate for themselves.[47] Both scholars had a rich seam of ego- documents to draw upon and King, in particular, has developed useful methodological frameworks for analyses. While Tim Hitchcock identifies 'County of England and Wales archives stuffed to overflowing with records of the old poor law'[48] no cognate calendars of pauper letters exist for Ireland for the period Sokoll and King analyse.[49] The Elizabethan Poor Law, which established a national framework for poor relief in England and Wales, did not apply to, nor did the Act of Settlement apply in, Ireland. Both produced discrete bodies of records.

How Ireland differed in statutory terms regarding the poor does merit further clarification. David Dickson argues that the Vagabonds Act introduced in 1530 laid the framework for how vagrancy was managed parochially. Under the act, a

---

[45] Thirty-seventh detailed annual report of the Registrar-General (Ireland), containing a general abstract of the numbers of marriages, births, and deaths registered in Ireland during the year 1900 [Cd. 697], p. 2.

[46] E.P. Thompson, *The Making of the English Working Class* (London, 1963).

[47] Thomas Sokoll, *Essex Pauper Letters, 1731–1837* (Oxford, 2001); Steven King, *Writing the Lives of the English Poor, 1700s–1830s* (Montreal, 2019).

[48] Tim Hitchcock, 'A new history from below', *History Workshop Journal*, 57 (2004), pp. 294–8 at 294.

[49] I am grateful to Dr Susan Hood, archivist, Representative Church Body, Dublin, for advice on this matter.

rudimentary form of biopower emerged with parishes of the Established Church being charged with the maintenance of lists of beggars, the issue of licences to distinguish between vagabonds and genuine poor, and with giving alms as appropriate.[50] While there was a bias towards co-religionist poor, Dickson states that Church of Ireland vestries allocated monies to Catholics, whose recipient numbers often surpassed the Protestant poor.[51] These measures relied totally on philanthropic sentiments and even if 'Irish property could resolve Irish poverty' there was no legislative instrument to levy a tax for such purposes. Instead, an informal system of welfare supports existed. It relied on what Laurence M. Geary terms 'religion, compassion and custom', which in national terms 'devolved on shopkeepers, tradesmen, small and middling farmers, many of whom were on the verge of beggary themselves'.[52] The 1772 act to establish workhouses and houses of industry only resulted in eleven institutions and the attempt of a system was, as Geary argues, ineffective.[53]

The panoply of houses of industry and philanthropic endeavours amounted to a quasi-Poor Law system, but each had their own individual character and how the people negotiated access and relief was unique to the type of institution they resorted to. According to Ciarán McCabe, the pre-Famine poor 'deployed agency in their engagement with individuals and relief mechanisms' but his evidence suggests that they did so in different ways, and more so in person and in oral testimony.[54] Although he does note an instance of a woman in 1820s Dublin who subsisted through writing 'begging petitions', it seems to be a fairly isolated incidence.[55] The salient fact is that the Irish poor had no legal entitlement to relief and Geary reminds us how that did not change on the passing of the 1838 Poor Law, which he states was 'grudging and demeaning, intended to degrade and deter, and was unreservedly hated by those it was supposed to relieve'.[56] The long tradition of seeking poor relief in writing and the skills that were shored up over decades of experience of the Elizabethan Poor Law gave rise in England and Wales to what King terms a 'rhetorical and strategic approach to negotiation', but it simply did not accrue to the same extent in Ireland in the pre-Famine period.[57]

While the poor leave a faint impression on the Irish historical record, save cursory personal metadata documented in the admission registers of various

---

[50] Vagabonds Act 1530, 22 Hen. VIII, c. 12.
[51] David Dickson, 'In search of the old Irish poor law', in Rosalind Mitchison and Peter Roebuck (eds), *Economy and Society in Scotland and Ireland, 1500–1939* (Edinburgh, 1988), pp. 149–55 at 152.
[52] Laurence M. Geary, 'The whole country was in motion: mendicancy and vagrancy in pre-Famine Ireland', in Jacqueline Hill and Colm Lennon (eds), *Luxury and Austerity: Historical Studies XXI* (Dublin, 1999), pp. 121–36 at 124.
[53] Geary, 'The whole country was in motion', pp. 128–9.
[54] Ciarán McCabe, *Begging, Charity and Religion in Pre-Famine Ireland* (Liverpool, 2018), p. 10
[55] McCabe, *Begging, Charity and Religion in Pre-Famine Ireland*, p. 239.
[56] Geary, 'The whole country was in motion', p. 121.
[57] King, *Writing the Lives of the Poor*, p. 7.

Poor Law unions and cases made on their behalf by relieving officers after 1847, there are of course, exceptions.[58] Landed estate papers contain a certain degree of information about the lives of tenants but less from an ego-documentation perspective. More is written about and for, than by, the Irish poor. R.A. Houston cautions in his analysis of 'peasant petitions' of their highly formulaic nature and contends that they were the collaborative efforts of tenants, family members, and scribes.[59] There is ample evidence of clergy, of all denominations, and philanthropists who wrote prolifically on behalf of the poor in Ireland.[60] Oral testimony of straightened circumstances, both urban and rural, can be found in letters to newspapers and pamphlets but these were generally penned by the more well-to-do community representatives or clergy of all denominations from poor regions. Personal attitudes towards seeking alms changed little from pre-Famine times where Geary notes the sense of shame associated with begging and how people did so away from their place of origin for the sake of anonymity and pride. Varying degrees of literacy nationally and monoglottism in Irish-speaking regions undoubtedly played a part in this dearth of ego-documents, but in accordance with tradition, the performance of poverty was intended to be oral and ephemeral, and was unlikely to be committed to paper.[61]

Under the Union (1801–1922), several administrative structures were put in place and all Irish institutions from the overarching Chief Secretary Office, which was at the helm of over fifty Irish departments, committees, and boards, to the General Prison Board, the Poor Law Unions, and individual asylums, kept letter books and these survive to varying degrees.[62] Their incomplete nature is owing to the fire at the Public Records Office in 1922. I am not suggesting that Irish archives are bereft of poor voices, but they are certainly harder to locate and contextualise. For example, Brendan Kelly, Oonagh Walsh, and Catherine Cox have all found various patient and their relatives' voices in their work on the district and criminal lunatic asylums.[63] In sole and co-authored pieces with Elaine Farrell

[58] Virginia Crossman, *Poverty and the Poor Law in Ireland, 1850–1914* (Liverpool, 2013), p. 66.

[59] R.A. Houston, *Peasant Petitions: Social Relations and Economic Life on Landed Estates, 1600–1850* (Basingstoke, 2014).

[60] Clara Breathnach, 'The triumph of proximity: the impact of district nursing schemes in 1890s rural Ireland', *Nursing History Review*, 26 (2018), pp. 68–82; Ciara Breathnach, '"...it would be preposterous to bring a Protestant here": religion, provincial politics and district nurses in Ireland, 1890–1904', in Donnacha Seán Lucey and Virginia Crossman (eds), *Healthcare in Ireland and Britain 1850–1970: Voluntary, Regional and Comparative Perspectives* (London, 2015), pp. 161–80. Martyn Lyons, *The Writing Culture of Ordinary People in Europe, c.1860–1920* (Cambridge, 2012), p. 9 takes the meaning of ordinary as lower orders and primarily 'the peasantry'.

[61] Margaret Kelleher, *The Maamtrasna Murders: Language, Life and Death in Nineteenth-Century Ireland* (Dublin, 2018); Nicholas Wolf, *An Irish-Speaking Island: State, Religion, Community, and the Linguistic Landscape in Ireland, 1770–1870* (Madison, 2014).

[62] Kieran Flanagan, 'The Chief Secretary's Office, 1853–1914: a bureaucratic enigma', *Irish Historical Studies*, 24:94 (1984), pp. 197–225.

[63] Kelly is a prolific author but his most relevant publications in this context are Brendan D. Kelly, *Hearing Voices: The History of Psychiatry in Ireland* (Dublin, 2016) and Brendan D. Kelly, 'Searching for the patient's voice in the Irish asylums', *Medical Humanities*, 42:2 (2016), pp. 87–91; see also

and Laurence M. Geary, I have shown how aspects of convict agency can be gleaned from General Prison Board files.[64] In the latter research we found that in times of unrest, when so-called 'Whiteboys' (those accused of agrarian crimes) were convicted of criminal offences, they were given disproportionately long sentences.[65] Petitioning the Lord Lieutenant for clemency emerged as a particular genre of writing in the late nineteenth century, and, as Elaine Farrell's work has shown, it was not unusual for convicts to self-advocate.[66] Those that emerged in response to men incarcerated on Whiteboy charges in the 1880s were usually instigated by relatives and mediated by a local legal representative or by a priest.[67] Emigrant letters are another hugely important source of Irish ego-documents and while some express the experience of poverty they predominantly reflect the purview of the upwardly mobile in a socially enabling, if often challenging, host environment and therefore constitute different forms of expression. Hope as opposed to despair characterised emigrant letters, and in instances where potential chain migration was concerned there was usually a very positive or indeed embellished perspective on life in the New World.[68]

Scholars of poverty letters argue that while problematic, they are authentic. They also make distinctions between those that were personally written or transcribed on behalf of a poor person. Steven King posits that pauper letters 'provide us with an—or perhaps the—authentic voice of the poor, we can have confidence that they represent and embody a set of rhetorical and strategic models and approaches to agency'.[69] If we are to trace agency in the 'heritage of the pauper letter'[70] then the formulaic letters written by the poor themselves emerges much later in Ireland than in England and Wales. In fact, Lindsey Earner-Byrne traces it to post-independence Ireland. Like King, she rightly makes the case that the poverty letters she explored contain authentic voices, because the recipient, the Roman Catholic Archbishop of Dublin, was adept at weeding out the

---

Oonagh Walsh, 'Cure or custody: therapeutic philosophy at the Connaught District Lunatic Asylum', in Margaret Preston and Margaret Ó hÓgartaigh (eds), *Gender and Medicine in Ireland, 1700–1950* (Syracuse, 2012), pp. 69–85; Catherine Cox, *Negotiating Insanity in Southeast of Ireland, 1820–1900* (Manchester, 2012), chapter 4 in particular.

[64] Ciara Breathnach, 'Medical officers, bodies, gender and weight fluctuation in Irish convict prisons, 1877–95', *Medical History*, 58:1 (2014), pp. 67–86; Ciara Breathnach and Elaine Farrell, '"Indelible characters": tattoos, power and the late nineteenth-century Irish convict body', *Cultural and Social History*, 12.2 (2015), pp. 235–54; Ciara Breathnach and Laurence M. Geary, 'Crime and punishment: Whiteboyism and the law in late nineteenth-century Ireland', in Don MacRaild and Kyle Hughes (eds), *Crime, Violence and the Irish in the Nineteenth Century* (Liverpool, 2017), pp. 149–74.

[65] Laurence M. Geary, *The Land War in Ireland. Famine, Philanthropy, and Moonlighting* (Cork, forthcoming 2022).

[66] Elaine Farrell, *Women, Crime and Punishment in Ireland: Life in the Nineteenth Century Convict Prison* (Cambridge, 2020), p. 30.

[67] Breathnach and Geary, 'Crime and punishment: Whiteboyism', pp. 149–74.

[68] David M. Fitzpatrick, *Oceans of Consolation: Personal Accounts of Irish Migration to Australia* (Cork, 1994).

[69] King, *Writing the Lives of the Poor*, p. 46.   [70] King, *Writing the Lives of the Poor*, p. 47.

disingenuous.[71] Her analysis of 4,343 letters to Archbishop Edward Byrne dating from 1921 to 1940 shows the continued tradition of priests writing what might be termed advocacy letters; these form 23.8 per cent of her sample. She notes how they were 'usually in relation to a parishioner's letter', which marks a shift in line with rising literacy levels and a strategic coordination of effort.[72]

Whether or not we can elicit truth and authenticity from the coronial court records is really down to whether or not we have conflicting evidence to show that the testimony was falsified or deliberately misleading. As a court of record, facts relayed were treated precisely as such, and untruths, even in cases of clear criminality, were not usually challenged there. In Dublin, the coroner's court was intensely localised. Witnesses were identified in DMP reports; this brought people to the attention of their local DMP constables, so giving misleading information came with a degree of risk of falling foul of local surveillance mechanisms. Cases involving children increased the risk of coming to the greater attention of other authorities like, for example, the much feared 'cruelty man' or NSPCC inspector.[73] Pernicious life insurance schemes were singled out by medical officers as a particular risk to infant life and, as we shall see, was routinely investigated with respect to child deaths.[74] On occasion, Dr Byrne took it upon himself to warn mothers and guardians in cases of child neglect to remain silent in his court of record lest it be used to implicate them in later criminal proceedings (discussed in Chapter 3).

Verisimilitude was further achieved through the structured devices in the standardised court forms—names, addresses, and sometimes occupations grounded informants and made them accountable, which in turn provided juries (all of whom were supposed to be resident in the jurisdiction) with confidence in witness statements. Equally these structures offered witnesses an opportunity to establish their connections to the case at hand and gave them the authority to speak about the particulars of what they saw or heard. There are a number of examples of unknown persons in these data who through silence faded out of the official view (for example, those who actively refused to be identified or to volunteer information to investigators). Cases of fatal domestic violence often had silent witnesses, and these are covered more carefully in Chapter 4. Alias users, those of no fixed abode, and transients comprise perhaps the saddest cases in the data used here.[75] Taken together the twenty-five unknowns comprising seven

[71] Lindsey Earner-Byrne, *Letters of the Catholic Poor: Poverty in Independent Ireland* (Cambridge, 2017), p. 3.

[72] Earner-Byrne, *Letters of the Catholic Poor*, p. 6.

[73] Sarah-Anne Buckley, *The Cruelty Man: Child Welfare, the NSPCC and the State in Ireland, 1899–1956* (Manchester, 2013).

[74] Anthony D. Buckley, '"On the club": Friendly Societies in Ireland', *Irish Economic and Social History*, 14 (1987), pp. 39–58.

[75] NAI/1900/83 Inquest on the body of Daniel Lyons who was of no fixed abode (NFA), 30 July 1900.

adults (six men and one woman, all drowning victims) and eighteen unknown infants (where parentage was not ascertained), offer an important window on the history of the depths of Irish social inequality and, apart from family breakdown, evidence of continued distrust in biopower and its agents.

A whole system of checks and balances was managed initially by the DMP and subsequently the court clerk documented statements verbatim. Most witness statements were signed with an X (their mark) as opposed to a signature, indicating low literacy levels in the cohorts represented here. This added to the burden of responsibility on the court clerk for carefully documenting the narrative recounted. There are wonderful examples of tell-tale Dublin colloquialisms, like the 'murder of children' that distracted H-car driver Edward Byrne prior to a fatal road accident[76] or the threat to 'get away out of that you cow' by an abusive man to his wife. She later had to recount the domestic abuse and violent events leading to her son's death (the case will be discussed further in Chapter 4).[77] Inverted commas both in the DMP reports and in witness statements were used deliberately to distinguish between the official's paraphrase and the direct voice of the informant. These direct voices echo those found in the autobiographical works of Seán O'Casey and the Dublin of his youth, which differed greatly from the writings of James Joyce and his opposing middle-class world view.[78] In sharp contrast with Joyce's voyeurism of 'Dear Dirty Dublin',[79] John Casey as he was known in the 1901 census, lived in the solidly working-class East Wall area of the Dublin docks at 4.2 Abercorn Road.[80] The geo-spatial conditioning of his childhood, as Michael Pierce has shown, had a profound impact on his *oeuvre*.[81] Murray argues that, in his early plays, O'Casey 'achieved mimesis of Dublin speech in its liveliness and rhetorical flourishes', sounds and turns of phrase that he absorbed from the streetscape.[82] In this book I aim to tease out these voices, which were such an intrinsic part of the 'soundscape', or what R. Murray Schafer terms the 'sonic environment' of O'Casey's childhood Dublin, that can be gleaned from these rich sources.[83]

---

[76] NAI/1901/179 Inquest on the body of William O'Brien, 3 July 1901.

[77] NAI/1900/124 Inquest on the body of Joseph McCabe, 2 October 1900.

[78] I am grateful to Dr Laurence M. Geary for this insight and guidance.

[79] 'Does a fellow good a bit of a holiday. I feel a ton better since I landed again in dear dirty Dublin...' James Joyce, 'A little cloud', in *Dubliners* (Dublin, 2012), pp. 81–96 at 86.

[80] See http://www.census.nationalarchives.ie/reels/nai003681229/ (accessed 12 August 2020). He lived with his mother, Susan, then a widow aged 66, and his brothers Michael and Thomas. All three sons were gainfully employed; John as a junior delivery clerk, Michael as a telegraph labourer, and Thomas as a postman.

[81] Michael Pierce, 'The shadow of Seán: O'Casey, commitment and writing Dublin's working class', *Saothar*, 35 (2010), pp. 69–85 at 74.

[82] Christopher Murray, 'O'Casey and the city', in Nicolas Green and Chris Morash (eds), *The Oxford Handbook of Modern Irish Theatre* (Oxford, 2016), pp. 183–200 at 187.

[83] R. Murray Schafer, *The Soundscape: Our Sonic Environment and the Tuning of the World* (New York, 1993).

Analytical Frameworks

Power and gender are the primary analytical frameworks used in this book, as both had a profound impact on the way in which blame was constructed and allocated in the 611 verdicts discussed here. As scholars of gender theory have cogently argued 'gender is in no way a stable identity or locus of agency from which various acts proceed; rather, it is an identity tenuously constituted in time—an identity instituted through a stylized repetition.'[84] Within this framework of instability in culturally produced gendered practices I bolster my case for looking at a short timeframe of relative stability in socio-economic terms. The instruments of biopower in turn produced new gendered repetitions of engagement or detachment, and consequently women and men experienced city life in very different ways. While institutions like Church and state could stake claims over overarching structures, their social affect was dictated by accepted gendered behaviours. Social control was maintained primarily by the people, who were swift in judgement and chose who they protected or 'delivered' up to the DMP or other institutional control mechanisms like the judiciary, the Poor Law union, or the asylum.[85] Odd behaviour was tolerated in working-class communities, but only to a certain threshold. Tolerance levels were determined by gender, social standing, and respectability.

Feminist geographers have long contended that because cities are patriarchal by design they exclude women.[86] While recognising the changing values of gendered social constructs over time, Maureen A. Flanagan posits that the built environment of Dublin, like London, Toronto, and Chicago, reinforced male power through the routinisation of the normativity of male values. All aspects of city life bore heavily upon women; for example, the ramifications of major infrastructural projects had little consideration for the impact on family life and reinforced '"a version of patriarchy" in which the values and behaviours of men are presumed normative and thus embedded in urban institutions and structures to privilege male control.'[87] New transport innovations, particularly the tram network, contracted the amount of space available to those who were more bound to domestic settings, like women, children, and older people. By day the streets were the preserve of women and children. Drew Gray argues how, in the London slums, rooms were multifunctional 'as bedrooms, living rooms and workrooms and if any attempt was going to be made to keep them clean…then houses had to

---

[84] Judith Butler, 'Performative acts and gender constitution: an essay in phenomenology and feminist theory', *Theatre Journal*, 40:4 (1988), pp. 519–31 at 520.

[85] Micheal Ignatieff, 'State, civil society, and total institutions: a critique of recent social histories of punishment', *Crime and Justice*, 3 (1981), pp. 153–92 at 187.

[86] Leslie Kern, *Feminist City: Claiming Space in a Man-Made World* (London, 2020).

[87] Maureen A. Flanagan, *Constructing the Patriarchal City: Gender and the Built Environments of London, Dublin, Toronto, and Chicago, 1870s into the 1940s* (Philadelphia, 2018), p. 3.

be vacated during the day'. He contends that this necessity to find space during daylight hours was part of the reason why photographs of late nineteenth-century streetscapes were always crowded.[88] Streets were really important spaces for children's play but were also where they competed with several physical dangers that philanthropic reformers later tried to address through specially designated play areas.[89] Modernity pushed their lived experiences into daylight, or specific artificially lit spaces during certain 'decent' hours. With street lighting, 'One was lit but did not light. One was identified but did not identify'; it aided policemen on their beat or, what Joyce terms, 'the organised passage' through the streets.[90] Artificial light did not confer the same levels of public safety to women as it did to men.

Thresholds of public and private lives had different boundaries for tenement dwellers. The classic 'public/private' spheres model used to categorise the lived experiences of ordinary men and women finds no traction in urban working-class settings. Building on Davidoff and Hall's classic text on the middle-class construction of space, Martin Hewitt has argued that for the English working classes domestic space was not private and the home 'was constructed not only with permeable walls but also without thresholds and even without doors'.[91] Kleinberg flatly rejects the idea of a neat public/private dichotomy and reinforces how classist the lines were, especially given how some women earned their living through and in their homes, thus making them public as well as private sites.[92] She also argues that it is not applicable to 'different race, age, regional, and ethnic groups'.[93] In her study of nineteenth-century America, Boylan notes that the 'chameleon-like qualities of terms such as "public" and "private", or "home" and "work", underscore the extent to which nineteenth-century dichotomies were fluid'.[94] For such reasons the public/private spheres debate, which differentiates between the lives of middle- and upper-class women and men, is not applicable to early twentieth-century Dublin City either; instead, there is definitely a sense of how the built environment worked in tandem with the political apparatus to shape the boundaries of acceptable behaviours, be they social or medico-legal.

---

[88]   Drew Gray, *London's Shadows: The Dark Side of the Victorian City* (London, 2010), p. 126.

[89]   Vanessa Rutherford, 'Muscles and morals: children's playground culture in Ireland, 1836–1918', in Leeann Lane and William Murphy (eds), *Leisure and the Irish in the Nineteenth Century* (Liverpool, 2016), pp. 61–79.

[90]   Joyce, *The Rule of Freedom*, p. 110.

[91]   Martin Hewitt, 'District visiting and the constitution of domestic space in the mid-nineteenth century', in Inga Bryden and Janet Floyd (eds), *Domestic Space: Reading the Nineteenth-Century Interior* (Manchester, 1999), pp. 120–41 at 127.

[92]   S.J. Kleinberg, 'Women's employment in the public and private spheres, 1880–1920', *DQR Studies in Literature: Leiden*, 45 (2010), pp. 81–103 at 103: 'the construct could only apply to those families wealthy enough to sustain a wife outside the labor force who did not generate some income, whether by taking in boarders, selling butter and eggs, or doing some remunerated labor.'

[93]   Kleinberg, 'Women's employment', p. 84.

[94]   Anne M. Boylan, 'Claiming visibility: women in public/public women in the United States, 1865–1910', in Janet Floyd, Alison Eastman, and R. J. Ellis (eds), *Becoming Visible: Women in View in Late Nineteenth-Century America* (Amsterdam, 2010), pp. 17–40 at 19.

Suzanne Mackenzie has argued that women operated at the intersections of the public and the private, and throughout this book the ways in which those associated with the coroner's court negotiated the spatial organisation of the city is brought to the fore.[95] Public and private are used in this study to denote life inside the home, which included shared landings, stairwells, and yards, and what Amanda Vickery terms, 'the world outside the front door'.[96]

Domestic violence precipitated by cramped living environments sometimes erupted into cases of manslaughter and murder, but far more common in the coroner's court were deaths of children, which put motherhood under intense scrutiny (as opposed to the grinding poverty, the weak positioning of labour rights, and the substandard accommodation which will be described further in Chapter 1). The adjudication of whether or not deaths were considered accidental or suspicious fell to the coronial courts and a network of police, medical professionals, and eye-witnesses, all of whom worked together to maintain biopower networks in the city. Biopower was implemented in Ireland through various instruments of census, civil registration, compulsory smallpox vaccination, and other forms of surveillance throughout the nineteenth century. Paradoxically, it was the inefficacy of the biopolitical structures that were supposed to safeguard the people that equally placed them in deep peril. For example, the extent of overcrowding in the tenements for Dublin's poorest inhabitants was not fully captured in the census and, because of informal letting practices, there was a fear of surveillance. A number of tragic cases discussed in Chapters 2 and 4 show greater numbers of people occupying properties than the official census counted in March 1901.[97]

Blame is an important conceptual framework for the analysis of any court records, but it has not been exploited thoroughly by historians. Despite the recent 'emotional turn' in the historical sciences, few advances have been offered to Mary Douglas's contention that social organisation is a strong determinant in how the legal system is applied and how blame is allocated.[98] Essentially, blame is a process where emotions are manipulated to cast aspersions on one person or group over another. Judith Rowbotham argues along similar lines to Douglas and adds that as modernity progressed the criminalisation process expanded, which in turn had a profound impact in how shame and blame were conceived. She used the English criminal justice system to contend that the 'terminology of shame and blame describes essentially emotionally grounded and publicly revealed moral judgements that are invoked to add texture to a legal decision, aiding the explana-

[95] Suzanne Mackenzie, 'Women in the city', in Richard Preet and Nigel Thrift (eds), *New Models in Geography: The Political-Economy Perspective* (London, 1989), pp. 109–26.

[96] Amanda Vickery, 'Golden age to separate spheres? A review of the categories and chronology of English women's history', *The Historical Journal*, 36:2 (1993), pp. 383–414 at 412.

[97] NAI/1900/146 Inquest on the body of Kate Anderson, DMP report, 25 October 1900.

[98] Mary Douglas, *Blame and Risk* (London, 1994), p. 6.

tory and justificatory processes that are an essential part of the law's public performativity'.[99] Blame and its closely associated concept of shame, while grounded in the law, operated, as Rowbotham contends, at the intersection of the people and the law.[100] She notes a definite shift and a more concerted use of stigmatisation at the beginning of the twentieth century even for what we might term ordinary crimes.[101]

Although it was modelled on the English system, the modern Irish coronial courts quickly became very localised in how they interpreted the law. Peter King traces similar patterns with English criminal courts and argues that while acts were centrally orchestrated, the law was 'remade on the margins'.[102] This is true to a degree, with respect to Dublin, but there are marked differences in the ways urban and rural Irish coronial courts operated, and whether or not the coroner was a medical or a legal professional also dictated how verdicts and riders were shaped.[103] Blame allocation was not the remit of the coroner's court; its core function was to ascertain cause of death, but jurors often took it upon themselves to advocate for victims or clearly identify perpetrators in riders, which were basically opinionated statements reflecting the personal values of all-male panels. Riders or addenda allocating blame in the coroners' courts cannot be fully understood unless they are located in their wider socio-economic, political, and cultural contexts. Blame was conditioned by the power structures that shaped the prevailing gendered norms and I discuss its contours in the thematic analysis of the cases. Riders, which Coen and Howlin define as jury 'statements…in addition to verdict', were attached to 193 of the 611 cases.[104] Although superfluous to the requirements of the court and holding no legal weight, they could have lasting ramifications, operating as they did in an interpretative space between medico-legal expertise and the people. In 1891, even after the 1876 and 1881 Coroners Acts (discussed further in Chapter 1), the authors of the judicial statistics' report opined that coroners' courts still retained a great deal of control over criminal cases through 'verdicts implicating or exonerating certain persons in cases of homicide'.[105] These statements held no legal weight, but they capture the essence of middle- and lower middle-class attitudes towards the working classes, the poor,

---

[99] Judith Rowbotham, 'The shifting nature of blame', in Judith Rowbotham, Marianna Muravyeva, and David Nash (eds), *Shame, Blame, and Culpability: Crime and Violence in the Modern State* (London, 2013), pp. 64–79 at 65.

[100] Rowbotham, 'The shifting nature of blame', p. 71.

[101] Rowbotham, 'The shifting nature of blame', p. 72.

[102] Peter King, *Crime and Law in England 1750–1850: Remaking Justice from the Margins* (Cambridge, 2006), p. 2.

[103] Niamh Howlin, *Juries in Ireland: Laypersons and the Law in the Long Nineteenth Century* (Dublin, 2017), pp. 78–83 provides an overview of the function of the jury at all levels of the judicial system. Shane Ewen, *What is Urban History?* (Cambridge, 2016) provides a very helpful overview of the state of the art in the field.

[104] Mark Coen and Niamh Howlin, 'The jury speaks: jury riders in the nineteenth and twentieth centuries', *American Journal of Legal History*, 58:4 (2018), pp. 505–34 at 505.

[105] Criminal and judicial statistics, Ireland, 1891 [C. 6782], pp. 24–5; Coroners (Ireland) Act 1881 (44 & 45 Vic.), c. 35; Coroners (Dublin) Act 1876, c. xciii.

and the destitute. Conspicuous consumption of alcohol, for instance, was routinely used as part of the framework of blame. Any evidence of drink taken could sully the reputation even of victims of grievous bodily harm and instead render them into agents active in their own demise. Levels of suspicion and the allocation of blame were conditioned by prevailing social convention and, in the coroner's court, both were highly gendered. For example, a married woman whose child died through accidental burning or scalding was less likely to be accused of neglect than an unmarried mother. Each case is punctuated by a set of social constructions: the repeated use of Mrs (and its implied respectability) in a DMP report and/or a coded recommendation of 'there is nothing to see here' could halt the process at preliminary inquiry stage and spare the bereaved the difficulties associated with an inquest.

Riders allocating blame in the coroner's court could be a powerful determinant in the legal course of action that followed, and it operated in tandem with shame. David Nash contends that shame was more of a collective phenomenon in the past compared to guilt in modern times, which is more of an intensely personal emotional response.[106] While he draws distinctions between primitive and civilised society, Nash also argues that shame is not a linear concept and suggests that Nobert Elias's 'shifting thresholds of repugnance' be used to unpick its history.[107] Shame in early twentieth-century Dublin City was not limited to the culpable; if a witness cooperated with the police on a matter that levied blame on another person, they risked their own ability to continue living in that neighbourhood. The case of 12-year-old Elizabeth McKenna, who died following what appears to have been a bullying incident near Glorney's Buildings off Lower Gloucester Street in the north inner city, illustrates this point. She went to fetch water after school and was struck in the stomach with a brick by a girl named Molly Dooley in March 1901. It was revealed at the coroner's court that 'the father and stepmother of the deceased knows where she lives but are reluctant to tell'; instead, they reconciled the situation in their own minds with the sense of inevitability of a premature death because the 'deceased was delicate from birth'.[108] Elizabeth McKenna's inquest received no newspaper coverage and no charges followed.

Sources and Methodology

The parameters of the timeframe for this study are dictated by statute, namely the 1876 act laying out new rules for the coroner's court for Dublin only, and the run of related source materials. Up until that act, the county of the city of Dublin was

---

[106] David Nash, 'Towards an agenda for the wider study of shame: theorising from nineteenth-century British evidence', in Judith Rowbotham, Marianna Muravyeva, and David Nash (eds), *Shame, Blame, and Culpability: Crime and Violence in the Modern State* (London, 2013), pp. 43–60 at 44.

[107] David Nash, 'Towards an agenda for the wider study of shame', pp. 51–2.

[108] NAI/1901/75 Inquest on the body of Elizabeth McKenna, 15 March 1901.

served by two coroners whose offices operated on alternate months. As it happened, in the bill stage Dr William White, one of the city coroners died— section 4 of the act amalgamated both offices and the surviving coroner Dr Nicolas C. Whyte was nominated as sole office holder.[109] In this study I adopt a case study approach to a complete two-year run of original inquest reports. Original inquest reports can include the form of inquisition, the post-mortem report, the DMP report, and witness statements. In only one case is the inquisition form missing, but the verdict is recorded elsewhere in the report.[110] The form of inquisition was not described in Irish law but it adopted elements of the version described in the English 1887 act. It is not possible to build a case study around the socially more probing 1911 census as a mere seven inquests survive for that year and nine for 1910.[111] The dataset is bookended by the start of Dr Byrne's thirty-two-year career as coroner to Dublin City and the twelve-month period after the 1901 census, which allows for a more detailed discussion of domestic life and household composition. It is sensitive to the fact that most of the court's subjects were people who were hardly documented during their lives. Coroners' cases were entered into a register and, during Byrne's tenure, the inquest reports were numbered sequentially. The registers provide a very high level view of the cases in hand (number, name, address, date of inquest, where it was held, and the verdict). Irrespective of where the inquest was held, all cases were also logged in the city morgue register, which was maintained from 1871. Among the additional details it holds are, 'time of admission' to the morgue, by whom identified, whether the deceased had property on their person and its value, and how the body 'was disposed of', meaning where it was buried and by whom (family, friends, or the poor rate, for example).[112] Admission for the purposes of the morgue register was metaphorical in instances of institutional deaths, as many were buried directly from the asylum or hospital as the case might be.

While I am fortunate that Dr Byrne's records have a complete survival of three coroner's registers dating from 1901 to 1927,[113] unfortunately, there is an incomplete set of corresponding original inquest reports. The records of

---

[109]   Huband, *A Practical Treatise on the Law*, pp. 257–60.

[110]   Huband, *A Practical Treatise on the Law*, p. 260. Only one inquisition form is missing, but the medical report is extant: NAI/1900/132 Inquest on the body of Francis Dignam, 8 October 1900. There is an anomaly in the numbering in 1901, NAI/1901/301.5 Inquest on the body of a child named Kathleen Clune held on 5 December 1901. It is unclear why it escaped administrative notice—the previous case was 3 December and an inquest was held on 6 December.

[111]   The surviving records for 1910–12 are at locational reference NAI/1C/67/41; this is subject to change.

[112]   On 23 May 1900 Edmond Ryan the clerk of the court wrote to Byrne to apologise profusely for 'this my first error' in the administration of the records associated with the case of NAI/1900/11 Inquest on the body of an Unknown Male Infant, 1 May 1900. 'I had no police report, no entry and did not know where it was found nor the verdict. This is a poor excuse as I could get all that from you': letter dated 23 May 1900. He had proposed making the case 10B, which Byrne did not permit.

[113]   NAI/G2/650/2 2004/75 Dublin City Coroner's Registers, 1900–27, Volume 1, 21/4/1900–13/7/1907; Volume 2, 15/7/1907–9/6/1916; Volume 3, 10/6/1916–12/9/1927.

Dr Joseph E. Kenny, Byrne's predecessor, who was coroner from 1891 until his own 'unexpected death' in April 1900[114] may have fallen victim to the fire in the Public Records Office in 1922, which wreaked particular devastation on pre-1900 court records.[115] Deaths associated with the Easter Rising of 1916 are not part of Byrne's corpus: as martial law prevailed, no civil inquests were held from 22 April 1916 until 8 May 1916, as the register shows.[116] For this study I have collated the data contained in the original inquest reports over a two-year timeframe and arranged them into fields of surname, name, age, occupation, cause of death, location of inquest, name of medical expert, verdict, whether or not alcohol was involved, and other miscellaneous medico-legal information. The result of my harvesting exercise is a dataset comprising 611 cases dating from 21 April 1900 to 30 April 1902.[117] This dataset of continuous records is robust and prioritises qualitative over quantitative analysis; it makes no claims whatsoever to a statistical representation of overall trends. Within the dataset, there are examples of all different types of deaths from natural causes to murder and, while its extension by another few years would serve to bulk out numbers, it would diminish the value of wrapping a case study around a census year especially in the context of ordinary lives and the uneasy relationship people had with the instruments of biopower.

Very often, as shown in the case of John Healy, coronial court records are the only evidence of ordinary lives and how they were lived. William Reddy has shown how court records can be fruitfully mined to give voice to intimate histories, but to maximise their capacity to reveal a history from below, one of my aims here, they need to be combined with other sources like the census and civil registration records to provide fuller contexts.[118] A data-matching exercise between the coroner's cases and the census returns affirm evidence of family structures and living arrangements as well as several irregularities in tenement life, family breakdown, and the precarious lives the poor lived. These matters receive thorough discussion throughout the book and specific attention in Chapters 2 and 4. With this sample quantitative dataset I aim to advance the ways in which scholars of modern Irish history can apply qualitative methods, for example, prosopography (collective biography) to coronial court records. Prosopography, as Laurence Stone argues, can elucidate 'social structure and social mobility' and it is

---

[114] *Freeman's Journal*, 12 April 1900.

[115] A sample of Dr Joseph E. Kenny's inquest reports survive, dating from January and February 1900—his numbering system was slightly odd compared to Byrne's systematic method. For example, Margaret Murphy's inquest which took place on 27 January is numbered 2301 and is contained in the same envelope as Mary Sharkey, 2302 also held that day. It figures that they are numbered sequentially from the beginning of his tenure in 1891. See Ciara Breathnach and Ian Walsh (eds.), *Original Inquest Papers of Dr Joseph E. Kenny, Dublin City Coroner, 1900* (Forthcoming, Dublin, 2022).

[116] Colm Campbell, *Emergency Law in Ireland, 1918–1925* (Oxford, 1994); NAI/G2/650/2 2004/75 Dublin City Coroner's Registers, 1900–27, Volume II.

[117] The last case prior to 21 April 1902 was held on 19 April—up to that point there were a total of 603 cases; no cases came before the court on 20 or 21 April 1902. I have simply rounded off the month.

[118] Reddy, *The Navigation of Feelings*, analyses court records through a history of emotions lens.

an appropriate lens with which to examine the Dublin City coroner's court records.[119] In the context of modern history the approach has its origins in the *Dictionary of National Biography*, predominantly a history of 'great white men'. But in more recent historiography it has offered opportunities to explore ordinary lives through collective experience.[120] Pioneering work by digitisation projects like the Old Bailey Online and related projects like London Lives, provide ready and excellent sources for the application of prosopographical methods to ordinary lives.[121]

That the Irish actively resisted the earlier censuses has been well described, but scholars are in agreement that by the time the 1901 census came about, most people in the Dublin metropolitan area cooperated with enumerators.[122] Data linkage, albeit manual, forms an important methodological device in this research; fortunately, the 1901 manuscript census returns have a full survival rate and are readily available online.[123] The census offers what I am terming an important data verification touch point of 'biological citizenship', for lives that otherwise leave a faint impression on the historical record. Apart from commonalities in names, Dublin had a large influx of internal Irish migrants; therefore, finding ordinary people can be extremely challenging. Death registration rates improved in Dublin following the 1878 Public Health Act, which enabled the Registrar General to use burial returns to correct the official figures. Birth registration posed other problems, especially if birthing occurred in domestic environments without medical attendants. Poor mothers were often reticent to engage with the authorities and thus unattended births could escape attention.

Like in England, the minutiae of how the poor lived and died provided the middle-class readership of national and provincial newspapers with a source of sensationalist headlines and stories, which offers social historians plenty by way of surrogate copies of inquests that are no longer extant. Similar accounts of cases can be found in the Irish newspapers, where there are abbreviated but verbatim excerpts, which apart from the odd captivating headline offered little by way of opinion or commentary. In the absence of original inquests, Vicky Holmes's

---

[119] Lawrence Stone, 'Prosopography', *Daedalus*, 100:1, *Historical Studies Today* (Winter, 1971), pp. 46–79 at 46.

[120] K.S.B Keats-Rohan, *Prosopography Approaches and Applications: A Handbook* (Oxford, 2007). On the limitations of histories of 'great men', see Christine MacLeod and Alessandro Nuvolari, 'The Pitfalls of Prosopography: Inventors in the "Dictionary of National Biography"', *Technology and Culture*, 47:4 (2006), pp. 757–76.

[121] See https://www.oldbaileyonline.org/; https://www.londonlives.org/ which examines crime, poverty, and social policy; and UNESCO site of memory, http://www.foundersandsurvivors.org/, which uses the history of the Australian convict prison as a focal point (all accessed 16 March 2022).

[122] Joel Mokyr, *Why Ireland Starved: A Quantitative and Analytical History of the Irish* (London, 2005); E. Margaret Crawford, *Counting the People: A Survey of the Irish Censuses, 1813–1911* (Dublin, 2003); Joseph Lee, 'On the accuracy of the pre-Famine Irish censuses', in J.M. Goldstrom and L.A. Clarkson (eds), *Irish Population, Economy, and Society: Essays in Honour of the Late K.H. Connell* (Oxford, 1981), pp. 37–56.

[123] See http://www.census.nationalarchives.ie/search/ (accessed 18 July 2018).

research on Ipswich, England, has exploited newspapers to show how working-class subjects were not afforded any degree of privacy or dignity in death. She describes how the sanitary state of homes was often laid bare in the inquest reports, described as 'filthy' or too small to contain a jury for the viewing of the body.[124] These class indicators were usually more subtly put in DMP records; for example, in the case of James Ryan (and several others), which concluded with 'the deceased lives in a tenement house'.[125] These comments were used in a codified way to mean that it was too small to contain a jury. A combined expression of grief and pride probably led Thomas Malone's mother to request that the inquest be held at their home at 50a Amiens Street in May 1900.[126] Her request was honoured as the DMP report stated the location was suitable, but it was a rare occurrence.

Newspaper coverage of the Dublin City coroner's court is inconsistent—it was often used as a content filler and was sensitive to competing interests. Libel laws and their legacy in Ireland strictly controlled the ways in which newspapers could conduct business. According to Ann Andrews, they were used as a detterent to would be agitators and were 'enforced more strictly in Ireland than in Great Britain'.[127] Robert Munter traces this censorship to the early eighteenth century and stressed that 'the government could and did rely on the fear of their investigations and prosecutions to control the press'. The Irish press continued for the centuries that followed to 'play safe', which is another reason why newspapers can only be used in a limited way for the purposes of this study.[128] Newspapers were liable to criminal prosecution if they published 'an ex parte statement of the evidence at a coroner's inquest tending to prejudice the fair trial of a person suspected of having caused the death'.[129] Citing editorial bias and imprecise information as primary drawbacks Alecia Simmonds has recently cautioned about using newspapers and gazettes for the purposes of research on the history of emotions in legal history. She also advises that it is important to draw clear lines between adversarial hearings, where the purpose was to establish an unambiguous narrative of truth and, as a consequence, innocence or culpability or blame via cross-examination, and inquisitorial ones, 'where the primary purpose is not to win the case, but to discover the truth'.[130] Apart from this, newspaper reporting of coronial inquiries posed risks for future criminal cases and paradox-

---

[124] Holmes, 'Home cultures', p. 310.

[125] NAI/1900/142 Inquest on the body of James Ryan, 19 October 1900.

[126] *Belfast Newsletter*, 11 May 1900; NAI/1900/19 Inquest on the body of Thomas Malone, 10 May 1900. Malone, aged 29, died of valvular heart disease.

[127] Ann Andrews, *Newspapers and Newsmakers: The Dublin Nationalist Press in the Mid-Nineteenth Century* (Oxford, 2014), p. 6.

[128] Robert Munter, *The History of the Irish Newspaper, 1685–1760* (Cambridge, 1967), pp. 100–1.

[129] Huband, *A Practical Treatise on the Law*, p. 289.

[130] Alecia Simmonds, 'Legal records', in Katie Barclay, Sharon Crozier-De Rosa, and Peter N. Stearns (eds), *Sources for the History of Emotions: A Guide* (London, 2020), pp. 79–90 at 82.

ically they provided a measure of the public appetite for punishment. Judith Rowbotham contends that in England and Wales the national press played a central role in educating the public about the criminalisation process as well as reinforcing the reasons for the allocation of blame. She noted that 'opinionated commentary that contextualised this reportage could also indicate and steer the approved forms of community shaming or stigmatisation that could acceptably accompany a formal sentence.'[131]

A further problem with using Irish newspapers in this study is their inherent political biases, which had an enormous impact on content. For example, the *Irish Times*, established in 1859, was what Michael Foley describes as a liberal unionist newspaper, and rarely, if ever, reported anything from the coroner's court.[132] Of the national dailies, the *Freeman's Journal* and *The Nation* were solidly national-ist—both published infrequent accounts of the coroners' court proceedings, and the latter published far fewer articles than the former. To illustrate the point of newspaper bias, David Nash uses a peculiar case of a man convicted for extreme cruelty in 1870 (he placed his wife in a mask) to juxtapose the London versus regional newspaper coverage. Nash shows how the former 'played upon the discourses of the uncivilised Celtic fringe', while the latter 'focused on the 'uncivilised behaviour of a foreign "French husband"'.[133]

For such reasons, I have not (yet) endeavoured to match the coroner's register entries from 1900 to 1927 to the newspapers as they were not part of a regular reporting system. The most consistent presence was the *Evening Herald*, a Dublin daily that ran Monday to Saturday, and while it invariably carried coverage of the proceedings of the day in the coroner's court it was not a guaranteed inclusion. If a case was mundane, like an all too common cardiac-related death of what was then considered a middle aged (between 40 and late 50s) or elderly (over 60) person, then it was unlikely to have been reported unless it was a particularly slow news day.[134] Controversial cases were more likely to appear in national and provincial newspapers. Sometimes verdicts and riders were used, in whole or in part, verbatim as headlines when they were sensational. Social class dictated content too; some elements of working-class Dublin life were at odds with early twentieth-century Irish nationalism, and for reasons I explore throughout the book, I believe that it is better to take advantage of the full inquest reports and work systematically from them to other sources rather than trying to establish and resolve the complicated relationship between the coroner's register, the morgue

---

[131]   Rowbotham, 'The shifting nature of blame', p. 74.

[132]   Michael Foley, 'Colonialism and journalism in Ireland', *Journalism Studies*, 5:3 (2004), pp. 373–85 at 377.

[133]   David Nash, 'Towards an agenda for the wider study of shame', pp. 43–60 at 51.

[134]   Sarah McHugh, 'The institutional care of Ireland's elderly women, 1845–1908' (unpublished PhD thesis, Queen's University Belfast, 2021). I had the pleasure of examining this excellent thesis—it discusses the matter of old age and how it was defined in Ireland.

register, and potential newspaper articles. Juror questions were not captured by the court's clerk, as they were beyond his remit, but answers were often denoted as 'to a juror'. If a case was of wider public interest, newspapers sometimes printed these questions and I have garnered them where possible.

Judicial court proceedings have received attention from scholars of Ireland and while these studies explore ordinary lives to an extent, it is predominantly from the perspective of deviant behaviour.[135] Unlike the petty sessions or the criminal courts where the subjects were either perpetrators or victims of crime, this sample shows that less than 10 per cent of cases coming before the coronial courts involved criminality. Furthermore, from 1846 the function of the Irish coronial court system was purely inquisitorial—to establish the identity of the deceased, determine the facts surrounding the death, and from 1864 to issue a verdict that was subsequently documented as the registered cause of death by the local registrar. It was primarily a court of record. The coroner also had power to put the prisoner on trial in cases of suspected foul play from 1828 to 1962.[136] Bail was permitted to those found guilty of manslaughter by the coroner's jury but not in Dublin after the 1876 act.[137] Four cases in 1878 brought clarity to the matter of overlapping jurisdiction between the coronial and criminal courts in homicide cases. Police in Ireland and England could initiate both processes simultaneously but difficulties arose when the presence of prisoners on remand by magistrates was requested or required at the inquest. In such instances attorneys could apply for a writ of habeas corpus to insist that prisoners be present at a coroner's case. Decisions in three Irish and one English case clarified the matter and decreed that the accused did not have to be produced before the coroner.[138] This effort to create a clear

---

[135] Vaughan, *Murder Trials in Ireland*; Elaine Farrell, 'A Most "Diabolical Deed"': *Infanticide and Irish Society 1850–1900* (Manchester, 2013).

[136] Criminal Law (Ireland) Act, 1828 (9 Geo. IV), c. 54. Section 6 remained in place until the Coroner's Act 1962:

> That every Coroner, upon any Inquisition taken before him, whereby any Person shall be indicted for Manslaughter or Murder, or as an Accessory to Murder before the Fact, shall put in Writing the Evidence given to the Jury before him, or as much thereof as shall be material; and shall have Authority to bind by Recognizance all such Persons as know or declare anything material touching the said Manslaughter or Murder, or the said Offence of being accessory to Murder, to appear at the next Court of Oyer and Terminer or Gaol Delivery, or other Court at which the Trial is to be, then and there to prosecute or give Evidence against the Party charged; and every such Coroner shall certify and subscribe the same Evidence, and all such Recognizances, and also the Inquisition before him taken, and shall deliver the same to the proper Officer of the Court in which the Trial is to be, before or at the opening of the Court.

Vaughan, *Murder Trials in Ireland*, p. 41 cites the case of Andrew Carr, who was 'committed on a coroner's warrant' and subsequently executed in 1870 for the brutal murder of Margaret Murphy. He had been drinking heavily at Crinion's Public House, prior to the fatal attack and the inquest was held there. Dr N.C. White was the city coroner, the jury returned the verdict of 'willful murder', and the 'prisoner was fully committed on the coroner's warrant to stand trial at commission': *Mayo Examiner*, 20 June 1870; *Drogheda Conservative*, 18 June 1870; *Irish Examiner*, 20 June 1870.

[137] Huband, *A Practical Treatise on the Law*, p. 282.

[138] Huband, *A Practical Treatise on the Law*, pp. 246–9.

separation of concerns meant that the coroner's jury remit was confined to cause of death only.[139] It was still noted as a welcome endeavour in the judicial reports in 1891.[140] This matter of separate domains was reiterated in cases of workplace accidents and extreme inter-personal violence discussed in Chapters 3 and 4, where legal counsel tried to enter matters on the record in order to sway riders and, to a lesser extent, verdicts to their advantage for future litigation purposes. Dr Byrne swiftly recognised and did not countenance any cynical ploys.

A further point to note with regard to the Irish coronial records is that from 1878 the number of coroners' inquests held in Ireland were no longer recorded in the judicial statistics. This was at the behest of the Registrar General who contended that they did not belong there, as most coroners' cases were non-criminal. But thereafter, the Registrar General did not report these figures annually discretely nor did the local government board, which only recorded salaries paid to the coroner and associated staff.[141] There were isolated incidents of decennial aggregates, for example a supplement to the ARRGs in 1901 reported that a total of 2,930 inquests occurred in the Dublin Registration area from 1891 to 1900.[142] The 1894 DMP report to parliament noted how 314 coroners' inquests were held in 1894, '286 in 1893 and 282 in 1892'.[143] The 1895 judicial statistics report affirmed the relationship between the DMP and the coroners' courts but stated that no returns of proceedings were included in its reporting mechanism for statistical purposes.[144] Police reports form another very important source for my study but again the reporting of DMP activity is difficult to correlate with annual reports. For example, the ARRG provides aggregate figures to provincial level and quotes a figure of 316 inquests that took place in 1900 in the 'Dublin Registration District', which was not coterminous with the city coroner's jurisdiction (Map 0.2).[145] Reports of all 208 cases conducted by Dr Bryne are extant for that year, as are sixty-three inquest reports from his predecessor Dr Kenny; the morgue register for that year shows that a further sixteen were conducted by Christopher Friery in his caretaker ministry (none of whose inquest reports survive), making a total of 287 in that year.[146] Kenny's reporting is confusing and

    [139] Criminal and judicial statistics, 1880, Ireland, Part I, Police—criminal proceedings—prisons; Part II, Civil proceedings in central and larger and smaller district courts [C. 3028], p. 13.
    [140] Criminal and judicial statistics, Ireland, 1891 [C. 6782], pp. 24–5: 'It is not, however, the custom now to bring prisoners charged with homicide, &c before the Coroners' Courts, and in a large number of cases the finding of the Jury relates merely to the cause of death.'
    [141] Annual report of the Local Government Board for Ireland, for the year ended March, 1900 [Cd. 338].
    [142] Supplement to the thirty-seventh report of the Registrar-General of Marriages, Births, and Deaths, in Ireland, containing decennial summaries of the returns of marriages, births, deaths, and causes of death in Ireland, for the years 1891–1900 [Cd. 2089], p. 21.
    [143] Statistical Tables of Dublin Metropolitan Police, 1894 [C. 7734], p. viii.
    [144] Return of Judicial Statistics of Ireland, 1895 [C. 8616], p. 24.
    [145] 2,320 nationally and 802 in Leinster, ARRG, 1900, pp. 20, 166.
    [146] NAI/G2/649/43 Corporation of Dublin, Coroner's Court and Morgue Register. From January 1900 to 9 April 1900 Kenny conducted fifty-four inquests numbered consecutively from 2,316 to 2,369. From 9 April to 18 April, County Coroner Christopher Friery as acting Coroner to the City

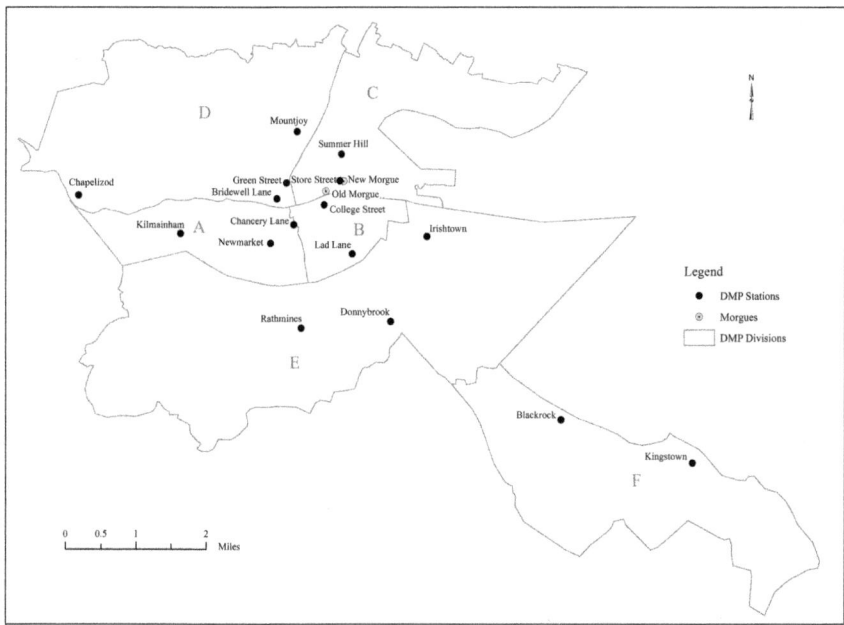

Map 0.2 Map of the DMP divisions and stations in Dublin City

Source: Dublin Metropolitan Police Committee of Inquiry 1883 [C. 3576, C. 3576-I], p. 25 and
Statistical Tables of the Dublin Metropolitan Police for the Year 1901 [Cd. 1166], p. 33. OSi historic
25-inch basemap © Ordnance Survey Ireland/Government of Ireland, Copyright Permit No. MP 006821.
Cartography: Dr Rachel Murphy.

none of the sixty-three original inquests that survive from his tenure include the
DMP report. Byrne introduced a systematic recording mechanism and a large
proportion of the inquests included here have a DMP report. At time of writing, it
is unclear if the corresponding (or indeed duplicate) files can be found in the
police administrative records.[147] Essentially, the extant records of the Irish system,
despite coming under the Crown and Peace files in broader administrative terms,
were municipal records with no clear reporting mechanism to local or central
government after 1878. This places my study at a slight disadvantage in comparative terms. It is not possible to track coronial court activity in other major urban
centres like Belfast, Cork, Galway, Limerick, and Waterford without conducting
similar case studies and creating datasets for each; furthermore, the inquests for
those cities have a similarly patchy survival. By January 1901 the DMP district
included divisions E (Donnybrook) and F (Kingstown), and incorporated the
extensions decreed under the city boundary extension.[148]

---

conducted sixteen numbered 1–16. Dr Byrne began a new system on 19 April with John Healy's case
numbered 1.

[147] The Gárda Síochána Museum archives have been closed to public access for a few years.

[148] Dublin Metropolitan Police, Report of the Committee of Inquiry, 1901 [Cd. 1088]; Dublin
Corporation Act 1900 (63 & 64 Vic.) c. cclxiv.

Fragmentary evidence beleaguers the pursuit of the history of ordinary lives and, to fully exploit the richness of the inquests, it is necessary to approach the records from a number of thematic perspectives to enable analyses of the aggregate data. The built environment is another very important source for this work.[149] By the 1890s the north side contained most of the warehousing and docking facilities for the import and export of goods.[150] Compared to the south side of the city it was disproportionately and heavily populated with tenement housing located adjacent to industrial critical mass. Health inequality did not end there— the north side which was divided into four registration districts (North City No. 1 West, North City No. 1 East, North City Nos 2 and 3) containing abattoirs and factories that created harmful pollution and effluvia. The south side had four registration districts numbered 1 to 4. North City No. 3 civil registration district (RD) had the ignominy of having the highest death rate from enteric fever, with South City No. 4 and No. 2 RDs following behind.[151] All three districts had the highest rates of respiratory disease indicating that air and water pollution played a major role in the poor health outcomes that are recurrent in the coronial court records. Despite the tireless efforts of sanitarian reformers like Sir Charles Cameron, the city suffered from a distinct lack of infrastructural development to improve public health (Map 0.3).[152]

The city boundaries were themselves a source of controversy but, despite opposition, by 1901 they had expanded to include the townships of New Kilmainham, Drumcondra, Clonliffe, Glasnevin, and Clontarf.[153] Affluent townships of Pembroke and Rathmines mounted a fierce resistance to the perceived 'Nationalisation' of the City Council from the 1880s onwards, and as Ciarán Wallace has argued both escaped the city taxation net for a further thirty years.[154] The *Freeman's Journal* boasted how in 1902 the South City Ward was avowedly nationalist: 'now that the ward has been recaptured in the nationalist interest…it only remains with its organisation to hold it'.[155] Political persuasions aligned to social class had an enormous impact on the lives of ordinary people. When the

---

[149] Susan Galavan, *Dublin's Bourgeois Homes: Building the Victorian Suburbs, 1850–1901* (London, 2017); Susan Galavan, 'Building Victorian Dublin: Meade & Son and the expansion of the city', in Ciarán O'Neill (ed.), *Irish Elites in the Nineteenth Century* (Dublin, 2013), pp. 51–67.

[150] 'Does a fellow good a bit of a holiday…', Joyce, 'A little cloud', p. 86.

[151] Report of the committee appointed by the Local Government Board for Ireland to inquire into the public health of the city of Dublin, 1900, Cd. 243, Cd. 244, p. 7, hereafter Dublin Report, 1900.

[152] Michael Corcoran, *Our Good Health: A History of Dublin's Water and Drainage* (Dublin, 2005), pp. 43–4. Corcoran credits Professors Mapother and Cameron and their contemporaries with many extraordinary contributions to Dublin life, primarily in public health. Mapother became the first Professor of Hygiene at the RCPI in 1864 and Chief Medical officer of the city—he was succeeded by Cameron in 1880.

[153] Dublin Corporation Act 1900 (63 & 64 Vict.) c. 264. It was enacted on 15 January 1901.

[154] For discussion of Nationalisation in Dublin City, see Ciarán Wallace, 'Civil society in search of a state: Dublin 1898–1922', *Urban History*, 45:3 (2018), pp. 426–52; see also Local Government (Dublin) Act, 1930.

[155] *Freeman's Journal*, 31 May 1902.

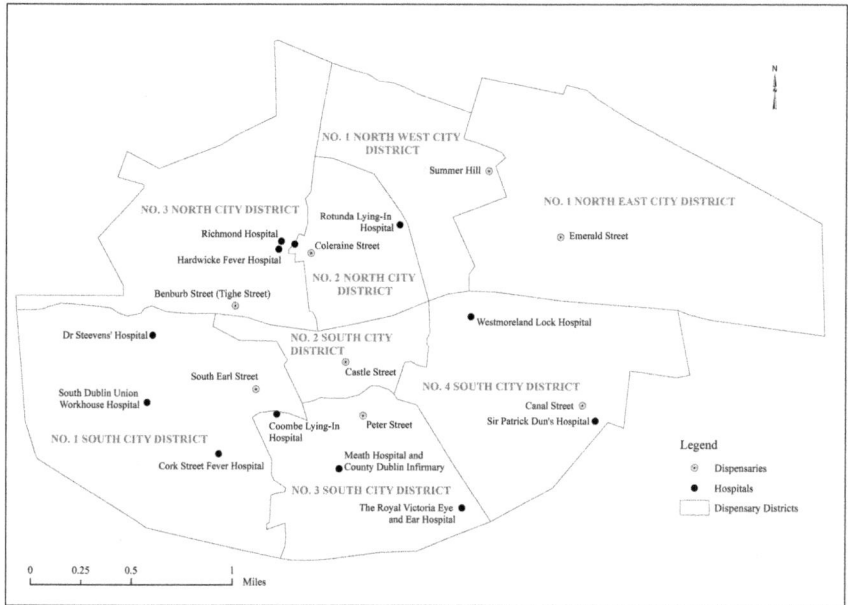

Map 0.3 Map of the hospitals and dispensaries in Dublin City

Source: Map derived from the Report of the committee appointed by the Local Government Board for Ireland to inquire into the public health of the city of Dublin, 1900 [Cd. 243, Cd. 244], see appendices, no page numbers. OSi historic 25-inch basemap © Ordnance Survey Ireland/Government of Ireland, Copyright Permit No. MP 006821. Cartography: Dr Rachel Murphy.

Committee on Public Health reported in 1900, Dublin City comprised a mere 3,733 statute acres, which contained a population of almost 250,000 and some of the country's poorest ordinary people.[156] As the satirical cartoons of Thomas Fitzpatrick illustrated (Figure 0.2), it was not a healthful place—fundamental matters of clean water and safe sewerage disposal were not given enough priority in the preceding decades, and these environmental matters combined with poverty to limit life expectancy for the poor in particular.[157]

Apart from establishing vulnerability among certain cohorts in particular life cycles, this book combines evidence presented at the coronial courts with contemporary maps to exploit the potential of the rich socio-economic and geographical data, exemplified in John Healy's case. Throughout the book, and where possible, I graft the details and the final journeys of the cases to Ordnance Survey and extant 1893 'Goad Maps' a section of which is shown in Map 0.1. Charles A. Goad was a civil engineer who drew Fire Insurance Plan (FIP) maps for major urban centres. Having previously conducted similar work in Canada,

---

[156] Dublin Report, 1900, p. 2.

[157] James Curry and Ciarán Wallace, *Thomas Fitzpatrick and 'The Lepracaun Cartoon Monthly', 1905–1915* (Dublin, 2015).

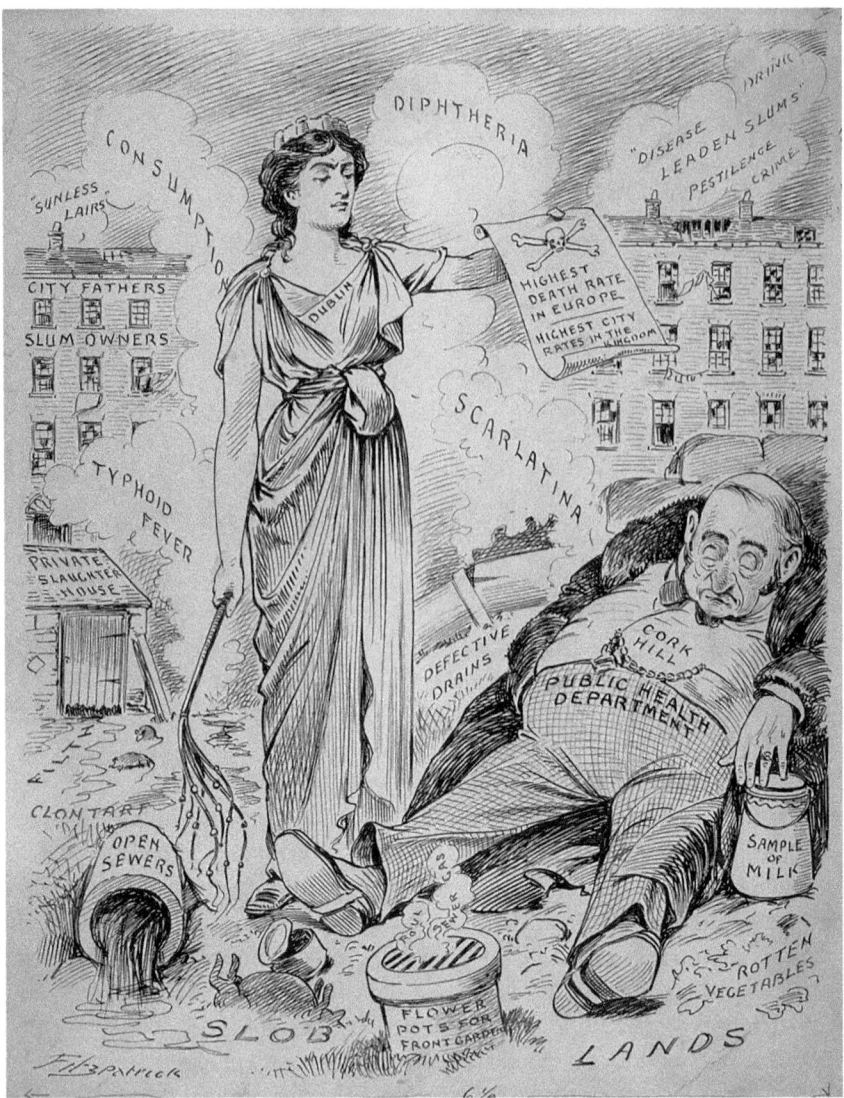

Figure 0.2 Thomas Fitzpatrick cartoon 264—highest death rates in Europe?
Source: (TF/4) Image Courtesy of the Royal College of Physicians of Ireland.

his reputation was well established when he commenced this work in the United Kingdom in 1885. Goad's business model was based on a leasing system to relevant industries. A primary volume was provided and, once updates were available, clients would return their originals and the new colour-coded information was pasted on top. Wonderfully detailed to building purpose level, the function of the maps was to service the burgeoning insurance industry of the late nineteenth century in risk assessment. Not only did the hand-painted maps cover the central business district of each major city, they also showed ancillary services associated with industry and trade; for example, warehouses and ports located to the east of Dublin City centre were important for the purposes of insurance surveying. Goad Ltd developed an excellent reputation for its work and applied the same template to each city. The key plans for the City of Manchester included an 'explanation of signs used': buildings were colour-coded as follows: yellow signified high-risk wooden structures, red was for brick, light blue denoted skylights on lower build- ings, and purple for higher buildings with skylights.[158] Water courses, building heights, and the level of fire brigade support were fundamental to the FIPs and they were drawn in collaboration with the local fire brigade.[159] Dublin Fire Brigade (DFB) was established in 1862 and, by 1901, it was accessible via a tele- phone network and fire hydrants were located throughout the densely populated inner city.

Reflecting the industrial and commercial contours of the city in 1893, the key map (Map 1 of nineteen, scale of 600 feet to 1 inch[160]) divided Dublin into eight- een FIP districts (each mapped to a closer scale of 40 feet to 1 inch), or twelve maps (numbered 2–13) north of the Liffey and six (numbered 14–19) to the south. Each of the smaller maps carries an excellent level of detail that can be cross-referenced with street directories or what Patrick Joyce calls the 'silent agents' of 'quasi-governmentality' containing as they did statistics about popula- tion and crime.[161] Together with my colleague Dr Rachel Murphy, we have used Ordnance Survey maps of Ireland to plot the boundaries of city wards, the agents of biopower, and some of the more controversial cases in this sample, conveyed in Chapter 4. Further to maps, I make use of historical photographs from a few col- lections held at the National Library of Ireland (Figure 0.1) and the Royal Society of Antiquaries of Ireland's 'Darkest Dublin' collection, which provide an import- ant visual register to the Dublin presented in this book.

Book Structure

Microhistorians have long since argued that smaller data have the ability to eluci- date the ordinary and the everyday in ways that macrohistory and demographic

---

[158] See http://www.bl.uk/onlinegallery/onlineex/firemaps/england/northwest/goadlegendmanchester. html (accessed 30 January 2019).

[159] Gwyn Rowley, 'British fire insurance plans: the Goad productions c.1885–c.1970', *Archives*, 17:74 (1985), pp. 67–78. Rowley notes that once prepared the maps were bound into a large atlas and individual sheets generally measured 25 1/4 inches (63.7 cms) by 21 inches (54 cms).

[160] See http://www.bl.uk/onlinegallery/onlineex/firemaps/ireland/largeimage146585.html (accessed 30 January 2019).

[161] Patrick Joyce, *The Rule of Freedom: Liberation and the Modern City* (London, 2003), p. 198.

models cannot.[162] Peter King's contention, from his work on the English judicial courts in the long eighteenth century, that 'the justice delivered by the courts was shaped and remade as much from below, from within and from the margins as it was from the centre' is relevant too as coronial courts quickly adapted to their locality.[163] David Nash and Anne-Marie Kilday, historians of crime and criminality, both advocate a microhistory approach to judicial court records, and for good reason—the devil is in the detail.[164] Taking example from historians of criminality and microhistorians, in the following chapters I examine the coronial records in three ways: as a corpus to outline overall trends in cause of death in Dublin City, spatially and thematically to create critical mass in cause of death and, individually, to provide a richer socio-cultural perspective on mortality at the turn of the century. In so doing, I adopt a combination of urban history, prosopography, and microhistory approaches to the circumstances surrounding particular causes of death, like fires in tenements or deaths in waterways.[165]

In order to understand the individual inquests it is necessary to outline the history of the Irish coronial system, its relationship with the judiciary and how the Dublin City coroner's court developed its own unique character. Adding to work by Ian Burney, which has focused on the administrative and operational features of the English system,[166] my aim is to deepen the reader's understanding of the court's power and positioning in the Irish medico-legal landscape. Chapter 1 charts how the coroner's court operated in a wider municipal framework of local government and the emergency services, some of which were well established, like the DMP; the DFB was achieving more prominence by 1900 and the Dublin Corporation Ambulance, established in 1899 was relatively new.[167] Through a discussion of gender, institutions, religion, and medico-legal dictates this book outlines how the coroner's court worked in tandem with the complicated network of medical, legal, and municipal services in Dublin City.

The rest of Chapter 1 provides contextual information to aid readers in understanding the socio-economic contexts of the coroner's cases. For example, it is important to consider the insanitary and dilapidated state of Dublin City, which,

---

[162] Sigurður Gylfi Magnússon and István M. Szijártó, *What is Microhistory?: Theory and Practice* (London, 2013). For example, microhistory has been fruitfully employed by Barry Reay in his work on English rural society: Barry Reay, *Microhistories: Demography, Society, and Culture in Rural England, 1800–1930* (Cambridge, 1996).

[163] King, *Crime and Law in England 1750–1850*, p. 2.

[164] David S. Nash and Anne-Marie Kilday (eds), *Law, Crime and Deviance Since 1700: Micro-Studies in the History of Crime* (London, 2016), Introduction, pp. 1–16 at 2.

[165] Carlo Ginzburg, John Tedeschi, and Anne C. Tedeschi, 'Microhistory: two or three things that I know about it', *Critical Inquiry*, 20 (1993), pp. 10–35; Ewen, *What Is Urban History?*

[166] Burney, *Bodies of Evidence.*

[167] Dukova, *A History of the Dublin Metropolitan Police*, p. 59; Tom Geraghty and Trevor Whitehead, *The Dublin Fire Brigade: A History of the Brigade, the Fires and the Emergencies* (Dublin, 2004); Dublin Corporation Fire Brigade Act, 1862 (25 & 26 Vic.) c. 38. No study of the ambulance service has emerged to date.

as several contemporary experts argued, gave rise to an excess mortality from the 1860s right up until the turn of the century. It is also necessary to understand the evolution of the Dublin tenements to foreground discussion in Chapter 2, which focuses on how the home was perhaps the most dangerous location for children. I provide examples of typical family income and expenditure to put vulnerability into a wider socio-economic context. There was rarely, if ever, anything left over for what middle-class reformers would have considered luxury expenditure on alcohol. I outline when and where it was available for purchase and why drinking culture was so embedded in urban life. The final section of Chapter 1 focuses on gender and how a gendered framework can assist in the reading of coroner's inquests, particularly in those involving criminality.

Using the quantitative data collated from the coroner's records, and adopting a mixed methods approach it is possible to empirically re-categorise the inquests in spatial terms into deaths occurring in domestic and public settings. Within these broad categories an unsurprising majority, or 307 deaths, occurred in domestic spaces, 260 occurred outside and forty-four died in institutions (prisons, asylums, and hospitals). As Figure 0.3 shows, of the 260 occurring outside the home, 109 occurred at or arose from accidents at work (twenty-six were in accidents related to work on waterways), a further forty-three drowned in the waterways in non-occupational terms, and I use the category of 'found' to describe sixty-seven deaths that occurred in 'in between' places, for example, bodies being discovered on streets, or the case of one adult male found in a public house. Vehicular traffic caused the deaths of thirty-seven people who were knocked down in non-work-related accidents; four people died as a result of unusual accidents that cannot be neatly classified; sixteen had no fixed abode (described in the records as someone who was sleeping rough or was simply spending a night in a lodging house). When the collapse of two tenements houses on Church Street claimed seven lives in 1913, it occasioned a report into the condition of working-class housing.

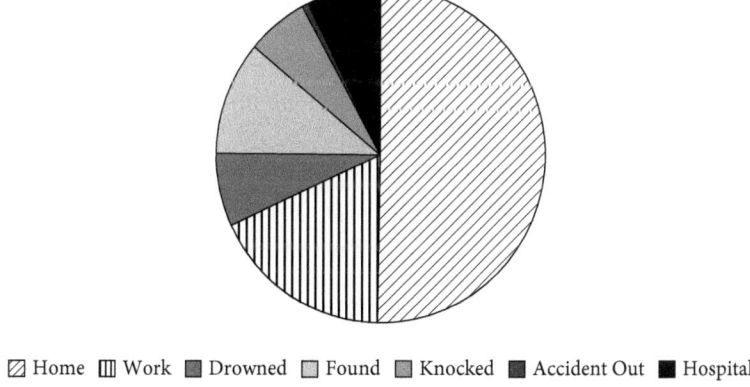

☑ Home Ⅲ Work ■ Drowned ▢ Found ▣ Knocked ■ Accident Out ■ Hospital

Figure 0.3 Locational categorisation of 611 cases

Published in 1914, it noted that most front doors were open and it was customary for people to wander in to houses to use the water closet.[168] It was not unusual for those of no fixed abode to occupy hallways at night. Thus a few bodies were discovered. 'Street dealer in fruit' Anne Rogers was found in the 'open hall' of 51 Beresford Street. Her husband last saw her alive the previous day in Monkstown. Dr Maughan found old standing disease in her left lung and considered the 'lower two tiers useless'. Her death was considered to be a combination of heart and lung disease accelerated by exposure.[169] Long after the Poor Law was established, the old tradition of charity and compassion identified by Geary is in strong evidence in these records.[170] While the front door of a tenement building might have been of great significance in keeping the prying eyes of biopolitics and the middle classes out, to the destitute such thresholds were permeable and they could rely on the poor for food and shelter.

I use the categories of inside and outside to shape my chapter structure and to assist in the thematic analysis of these data. In the case of public and domestic hazards (which taken together account for 64 per cent of deaths), much can be credited to the mixed fortunes of the city itself and how it shaped the construction of gender identities. Of the 611 cases, 205 were female and another two were gender unknown (both concerned infant bodies, one of which was decomposed and the other mutilated to such an extent that it was impossible to determine).

Reflecting the hazards of urban life and using the broad categorisation of the three locational types that find strongest representation in the data used here, deaths in domestic spaces, outside domestic spaces, and suspicious, violent deaths are the thematic focus of Chapters 2, 3, and 4, respectively. Taking this spatial and thematic approach it is possible to draw attention to tropes of social class and deviancy, as well as the language of medico-legal literacy.

The home was where many poor people spent their ailing years outside, and perhaps fearful, of 'modern' medical care. Chapters 1 and 2 raise questions about how ordinary people perceived and understood biopower, which for the most part was administered through the Poor Law and via the policing system, and through civil society to a lesser extent. Children aged 12 and under comprise 162 of the 611 cases, sixty-nine of whom were aged under 12 months—again, this is a small fraction of what was an appallingly high and localised urban infant mortality rate. This forms much of the focus in Chapter 2.

Inner-city dwellers lived in such close quarters that it was unavoidable that family life would spill out into the streetscape. The contours of Dublin City were shaped in large part by the North and South Circular roads and waterways, both

---

[168] Report of the departmental committee appointed by the Local Government Board for Ireland to inquire into the housing conditions of the working classes in the city of Dublin [Cd. 7273], p. 4.

[169] NAI/1902/28 Inquest on the body of Anne Rogers, 28 February 1902.

[170] Geary, 'The whole country was in motion', p. 124.

natural and manmade, namely the River Liffey and the Royal and Grand Canals.[171] Both the canals and the circular roads were constructed in the late eighteenth century and from 1861 until 1901 they marked the parameters of the city boundaries.[172] Within these confines, and by 1900, the Dublin United Tramways Company (DUTC) was operating several electric tram routes from the city centre to the suburbs.[173] Old transportation mediums jostled for space with new technological features of modernity, trams and trains, which meant that small streets unable to bear the burden of such traffic were congested with greater volumes of the unpredictability of horsepower.

Chapter 3 will pick up threads from the preceding chapters to discuss the impact of modernisation on life in the city and how domestic life, when it inevitably burst onto the streetscape, created a host of other causes of death. Urban historians like Erika Hanna, Ruth McManus, and Jacinta Prunty all cite physical nuisances as a primary reason for the upper-class flight to the suburbs and in this chapter I will draw attention to the levels of noise pollution in Dublin and how it may have contributed to child deaths.[174] Peter Hession argues that 'The "shricks", "oaths", [and] "imprecations"' of prostitutes were aural contamination of the urban soundscape, as much as the "rhetoric" of their physicality', but the same charge could be levied against the hawkers of Henry and Britain Streets, whose livelihoods depended on their ability to give voice to their wares.[175] Prior to the discovery of her body, the last recollection of Anne Carroll was of her singing and selling fish on 17 May 1901—she was found between 10 a.m. and 11 a.m. at 10 Spital Fields. The 50-year-old widow's death was from cardiac disease, and she was of no fixed abode. It was her contribution to the soundscape of the city that marked out her final movements.[176] With the gradual introduction of trains and later trams to the city streets, noise levels increased accordingly, which created a cacophony of competing sounds. In turn it increased risks, particularly for children who did not hear the impending danger of horse hooves, trains, and trams.

I make distinction here between non-occupation-related deaths occurring 'outside' in streetscapes and waterways, and those associated with work for rail and

---

[171] Christine Casey, *Dublin: The City Within the Grand and Royal Canals and the Circular Road with the Phoenix Park* (New Haven, 2005), p. 44.

[172] *Census of Ireland for the year 1861. Enumeration abstracts, showing, by provinces, counties, cities, boroughs, and towns,* 1861 [2865], p. 4. Dublin Corporation Act 1900, c. cclxiv, section 26 [63 & 64 Vic.].

[173] Dickson, *Dublin*, pp. 346–7; Francis J. Murphy, 'Dublin trams 1872–1959', *Dublin Historical Record,* 33:1 (1979), pp. 2–9.

[174] Joseph Nugent, 'The human snout: pigs, priests, and peasants in the parlor', *The Senses and Society,* 4:3 (2009), pp. 283–301. Nugent focuses on rural Ireland but notes how the olfactory register of Ireland was reordered with modernity.

[175] Peter Hession, 'Social authority and the urban environment in nineteenth-century Cork' (PhD thesis, University of Cambridge, 2018), p. 232. I am grateful to Peter for sharing, without hesitation, his unpublished thesis. Maith thú Peter.

[176] NAI/1901/144 Inquest on the body of Anne Carroll, 18 May 1901.

dock workers. Accidental deaths in the workplace were highly gendered. Only six of the 109 occupational deaths can be clearly classified as deaths of females at work outside the home, but there are others occurring in domestic settings that are debateable. Many women conducted paid work or outwork in their homes, several others took in lodgers and fed them for payment, and others kept 'nurse children'—these forms of female labour were not properly recognised by official instruments that devalued or excluded them. Men suffered the highest casualty rate in connection with transportation; there are numerous deaths associated with crushing and falling on train lines but for most part these were accidents linked to the workplace. These accidents were often very violent in nature, but none were suspiciously so. Although occupational deaths constitute over a sixth of the cases in the dataset, the limited survival of company records coupled with the precarious contractual nature of some work makes it difficult to conduct fuller research. For example, the records of the steam ship, tram, and rail companies are not extant. Many construction deaths were of workers employed in ad hoc gangs by 'third party' contractors who were unlikely to maintain records. Further to this, personnel records of the companies that are still going concerns are subject to embargoes. For such reasons, I have grouped occupational deaths under those occurring 'outside'. Workplace injury, and disability arising from it, is a research area that really merits further and deeper consideration by labour historians and is explored briefly here from the perspective of fatalities.

Chapter 4 examines suspicious and violent death. It is divided into three sections which move away from the locational focus of the previous chapters by taking a life-cycles approach. The first section deals with infanticide, the second examines cases of suspected suicide, and the final section examines interpersonal violence. The elevation of a case from accidental to suspicious hinged to a large degree on the discretion and intuition of the DMP constables. In all suspicious cases there was a strong medico-legal preoccupation with the conspicuous consumption of alcohol in both private and public spaces. Violent deaths were often as a result of the excesses of alcohol and that relationship will receive careful consideration in the final section of the penultimate chapter.[177] By tracing instances of foul play through to conviction, it focuses on the way in which verdicts and riders could have impact beyond the non-judicial coroner's court.

Evidence of the impact of blame and shame, and how both were socially constructed in a gender and class binary, is threaded throughout the book. The Conclusion provides a summary of findings and reiterates the importance of examining coronial court records from the perspective of power and to consider how they intersected with social class and gender. As my work with Eunan O'Halpin has shown, with regard to unknown and unnamed infant dead, the

---

[177] A theory of consumption put forward in 1899 by economist Thorstein Veblen, *The Theory of the Leisure Class: An Economic Study of Institutions* (New York, 1899).

coroner's court in returning verdicts of 'accidental' death and riders attaching 'no blame to anyone', even in the face of irrefutable evidence of foul play, had remarkable discretionary powers, which could in turn keep cases out of, or indeed place cases into, the criminal courts.[178] Using a wide social lens, aided by a mixed methods approach, the function of this court of inquiry and its relationship with the Irish judiciary will be clarified in this book.

---

[178] Ciara Breathnach and Eunan O'Halpin, 'Scripting blame: Irish coroners' courts and unnamed infant dead, 1916–32', Social History, 39:2 (2014), pp. 210–28.

1

Dublin, the City Coroner's Court, and the Everyday

Urban life operated within layered boundaries, some of which were physical and visible, but others were intangible, like legal, cultural, and social limits, and had to be learned. These boundaries were critical to the harmonious functioning of Dublin City and, from gendered and class perspectives, they laid the groundwork for the social determinants of health, life expectancy, and cause of death. This chapter begins by positioning the coroner's court within the medico-legal framework of the city; it provides an outline of how its associated biopower surveillance network was constituted and how all mobilised in tandem with respect to sudden deaths. It then turns to the city environment, daily life, and the powers that shaped the lives of those who were the natural constituency of the coroner's court—the poor. My analysis of the inquest dataset shows that because of the small confines of the home the parameters of ordinary lives naturally extended beyond the front door, to the streetscape and further to the public house, which became a recourse for many. As such, this book considers people moving in concentric circles moving outward from the home and how age, gender, and class shaped the experiences they had in domestic settings, in the streetscape, at work, or in institutions, as the case might be. These experiences shaped behaviours some of which in turn led them to become subjects of coronial court inquiries. Cases with alcohol abuse in evidence received careful attention in the coroner's court. The chapter concludes with a discussion of alcohol consumption both within and outside the home.

Why Dublin is worthy of discrete analysis is enveloped in the way in which the coroner's court itself evolved as an institution. Under the 1846 Act, Irish coroners were subject to a property qualification with minimum stated values but no professional markers were established.[1] Remuneration was a key aspect of how the system in Ireland deviated significantly from its English and Welsh counterparts; Irish coroners were not permitted to earn amounts (paid in fees of no greater than £1 10s. per case) in excess of £100. By contrast, coroners in England and

---

[1] Coroners (Ireland) Act, 1846 (9 & 10 Vic.), c. 37, section xvi. Either a freeholder of 'a clear yearly value of' £100 or the beneficiary of an estate worth at least £50 per annum.

Ordinary Lives, Death, and Social Class: Dublin City Coroner's Court, 1876–1902. Ciara Breathnach, Oxford University Press. © Ciara Breathnach 2022. DOI: 10.1093/oso/9780198865780.003.0002

Wales received an average payment of between £200 and £300 per annum.[2] Undoubtedly this had an impact on professional esteem and it was Dublin that initially saw a reversal of fortunes. Reflecting the middle-class composition of the medical profession in Dublin, it did not mention the property qualification; instead it was argued that the cap on salaries acted as a disincentive to attract the best possible candidates to the profession. Following a petition made by Irish medical licentiates to the Lord Lieutenant in 1871 about pay and conditions, some change was enacted in 1876 when an act applying to Dublin only was passed. It stipulated that coroners should be either legally (barrister or solicitor) qualified or medical professionals registered in accordance with the 1858 Act.[3] Apart from qualifications and payment, the 1876 Dublin Act amalgamated the two offices that had previously operated in alternate months. After one of the coroners, Dr William White, died in June 1876, the surviving officer holder Dr Nicolas Conlethus Whyte became solely responsible.[4] He was first appointed on 13 February 1868 and served until his death on 2 July 1891.[5]

In 1881 these professional requirements were extended to the entire country with an additional provision allowing justices of the peace of five years standing to hold office. This was a separate act that did not apply to Dublin, given its own act a few years prior. In Ireland, qualified doctors were paid to provide evidence in all cases but nationally, the coroners' service was dominated by legal as opposed to medical professionals.[6] Several professional gains were made in the late nineteenth century and when Dr Byrne took office the appointed salary was £500 per year and there was an allowance of £50 for the payment of a clerk. Together with other senior city officials, in late 1902 he petitioned the city council for an increase in salary owing to the increased jurisdiction with the city boundary changes that took effect in 1901.[7] Two coroners were employed by the County Council of

[2] Coroners (Ireland). Copy of a memorial addressed to the Lord Lieutenant by the coroners of Ireland, requesting that a measure on their behalf may be brought before Parliament early in the present session. [HC, 1871] (86).

[3] Medical Act, 1858 (21 & 22 Vic.), c. 90.

[4] Coroners (Dublin) Act (39 & 40 Vic.) c. xciii; Medical Act (21 & 22 Vict) c. 90), An Act to Regulate the Qualifications of Practitioners in Medicine and Surgery. Dr Whyte was MRCS (Eng.) 1853; *The medical directory for 1870 and general medical register, including the London and provincial medical directory, the medical directory for Scotland, the medical directory for Ireland, with a medical directory of the Army, Navy, and Mercantile Marine, a medical directory of registered practitioners resident abroad; also statistical and general information respecting the universities, colleges, schools, hospitals, dispensaries, societies, poor-law service, asylums for the insane, public services, &c., in the United Kingdom.* (hereafter *The Medical Directory*), p. 920. Thom's *Directories for Ireland* (Dublin, 1871), p. 1025. William White was LAH Dublin 1837; *The Medical Directory, 1870*, p. 921; *Weekly Irish Times*, 24 June 1876.

[5] *Irish Times*, 7 July 1891.

[6] For a discussion of the evolution of the Irish service see Clark, 'General practice and coroner's practice', pp. 37–56.

[7] *Irish Times*, 21 November 1902. Byrne stated in an inquiry into the petition that the additional duties' cost meant forty-two more cases in the year and additional time travelling, costing him appointments to the value of £175 in the eleven months since the boundary came into effect: Dublin City Council Printed Minutes 1900 (Dublin City Library & Archive), pp. 209–210. I am grateful to

Dublin, Christopher Friery and Henry L. Harty, at a salary of £200 per annum.[8] Byrne began his working life as a clerk at Power's Distillery and he later worked at Dublin Corporation, in the accountancy division. By night he attended the Ledwich School of Surgery and Medicine School. Academic snobbery prevailed in the late nineteenth century and 'night school' certificate holders were generally looked down upon; indeed, on his death in 1932 the *Medical Press and Circular* saw fit to mention in his obituary that he 'must have been one of the last survivors of those qualified from the "night schools"'.[9] Laura Kelly, also citing the *Medical Press and Circular*, notes inferences that the Ledwich School was among those considered guilty of inflating its student numbers. In the hierarchy of Dublin medical schools it was towards the bottom and the Irish system was generally accused of poor record keeping. This resulted in allegations of 'sham certificates' being issued to students who had paid fees for courses but may not necessarily have had a complete attendance record.[10]

Irrespective of his humble educational origins, Dr Louis A. Byrne became a licentiate in medicine, LM Coombe Hospital Dublin in 1884; he earned further accolades from the Royal College of Surgeons of Ireland, LRCSI in 1885; the Royal College of Physicians of Ireland, LRCPI in 1886; and his Fellowship in Surgery, FRCSI in 1889.[11] Although professionally a surgeon and the prenominal convention is now Mr, I refer to him throughout as Dr Byrne, which is how he is identified in most of the coronial court records. He began his forty-year career as surgeon at Jervis Street Hospital in 1890, and in the following year he married Isabella F. Willis of Ailesbury Road.[12] Isabella came from a very well-to-do and socially well-connected family—her father was the apothecary Dr Thomas Willis, who was renowned for his charitable works. Her sister Ada was married to Alderman Joseph Meade, son and heir to the family building company, which developed the exclusive homes of Ailesbury Road from 1863.[13] Little is known about Byrne's early life save that his marriage registration documents that his father John, was a perfumer.[14] On marriage, Dr Byrne gave his address as 20 High

---

Dr Mary Clark, City Archivist, Dublin City Archives and to Tara Doyle, Senior Librarian, Dublin City Libraries, for their assistance.

[8] Friery's term began 16 April 1894 and Harty's 18 July 1850: local government (Ireland) officials, Return to an order of the Honourable the House of Commons, dated 14 March 1901 [331], no page or table number. Image 177 of 322 on Proquest's House of Commons Parliamentary Papers.

[9] Kirkpatrick Index, Royal College of Physicians of Ireland (RCPI) Archive, clipping from the *Medical Press and Circular*, 7.xxi (1932); *British Medical Journal*, 2:1171 (1932).

[10] Laura Kelly, *Irish Medical Education and Student Culture, c.1850–1950* (Liverpool, 2017), pp. 21–2.

[11] Kirkpatrick Index, RCPI Archive, clipping from the *Medical Press and Circular*, 7.xxi (1932); *The Medical Directory, 1900*, p. 1604; Case NAI/1900/150 Inquest on the body of William Haskins, 31 October 1900. Death occurred at the Ledwich School.

[12] See https://civilrecords.irishgenealogy.ie/churchrecords/images/marriage_returns/marriages_1891/10685/5894060.pdf (marriage record, accessed 2 November 2021).

[13] See Galavan, *Dublin's Bourgeois Homes*, p. 40.

[14] He may have been the same John Byrne listed as a Hairdresser and Wigmaker in 1835 at 119 James' Street: *Dublin Almanac and General Register of Ireland* (Dublin, 1835), p. 392; *Gentleman's and Citizen's Almanack* (Dublin, 1842), p. 671.

Street, Dublin, which was occupied by Dr Abraham Tarleton in 1901 indicating that this was a well-trodden path for medical men.[15] By the 1901 census Dr Byrne, after ten years as an established city surgeon, was living at 79 Harcourt Street. At that point he had four young daughters, and Isabella had a nurse and a house-maid to assist with the household work.[16]

Coronerships, despite their relatively low remuneration, were undoubtedly prestigious and could add greatly to the professional reputation and the upward social mobility of both legal and medical office holders. Geary has convincingly argued that the true value of being a dispensary doctor, as the position was so poorly paid and the system was full of abuses, was the gravitas it lent to establish-ing private practice.[17] Representing something of a new breed of non-hereditary medical practitioner from humbler backgrounds, Byrne earned a reputation as an excellent surgeon and teacher. Coroners were not permitted to hold other public offices. Byrne's predecessor Dr Joseph E. Kenny came from a more solidly middle-class background and earned his qualifications in Dublin and Edinburgh.[18] A Roman Catholic and Irish Parliamentary Party 'Parnellite' MP, he continued his private medical practice during his tenure as coroner from 1891 until his untimely death in April 1900 from an infection that set in following a tooth extraction. In accordance with municipal legislation, an election had to be held within ten days of the vacation of office.[19] Twelve candidates presented themselves for election, of whom five were legally qualified. On the third count Dr Byrne was declared duly elected.[20]

Recognising the tension between medical and legal controls over the profes-sion, a *British Medical Journal* article commented how on Dr Byrne's election, it was 'satisfactory to find that the office of coroner again devolves on a medical man'.[21] In Dublin, more localised tensions were at play, and it was noted in the *Belfast Newsletter*, with a degree of salaciousness, that Byrne was brother-in-law of the Alderman Joseph Meade and that the runner up was Dr Robert D. Kenny, brother of the previous incumbent.[22] Indeed, the inquest into the death of William Caruthers exhibits the degree of professional rivalry and perhaps

---

[15] Tarleton lived alone. See http://www.census.nationalarchives.ie/reels/nai003721734/ (accessed 2 November 2021).

[16] See http://www.census.nationalarchives.ie/pages/1901/Dublin/Fitzwilliam/Harcourt_Street/1306577/. In 1911 they lived at 50 Merion Square, and had four servants: see http://www.census.nationalarchives.ie/pages/1911/Dublin/South_Dock/Merrion_Square__East/86066/ (both accessed 2 November 2021).

[17] Laurence M. Geary, 'The medical profession, health care and the poor law in nineteenth-century Ireland', in Virginia Crossman and Peter Gray (eds), *Poverty and Welfare in Ireland, 1838–1948* (Dublin, 2011), pp. 189–206.

[18] *British Medical Journal*, 21 April 1900; Ciara Breathnach and Ian Walsh (eds), *Original Inquest Papers of Dr Joseph E. Kenny, Dublin City Coroner, 1900* (Forthcoming, Dublin, 2022).

[19] The Borough Coroners (Ireland) Act 1860 (23 & 24 Vic.), c. lxxiv.

[20] Minutes of the Municipal Council of the City of Dublin, 1900, pp. 208–11.

[21] Anon, *British Medical Journal*, 28 April 1900, p. 1056: https://www.ncbi.nlm.nih.gov/pmc/articles/PMC2506001/pdf/brmedj08505-0046.pdf.

[22] *Belfast Newsletter*, 20 April 1900.

personal distrust between the old and the new guards in Irish medicine of Drs Kenny and Byrne, respectively. The DMP report stated that Kenny, who had treated Caruthers at the North Dublin Union (NDU), deemed an inquest unnecessary but requested the case be reported. Although the death had no indication of foul play, Dr Byrne held the inquest and found that Caruthers died following a fall while drunk at his employers yard Mr McGrane, 1 New Lisburn Street, and the verdict was, 'Delirium Tremens set off by intemperance and shock of fall, the immediate cause of death was cardiac failure'. There were two medical reports, that of Dr Ernest Moorehead of the Richmond Hospital where he was first treated, and Drs Kenny and Jackson of the NDU gave evidence to the DMP.[23]

The Coronial Network

The coroner's court and city morgue opened on the corner of Marlborough Street and Old Abbey Street on the North Side of the city in September 1871.[24] Prior to that, the Dublin City coroner's court was peripatetic. Dr Nicholas C. Whyte and Dr William White held inquests at houses or hospitals and when necessary, they requisitioned bigger spaces as permitted under the 1846 Act.[25] The 1866 Sanitary Act placed an onus on local authorities to provide suitable accommodation for the reception of dead bodies for the purposes of post-mortem and to pay the expenses associated with its upkeep as well as the costs associated with inquests. In Dublin that was to be funded from the Borough Rate.[26] City authorities did not take immediate action and when unknown bodies were discovered in streets and waterways the facilities in 1868 were still what Charles Cameron described as 'an insult to the dead'.[27] It was in fact what the Public Health Committee in 1870 admitted was a shed associated with a dairy yard, which was 'defective and discreditable'.[28] With the exception of the major cities, by the close of the nineteenth century the facilities for holding inquests were not properly developed. The precedent set under the 1846 Act, that publicans be compelled to make their

---

[23] NAI/1900/108 Inquest on the body of William Carruthers, 8 September. The only other case where Kenny was medical witness is NAI/1900/18 Inquest on the body of Sarah Sheffield, 7 May 1900.
[24] The Irish Times and Daily Advertiser, 29 September 1871.
[25] Freeman's Journal, 28 January 1869, report of Dr Whyte holding an inquest at a brush factory; Freeman's Journal, 17 March 1869, inquest at Ship Street Barracks; Freeman's Journal, 5 September 1869, inquest at Steevens' Hospital; Freeman's Journal, 23 November 1869, inquests held at 108 North King Street and York Livery Stables; Freeman's Journal, 18 June 1866, inquest held at the theatre of the Mechanics Institute.
[26] Sanitary Act 1866 (28 &29 Vic.), c. 90, s. 27.   [27] Freeman's Journal, 23 September 1868.
[28] 1900 Report, p. 184. The Public Health Committee of the Corporation was responsible for the provision of a mortuary house, morgue and coroner's court using funds from the Grand Jury fund: Royal Com. to inquire into Sewerage and Drainage of City of Dublin. Report, Minutes of Evidence, Appendix, Index [c. 2605], p. 169.

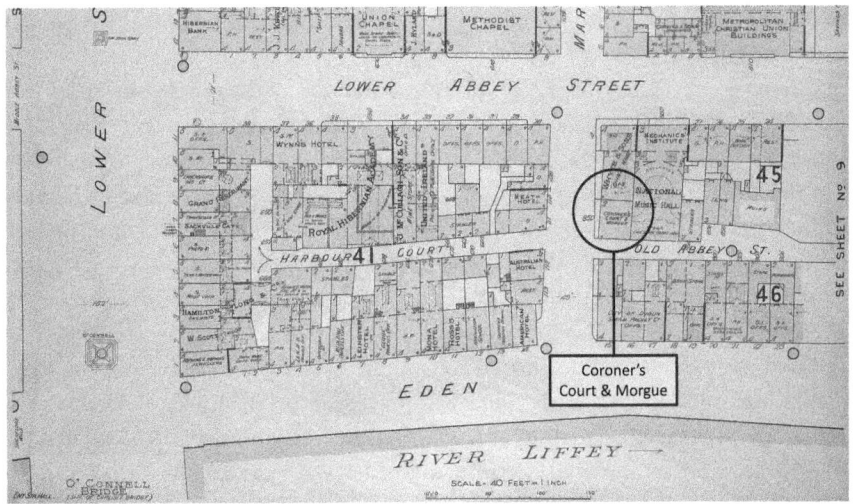

Map 1.1 Coroner's court and morgue, Dublin 1871–1902

Source: Goad Map, 1893, shelf 145.b.4.(2.), Vol. 1: sheet 8, enhanced and modified by author.
http://www.bl.uk/onlinegallery/onlineex/firemaps/ireland/largeimage146672.html (accessed 3
February 2019).

licensed premises available when necessary, continued for longer in rural
Ireland.[29]

Reflecting the legacy of the low esteem in which the system was initially held,
Map 1.1 shows how part of a mixed-use building was repurposed for the coroner's court in 1871. The same building included the National Music Hall, the
Mechanic's Institute and Whyte & Sons China Warehouse. Needless to add, it
quickly outgrew its purpose and during the summer months there was an unbear-
able stench. Inquests were held there until 1902 when a purpose-built coroner's
court opened on the junction of Store and Amiens Streets.[30] This was as a result of
mild professional gains, and the influence of medical power-brokerage in the city.
Dublin was what James H. Murphy terms 'just as much a British city as it was a
specifically Irish one' and in terms of example, it looked to cities of comparable
size in Britain to find best practice in 'questions of taxation, industry and
infrastructure.'[31] Following a visit to various purpose-built coroners' courts in
England, Dublin City Councillor Joseph Nannetti recommended that the plan of
the Prince's Dock Mortuary in Liverpool be used as a template for the proposed
new Dublin morgue. The site of the Custom House Flour Mills, which had

---

[29] Burney, *Bodies of Evidence*, pp. 80–106.

[30] 1, 3, 4 Amiens Street, entrance to morgue, 110l (rateable valuation), *Thom's Directory, 1903*,
p. 1411; 3 Store Street West, city morgue—Byrne, Louis, A., city coroner—res. 79 Harcourt Street;
O'Kelly, John, clerk 110l; Dublin metropolitan police barrack C division. *Thom's Directory, 1903*,
p. 1597.

[31] James H. Murphy, *The Politics of Dublin Corporation 1840–1900* (Dublin, 2020), pp. 12–13.

frontage at Amiens and Store Streets was recommended as a potential site in conjunction with the City Architect, Charles J. McCarthy.[32] The measure was described as 'absolutely necessary' and the condition of the existing facilities was described as being in a 'shocking condition'.[33] The old building became the site of the Irish National Theatre Society in 1904. It was later renamed as the Abbey Theatre. For reasons of proximity, and owing to the lack of capacity in tenements to facilitate a 'viewing of the body' by jurors, the majority of the Dublin metropolitan area inquests took place at the city morgue or at hospitals; for example, Christina Morrison's inquest was documented on the inquisition form as having been held 'at the dead house at Sir Patrick Dun's hospital'.[34]

From the inquests it is possible to recreate Dr Byrne's professional world as well as the final movements of his subjects; they also provide an overview of power hierarchy and brokerage in the coroner's court and in the city itself. Medical doctors, police, and witnesses all contributed to what was occasionally a medico-legal spectacle and, aided by daily newspaper coverage, its sphere of influence extended far beyond the confines of the court and its place in Irish social life was entrenched. The proceedings of the Dublin coronial courts provided a source of staple content for the *Evening Herald*, which was often syndicated to national and regional newspapers.

As the case of John Healy shows, coroners' inquests have an extraordinary level of topographical data, and when they are read as a corpus their spatiality becomes all the more apparent. Hospitals like Dr Steevens', Sir Patrick Dun's, Meath, Mercer's, Jervis Street (where Byrne worked as a surgeon), Adelaide, and the Richmond Asylum, all anthropomorphise into distinct characters, as do police stations like Store Street, Summerhill, Mountjoy, College, Lad Lane, Newmarket, Bridewell Lane, Green Street, Chapelizod, and Chancery Lane (Map 0.2), which are all referenced in the records of the coroner's court. DFB featured to a lesser extent, as did references to telegraphic services and water sources.

Medical attendants working at the aforementioned hospitals formed part of Byrne's professional network and indeed some of his colleagues exhibited considerable flair for conducting detailed anthropometrical readings in their post-mortem reports. In the early years, his Jervis Street Hospital colleague Dr John Burgess acted as Assistant Coroner. Drs John Begley, Abraham Tarleton, Carrol O'Sullivan, and George Taylor, who worked at nearby hospitals and conducted post-mortems for, and at, the city morgue, all provided very detailed reports. Of the 611 inquests used here, Tarleton and Begley were the medical witnesses in fifty-three cases each, and Burgess provided post-mortem reports for fifty cases.

---

[32] Report of the Finance and Leases Committee, *Dublin Corporation Printed Reports* (Dublin City Library & Archive), Volume 1, 1900, pp. 705–9.

[33] *Evening Herald*, 11 June 1900.

[34] Coroners (Ireland) Act, 1846 (9 & 10 Vic.) c. 37, NAI/1900/22 Inquest on the body of Christina Morrison, 12 May 1900.

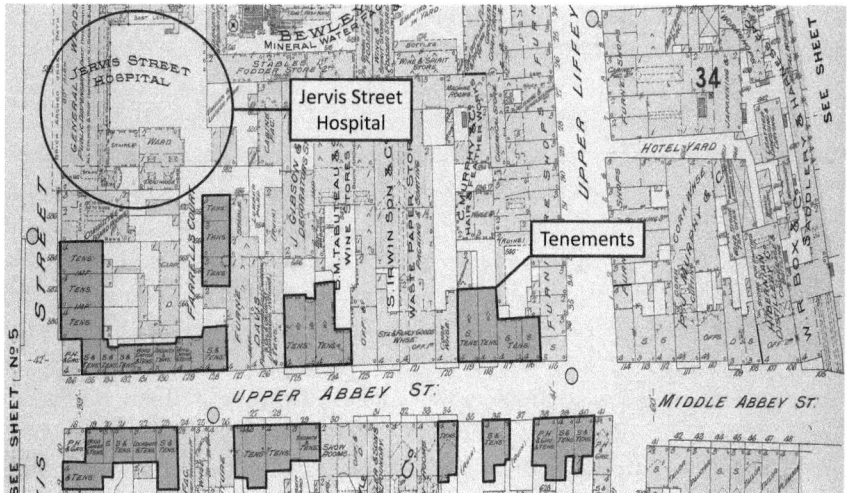

Map 1.2 Showing mixed usage buildings and tenements in inner-city Dublin
Source: Goad Map, 1893, shelf 145.b.4.(2.), Vol. 1: sheet 6, enhanced and modified by author.
http://www.bl.uk/onlinegallery/onlineex/firemaps/ireland/largeimage146665.html (accessed 3
February 2019).

Medical witness were paid £2 2s. in fees per post-mortem; for example, in the
quarter ending October 1900, Dr Begley was paid £14 14s. for seven, Dr James
Dunne was paid for five, and Dr Burgess for four cases.[35] In the previous quarter
ending July 1900, where there was an overlap between the Kenny and Byrne coronerships, Dr Robert D. Kenny received fees for six cases and Dr O'Sullivan for
five.[36] The practicalities of managing private practice alongside a busy court preoccupied Dr Byrne for the first few months and once he was established he never
used Dr Kenny again. Expert medical witnesses were naturally selected; if, as in
John Healy's case, a death occurred at Jervis Street Hospital then it followed that a
doctor from that location conducted the work. By 1900, £2 2s. was a nominal
sum, but being an expert witness carried other professional benefits and lent further weight to burgeoning and established careers alike.

With knowledge of individual competencies, Dr Byrne usually accepted their
evidence without question and guided his jury of between twelve and twenty-three
local men to do likewise.[37] By 1901, women had begun to make inroads to
employment in the city hospitals, like Dr Emily Martha Crooks who, according to
Kelly, was the first woman to hold the post of house surgeon at the Children's
Hospital. Dr Crooks conducted eight post-mortem reports on the bodies of

[35] Report of the Finance and Leases Committee, *Dublin Corporation Printed Reports* (Dublin City
Library & Archive), Volume III, 1900, p. 874.
[36] Report of the Finance and Leases Committee, p. 780.
[37] Coroners (Ireland) Act 1881 (44 & 45 Vic.), c. 35.

children.[38] Dr Kathleen Lynn, famed for her role in the 1916 Easter Rising and her subsequent establishment of the all-female-run St Ultan's Hospital, was mentioned in the admission records of cataract patient Mathew [sic] Smyth who was found dead in bed the morning after his admission at 7.25 a.m. by Nurse Mary Gilmor.[39] Opposition to the feminisation of the medical profession found expression in the coronial court records too: in one case, Samuel Davis, the landlord of 22 Island Street, sent a letter to the Coombe because 'a person was confined in the house and a Dr was wanted + A lady Dr came within an hour = I went myself to the Coombe and Dr Neill came within an hour'. Inherent in his commentary was his distrust of 'lady doctors', who in his view were not proper doctors.[40] Dr Bryne's court accepted Dr Crooks's evidence in the same way it accepted that of her male colleagues. The medical community was also very tightly knit. There were a few cases of what we might now consider to be cases of medical mismanagement/ misadventure in hospitals: Margaret O'Connor died after she received an anaesthetic. She was driving a horse and trap and when it hit a stone, she was thrown. Dr Michael Ballesty described in evidence how he administered the anaesthetic that caused heart failure.[41] Ballesty also conducted the post-mortem, which was not considered unethical or a conflict of interest at the time.

Class and local power brokerage again played a part in the composition of other aspects of the court, as it was a requirement that jurors be ratepayers of £4 per annum and resident in the coroner's district. Samuel Richardson, a barrister living in Clontarf,[42] was used repeatedly as a foreman and juror, as was James Farrell, a Spirit and Wine Merchant, 112 Marlboro Street.[43] With respect to both men, proximity triumphed and they appear with great regularity because there was often more than one inquest in a day, like on 18 March 1901 where Farrell acted in the cases of Margaret Hennessy and Frances Glynn.[44] Following a four-day reprieve in activity, on 17 September 1901 four cases presented at the coroner's court—Samuel Richardson was foreman for all of them.[45]

[38] Laura Kelly, *Irish Women in Medicine, c.1880s–1920s: Origins, Education and Careers* (Manchester, 2012), p. 169.

[39] NAI/1900/143 Inquest on the body of Mathew [sic] Smyth, 24 October 1900; Margaret Ó hÓgartaigh, *Kathleen Lynn: Irishwoman, Patriot, Doctor* (Dublin, 2006); Marie Mulholland, *The Politics and Relationships of Kathleen Lynn* (Dublin, 2002). Dr Lynn was not professionally implicated in this case.

[40] NAI/1900/32 Inquest on the body of a Female Infant, 28 May 1900.

[41] NAI/1900/130 Inquest on the body of Margaret O'Connor 5 October 1900: 'I had about a half a drachum of Chloroform, I had not reached full anaesthesia when Mr McDonnell reduced the dislocation the chloroform was discontinued and the patient seemed alright regaining consciousness when suddenly became cyanosed & died.'

[42] See http://www.census.nationalarchives.ie/reels/nai003674487/, barrister at law boarding in Clontarf (accessed 3 February 2020).

[43] See http://www.census.nationalarchives.ie/reels/nai003765542/ (accessed 27 November 2021).

[44] NAI/1901/76 Inquest on the body of Mary Hennessy and NAI/1901/77 Inquest on the body of Frances Glynn, both held on 18 March.

[45] NAI/1901/244-247 Inquests on the bodies of an Unknown Male (adult), Henry Farrelly, Mary Prendergast and Christina Reel, all held on 17 September 1901.

Niamh Howlin's work has used a selection of rural coronial court records and found similar patterns of convenience. She argues that of all courts, coroners 'could not afford to be fussy' because time was a paramount concern with regard to empanelling a jury.[46] While her examples are primarily drawn from areas of agrarian unrest, where she notes that it was not uncommon to have the full complement of jurors out of necessity, she also cites instances of potentially contentious and suspected cases of suicide, infanticide, and homicide as occasioning high numbers.[47] The jury was not indispensable either, as Howlin notes; a coroner could dismiss it if the members were unable to agree a verdict.[48] It should be noted that section 6 of the 1881 act, dealing with jury dismissal, did not apply to Dublin.[49] But custom and law were at variance and in what was described in a newspaper headline as a 'Strange Scene at a Dublin Inquest', Roman Catholic jurors refused to swear an oath on Protestant bibles. The jury was dismissed by the Roman Catholic Deputy Coroner Dr John Burgess, who was presiding that day.[50] Jurors could be fined for not showing up or for sending someone else in their stead.[51] Irrespective of their presence and, as other scholars have argued, an experienced coroner could sway a jury to his way of thinking. In most of the cases studied here the opinion of the medical witness was returned verbatim as the verdict. An important attribute of the inquest jury lay in its ability to attach a rider to blame or exonerate as it saw fit—this was common to the English courts too.[52] Although they were of no legal standing, they were important statements of opinion reached by majority consensus and could be used in subsequent criminal proceedings. As in the case of John Healy, his employer Mr James Maher was absolved of any wrongdoing and freed from any moral imperatives to compensate the mother of the deceased.

The DMP and the DFB

A system of mutual trust must have existed between the coroner, local dispensary doctors, and the DMP, as the city had a disproportionately high death rate and the average number of inquests was about 300 per year. It was estimated that the DMP was about 1,200 strong in 1901 and its jurisdiction extended to 32.15 square miles containing 380,000 people.[53] There was a considerable power imbalance

---

[46] Niamh Howlin, *Juries in Ireland: Laypersons and the Law in the Long Nineteenth Century* (Dublin, 2017), p. 81.

[47] Howlin, *Juries in Ireland*, pp. 81–2.   [48] Howlin, *Juries in Ireland*, p. 211.

[49] 1881 Act, section 6; Huband, *A Practical Treatise on the Law*, p. 255.

[50] *Weekly Irish Times*, 22 June 1901; *Freeman's Journal*, 18 June 1901.

[51] Juries Act (Ireland), 1871 (34 & 35 Vic.), c. 65; Petty Sessions Clerks and Fines (Ireland) Act, 1878 (21 & 22 Vic.), c. 100.

[52] Burney, *Bodies of Evidence*, p. 5.

[53] Dublin Metropolitan Police, *Report of the Committee of Inquiry, 1901* [Cd. 1088], p. 2.

between the various actors in the coroner's court. In a commission of inquiry into salaries of the various ranks of DMP personnel it was revealed that a detective constable, G Division, earned between £120 and £160 per annum. Ordinary rank-and-file policemen earned considerably less than detectives; in 1914, a review of pay and conditions, which had been the same since 1883, noted their financial embarrassment. Depending on the number of years of service, salaries ranged from 27s. to 37s. per week for constables. Resignations owing to inadequate pay were common and the matter of pay deductions for barracks accommodation was another sticking point. Individual pensions, pensions to widows, and children's allowances were also deemed inadequate.[54] Sanction for these pay increases was only received by the treasury in 1916, at which time the *Irish Times* described the situation as a crisis.[55]

By 1900, Dublin Corporation had a small network of fire stations located around the city; Tara Street was the biggest and it served the South East. Although regularly described in newspapers as men of 'zeal' and 'pluck', firemen struggled to reach parity of esteem with policemen or soldiers. While the DMP had a more established reputation than the DFB, lower grade officers in both groups were on similar salaries. Las Fallon notes the professional tensions between the DMP and the DFB when it was suggested that policemen should assist for free in erecting ladders at fire scenes.[56] The fire brigade services had their origins in the insurance industry and their purpose was to keep fire damage costs to a minimum.[57] The Royal Society for the Protection of Lives from Fire was established in Dublin but it was not until 1862 that the DFB Act was passed.[58] This brought the work under the remit of the corporation and granted powers to purchase the equipment necessary for a fully functioning fire service and removed any ambiguities about the lawfulness of such expenditures. The costs were to be met by the public water rates levied under the Waterworks Act 1861.[59] A new station was opened at Lower Buckingham Street and the corporation took over the running of the DFB in 1863. The Public Health Act 1878, the Waterworks Act, and the Local Government Acts permitted the extension and improvement of the service. The work of the DFB received considerable newspaper coverage—the speed in which they arrived and skill with which the valorised Captain Purcell and his men controlled the fires were all documented in newspaper coverage, as was the approximated value of the property lost and saved. 'Ceaseless', 'zealous', 'untiring' were among the

---

[54] Royal Irish Constabulary and Dublin Metropolitan Police, *Report of the Committee of Inquiry, 1914* [Cd. 7421], p. 28.

[55] *Weekly Irish Times*, 4 November 1916.

[56] Las Fallon, *Dublin Fire Brigade and the Irish Revolution* (Dublin, 2012), p. 9.

[57] Trevor Whitehead, *Dublin Fire Fighters: A History of Fire Fighting, Rescue, and Ambulance Work in the City of Dublin* (Dublin, 1970).

[58] *Irish Daily Independent*, 9 August 1900; Dublin Corporation Fire Brigade Act 1862 (25 & 26 Vic.) c. 38.

[59] Dublin Corporation Waterworks Act 1861 (24 & 25 Vic.), c. 172.

adjectives used to describe the 'efforts' as opposed to their working terms and conditions, which, like nursing, had an air of voluntarism associated with it, and it was paid accordingly.[60]

On 18 November 1899, George Leahy wrote in his capacity as Representative of the Firemen's Union to the Chair and members of the Dublin Corporation Waterworks' Committee to memorialise for better pay and general working conditions.[61] The Winetavern Street station team lived in substandard quarters located in Cook Street and Michael's Hill, which caused delays in getting them to the stationhouse and to emergency situations.[62] In 1899, Captain Purcell opined that most of his men lived in tenements and he only had quarters for eighteen men.[63] After years of lobbying, the Dublin Corporation Ambulance was established in 1899 as a branch of the DFB. A deputation report in 1897 recommended that an ambulance be established for accident cases, as well-meaning but unskilled people were using private vehicles to transport injured people to hospitals and in the process aggravating injuries.[64] In its first year of operation it dealt with 537 calls rising to 660 in 1900 and 808 in 1901.[65] Located initially at Chatham Row in the south side, the horse-drawn service expanded to two vehicles in 1901 and the second was located at Upper Buckingham Street in the north side.[66]

DMP constables lived in tenements too—four officers with service that varied from three to six years were 'retired on gratuity' in 1901, three of whom died shortly thereafter from phthisis.[67] According to the report of the Principal Medical Officer for the DMP, a total of twenty-two men took a combined number of 1,209 days in sick leave in 1901 owing to an outbreak of typhoid fever, four of whom succumbed to the illness and died.[68] Paradoxically, DMP constables who were uniformed, numbered, and therefore instantly recognisable were themselves subject to the gaze of biopower surveillance when they were 'on the beat'. The beat, which emerged in the early nineteenth century, itself gave rise to what Patrick Joyce terms circumspection which was a kind of 'social discipline', less about the observance of the law and 'a series of understandings, in effect nods and winks, that grew up between the police and city dwellers'.[69] To Joyce it was more

---

[60] *Evening Herald*, 17 January 1901.

[61] *Reports and Printed Documents of the Corporation of Dublin*, 1900, volume 1 (Dublin, 1901), pp. 468–80.

[62] *Evening Herald*, 13 August 1895.   [63] *Evening Herald*, 1 March 1899.

[64] Dublin City Archives, *Report of the Waterworks Committee, re Improvements in Connection with Fire Brigade and submitting Report of Deputation* (Dublin, 1898), p. 9. I am very grateful to Stephanie Rousseau and Clair Walton, Archivists, Dublin City Library for their advice and for their help in locating and scanning various documents during periods of prolonged closure 2020/21.

[65] *Annual Report from the Chief of the Dublin Corporation Fire Brigade Department, for the year ending 31st December 1909* (Dublin, 1910), no page number.

[66] Dublin City Archives, Dublin City Council/History/Ambulance Service/R1/01/03.

[67] Statistical tables of the Dublin Metropolitan Police for the year 1901 [Cd. 1166], p. 31.

[68] Statistical tables of the Dublin Metropolitan Police for the year 1901 [Cd. 1166], p. 32.

[69] Joyce, *The Rule of Freedom*, p. 111.

about learning to live with, as opposed to by, the law in the public domain. To a lesser extent, clergy of all denominations also held the role of biopower agents or, in the case of Roman Catholic priests, as disruptors to early efforts of imposing proper medico-legal processes. Chapters 2–4 will refer to the cases in which witnesses 'called for the Priest' as opposed to the doctor or the DMP constable when a relative was thought to be dying. Only eighteen of the non-institutional deaths concerned the demise of people who had been under medical care.

1900 Dublin City

Dublin's fall from grace in the nineteenth century has been well documented by historians, architectural historians, and historical geographers alike.[70] Following the Act of Union in 1801, it lost the status of the second city of the British Empire and was further degraded when it was overtaken by what Mary E. Daly terms 'upstart Belfast' in the 1830s.[71] Wealthier classes moved to London or to the suburbs in order to avoid tax and other nuisances. In the suburbs they found a more 'civil' society and, similar to what Hession found in Cork City, these new areas 'served as laboratories for more inclusive varieties of "polite" culture based on fresh permutations of symbolic, social and cultural capital'.[72] So unhealthy was the metropolitan area that it prompted a Royal Commission of inquiry into sanitation in 1879–80 and a Public Health Committee report in 1900.[73] Both provided comprehensive evidence of the degree to which appalling living conditions, precarious employment, and poor wages created serious health inequality and additional morbidity factors for certain cohorts.[74]

Despite the obvious dangers of urban living, it was the home that posed the most pervasive threat to life in Dublin at the beginning of the twentieth century. McManus and Brady assert that Dublin was experiencing 'a housing crisis with slums comparable to those of Calcutta'.[75] When the Local Government Board began its inquiry into the public health of Dublin City in 1900, its primary question was what caused the high death rate and it was tasked with providing a range of

---

[70] Christine Casey, *Dublin: The City within the Grand and Royal Canals and the Circular Road with the Phoenix Park* (New Haven, 2005), p. 4; Rob Goodbody, *Dublin, Part III, 1756–1847, Irish Historic Towns Atlas, no 26* (Dublin, 2014); Joseph Curran, 'Charity, finance, and legitimacy: exploring stateless-capital status in early nineteenth-century Dublin and Edinburgh', *Journal of Urban History*, 47:4 (2021), pp. 753–70.

[71] Mary E. Daly, *Dublin, the Deposed Capital: A Social and Economic History, 1806–1914* (Cork, 1984), p. 2.

[72] Peter Hession, 'Social authority and the urban environment in nineteenth-century Cork' (unpublished PhD thesis, University of Cambridge, 2018), p. 39.

[73] Sewerage and Drainage in Dublin 1879–80 [c. 2605]; Dublin Report, 1900.

[74] Dublin Report, 1900, p. 6.

[75] Joseph Brady and Ruth McManus, 'Dublin's twentieth-century social housing policies: tenure, "reserved areas" and housing type', *Planning Perspectives*, 35:6 (2019), 1005–103 at 1005.

recommendations to ameliorate the various problems. Following extensive investigation, it concluded that the state of the city's housing stock was the primary culprit in the mortality crisis. One witness described the majority of accommodation as

> Large tenement houses, each room occupied by a separate family: the house itself in a state of dilapidation; water supply inconvenient of access; dirty common staircases; inadequate water-closet accommodation in a foul state; back yards ill-paved and littered with refuse and excrement; are conditions of life in Dublin which we frequently encountered in connection with the dwellings of the poorer classes. These conditions tend to the production of a state of lowered vitality favourable to the contraction of disease and to fatal result of disease when contracted.[76]

For the purposes of the 1900 report, a tenement house was defined as a house let to two or more families.[77] Figure 1.1 depicts the rear view of the once grand Gardiner Street, which was part of the major urban development initiated by

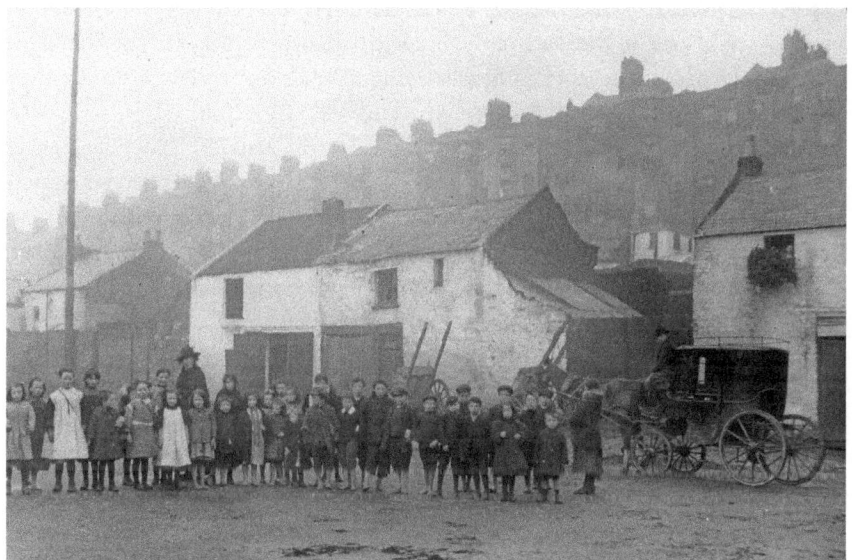

Figure 1.1 Summerhill, rear view of Gardiner Street

Note: I am grateful to Sarah Connaghan, Librarian, RSAI, for kind permission to reproduce here.

Source: Royal Society of Antiquities of Ireland, RSAI, BOX07_045. 'Street view, Summerhill, Dublin City, Co. Dublin, Ireland', http://rsai.locloudhosting.net/items/show/24371 (accessed 10 February 2019).

---

[76] Dublin Report, 1900, p. 10.   [77] Dublin Report, 1900, p. 2.

Luke Gardiner in the late eighteenth century.[78] As Ruth McManus, Erika Hanna, Jacinta Prunty, and Christine Casey's work has so ably shown, the grand houses of Georgian Dublin had degenerated to the status of tenement in the late nineteenth century.[79] By then the inner city was full of dilapidated housing stock (note missing window panes in Figure 1.1) owned predominantly by landlords whose interests found disproportionate representation in Dublin Corporation and other spheres of influence.[80] Unregulated, unchecked, and unfair, overcrowding was endemic in the Dublin housing sector and one-roomed tenancies rotated at a high frequency.

> ...the main factor—which is responsible for, at least, seven-eights of the whole excess in the death rate is the housing of the poor. I have a good deal of experience of foreign cities and of English cities, and I know no city where the overcrowding of the poor exists to the same extent as in Dublin.[81]

Thus Dr Joseph E. Kenny, coroner to the City of Dublin 1891–1900, replied when questioned at the Local Government Board committee about excess mortality. While an average of only one in every forty deaths materialised as a coroner's inquest, as a former NDU medical officer and MP, Dr Kenny was well-placed to make observations on the state of the inner-city housing stock. He continued his testimony by adding the fact that he was born in Dublin and had lived on Gardiner Street (Figure 1.1), which he identified along with Gloucester Street as having suffered considerable decline over the previous twenty years. By 1900, the class of people living in inner-city Dublin (see the proliferation of tenements on commercially busy streets, Map 1.2) shared a similar profile to what Hurren and King found in their study of the New Poor Law in Brizworth, Northamptonshire, who survived on 'persistently low wages and underemployment created a class of labourers always on the verge of crisis'.[82] Some progressive social housing schemes emerged in the late nineteenth century, but it was nowhere near enough to reverse the near century of neglect. Rents charged by the Dublin Artisans' Dwelling Company (DADC) (established to develop affordable housing in 1876) ranged between 2s. and 8s. per week, depending on the number of rooms in 1900.[83] Inspired in part by the Peabody Trust established in 1863 to build houses in London, the Third

---

[78] Goodbody, *Dublin, Part III*, p. 2.

[79] Erika Hanna, *Modern Dublin: Urban Change and the Irish past, 1957–1973* (Oxford, 2013); Jacinta Prunty, *Dublin's Slums 1800–1925: A Study in Urban Geography* (Dublin, 1998); Casey, *Dublin*, pp. 119–20; Ruth McManus, *Dublin, 1910–1940: Shaping the City & Suburbs* (Dublin, 2002).

[80] Cormac Ó Gráda, *Jewish Ireland in the Age of Joyce: A Socioeconomic History* (Princeton, 2006), pp. 42–3.

[81] Dublin rReport, 1900, p. 180.

[82] Elizabeth. T. Hurren and Steven A. King, '"Begging for a Burial": form, function and conflict in nineteenth-century pauper burial', *Social History*, 30:3 (2005), pp. 321–41 at 326.

[83] Dublin Metropolitan Police, *Report of the Committee of Inquiry, 1901* [Cd. 1088], pp. 9, 12.

Earl Iveagh began to develop housing schemes in the south city from 1894.[84] As Flanagan argues, the housing efforts of the Iveagh Trust and the DADC amounted to the 'remaking [of] Dublin's geography of poverty without confronting it'.[85]

While the nineteenth-century flight to the suburbs changed the social composition of Dublin City, many upper-class families retained ownership of their properties.[86] Much like what Sarah Wise found in London, the chain of slum property ownership in Dublin was difficult to establish. Wise's research on London has shown that 'the owners of the freeholds and leaseholds of these death traps included peers of the realm, churchmen, Bethnal Green vestrymen and several corpses: almost half the properties were managed by solicitors and other trustees to benefit the estates of the long deceased'.[87] Further to this, she noted that leaseholders in the Nichol area of East London acted independently to property owners and subdivided houses into weekly tenancies which in turn could be sublet by lodgers.[88] A different dynamic operated in Dublin and while property ownership shared the same social class profile like that of the Nichol in London, the ways in which Irish medical officers could challenge authority through campaigning was somewhat freer. In the transition from one to multiple family occupancy, sanitary conditions and water closet provisioning were not modified accordingly and these factors led in part to many deaths coming before the coroner's court from accidents and micro-epidemics of what contemporary experts categorised as 'communicable' diseases. Medical officers for health, Dr Edward D. Mapother (1835–1908) and later Sir Charles Cameron (1830–1921) openly criticised the property owners and, unlike their equivalents such as Dr George Paddock Bate in the Nichols, they did not need to worry about being dismissed.[89] In evidence to a Royal Commission in 1885, Cameron argued that the chain of ownership and responsibility in Dublin was easy to unravel. He blamed 'house farmers' or 'jobbers who live by screwing the largest amount of rent they can out of the tenants' for the awful state of housing, but when the local authorities tried to make them contribute to sanitary improvements the chain took no responsibility for basic repairs and upkeep.[90] By June 1900, there were four 'Lady Sanitary Sub-Officers' whose job it was to induce women in the lower-class tenement houses to keep their homes and the communal areas of the

---

[84] Dublin Improvement (Bull Alley Area) Act 1899 (62 & 63 Vict.) c. xi; F.H A. Aalen, *The Iveagh Trust: The First Hundred Years, 1890–1990* (Dublin, 1990).

[85] Maureen A. Flanagan, *Constructing the Patriarchal City: Gender and the Built Environments of London, Dublin, Toronto, and Chicago, 1870s into the 1940s* (Philadelphia, 2018), p. 150.

[86] Alvin Jackson, 'Ireland, the Union, and the Empire, 1800–1960', in Kevin Kenny (ed.), *Ireland and the British Empire* (Oxford, 2004), pp. 123–53 at 124.

[87] Sarah Wise, *The Blackest Streets: The Life and Death of a Victorian Slum* (London, 2009), p. 9.

[88] Wise, *The Blackest Streets*, p. 10.

[89] Wise, *The Blackest Streets*, p. 26; Obituary of Dr Mapother, *The British Medical Journal*, 1:2463 (14 March 1908), pp. 661–2.

[90] *Third report of Her Majesty's commissioners for inquiring into the housing of the working classes Ireland, 1884–5* [C. 4402], p. 22.

building in a sanitary state. Their purpose was to reinforce and aid the work of the male officers 'though not superseding'.[91] The rate at which buildings were condemned by the Public Health Committee was slow, and so substandard housing stock remained in perpetual use.

Life expectancy in the Dublin tenements is difficult to determine precisely; internal migrants from other counties accounted for 26.6 per cent of the population in 1901.[92] That aside, people moved with such great frequency that the touchpoints with statecraft, which relied heavily on individual engagement, were tentative. They are difficult to verify prior to the 1901 census, which is the first to have full surviving manuscript copy. The extent of underreporting of life events has yet to be determined and contemporary efforts to ascertain defaulters were not that comprehensive.[93] Using the 1821 census returns, Ó Gráda has estimated that life expectancy in the pre-Famine era was 37 to 38 years and that it rose steadily in the post-Famine era.[94] Walsh has determined that between 1901 and 1911, male life expectancy rose from 49.3 to 53.6 years.[95] These aggregate national estimates do not recognise regional variations, but in another study Ó Gráda shows the disparities in the life expectancy in Dublin, which for professional classes was between 53 and 60 years, when it hovered at 31 to 32 years for unskilled workers.[96]

Of the 87,606 deaths that occurred nationally in 1900, 72,322 deaths occurred in domestic settings, 11,181 in workhouses, and 2,850 in hospital or asylums.[97] That year, 9,976 people died in the Dublin registration area which included Pembroke, Rathmines and Rathgar, and Kingstown. Reflecting the better provision of hospital care in the metropolitan area, 1,744 deaths occurred in infirmaries, 190 in asylums, 1,724 in workhouses, and 6,318 in domestic settings.[98] Were all criteria for holding an inquest strictly applied, then a much higher number than circa 300 per annum should have come before the coroner—unfortunately, the DMP records of preliminary inquiries are not accessible and may not be extant. A partial survival of DMP reports can be found in the coronial court records, but there must have been a greater number of them, given the death rate and the predominantly domestic location of deaths.

---

[91] *Dublin Corporation Report*, Vol. 2, 1900, p. 696.
[92] *Census of Ireland, 1901. Part I* [Cd. 847], p. 234.
[93] *Thirty-seventh detailed annual report of the Registrar-General (Ireland), containing a general abstract of the numbers of marriages, births, and deaths registered in Ireland during the year 1900* [Cd. 697], p. 166. Hereafter ARRG, 1900.
[94] Cormac Ó Gráda, *Ireland Before and After the Famine: Explorations in Economic History, 1800–1925* (Manchester, 1993), p. 18.
[95] Brendan Walsh, 'Life expectancy in Ireland since the 1870s', *The Economic and Social Review*, 48: 2 (2017), pp. 127–43 at 135.
[96] Ó Gráda, *Jewish Ireland in the Age of Joyce*, p. 37.   [97] ARRG, 1900, p. 8.
[98] ARRG, 1900, p. 166.

Aside from sudden and accidental deaths, urban living took an insidious toll— lung disease was rampant, and the impact of physically demanding working lives is evidenced in the high numbers of non-specific heart conditions (cardiac syncope) between the ages of 40 and 60 in my sample. If marasmus as an ill-specified cause of death was too liberally applied for infants and young children, then its equivalent for sudden non-violent adult cause of death was 'fatty degeneration of the heart'. In this sample, cases were described in such terms; others were described as cardiac failure, syncope, valvular, ruptures, and mitral valve disease. The 1864 *Statistical Nosology* in its advice to coroners did not address sudden deaths with the same alacrity as it addressed violent ones, and the 1896 *Nomenclature of Diseases* offered few advances in knowledge with respect to cardiac deaths for clinicians.[99] The earlier volume remained in use even after revised editions were in circulation; it had a section devoted to coroners that encouraged the post-mortem examination of the organs to the extent that foul play could be ruled out and 'leave no more room for suspicion of innocence, than hope of impunity for crime'.[100] Vague and brief, the advice to coroners left plenty of room for manoeuvre. Diseases associated with the heart could be classified under 'sporadic diseases of uncertain or variable seat' or under organs of circulation numbers 58 to 66 in the original statistical nosology: carditis, disease of the cardiac valves, hypertrophy, aneurism, angina, fainting (syncope), arteritis, phlebitis, and varicose veins. Heart conditions could also be coupled with the respiratory organ range of laryngitis, laryngisimus stridulus, bronchitis, pleurisy, congestion of the lungs, asthma and phthisis (numbers 67–73, respectively).

Dangers of engaging in retrospective diagnoses notwithstanding, the most obvious culprit in the high mortality from lung complaints was the built and industrial environment of the city itself. Many city officials were landlords and therefore represented the status quo and thus the extraordinary efforts of public health crusaders like Sir Charles Cameron led to frustrating results and yielded very few dividends in terms of improvements to old housing stock. The selection of cases discussed in Chapter 2 exhibits the extent to which people were reticent to engage with medical services even when they were seriously ill. Old age accounted for 16,278 deaths nationally in 1900, and at the opposite end of the life course 11,088 infant and 17,161 child deaths (aged 1–5) occurred.[101] With respect to cause, 12,848 were attributed to all forms of tuberculosis of which 10,076 were pulmonary. The NDU had a death rate of 5.7 per 1,000 while the South Dublin Union (SDU) had a slighter lower rate of 5.5.[102]

Pulmonary tuberculosis was one of the leading causes of death in the city and it was at high levels of uncontrolled community transmission. Poor pulmonary health was tolerated; often people had no idea that they were suffering from the

---

[99] *Nomenclature of Diseases*, p. 97.   [100] *Statistical Nosology*, 1864, p. 66.
[101] ARRG, 1900, p. 20.   [102] ARRG, 1900, pp. 12–16.

disease and it was discovered only on post-mortem examination. For example, Michael Guilfoyle's brother testified that the 24-year-old railway porter had been 'suffering from an affection of his lungs' and was on sick leave when he was accidentally knocked down. The accident occurred between Moyvally and Kilcock stations: a priest and a doctor called to meet the train at Broadstone, no blame was attached to the driver, and post-mortem examination found longstanding tubercule of 'left lung almost entirely destroyed by tuberculous disease and almost useless functionally'.[103]

Household Economics

Even when seriously unwell, ordinary people could not afford to take time off work. As Table 1.1 shows, 14,604 Dublin City households were living on less than a pound a week in 1914; 13,244 of the total number paid less than 3s. a week in rent. Pitiful indeed was Dublin's positioning in the UK context: the report noted how it could not be compared to other manufacturing centres—alcohol, soda water, and biscuits were the limits of the city's products and it had 'no special trades of its own'.[104]

Communal budgets were common to most households, and they only worked if male breadwinners handed over their earnings to their wives. And, as Emma Griffin has contended, 'A mother's role was...to transform the husband's wages into a tolerably comfortable domestic existence for each and every member of the family'.[105] Scant evidence of household budgets survives for early twentieth-century Dublin save some observations made by Cameron for various annual

Table 1.1   Households and average income, 1914

Number of households	Amount in shillings
5,406	Less than 15
9,000	15–20
2,584	20–25
1,627	25–30

Source: Report of the departmental committee appointed by the Local Government Board for Ireland to inquire into the housing conditions of the working classes in the city of Dublin. [Cd. 7273], p. 8.

---

[103] NAI/1900/41 Inquest on the body of Michael Guilfoyle, 13 June 1900.

[104] *Report of the departmental committee appointed by the Local Government Board for Ireland to inquire into the housing conditions of the working classes in the city of Dublin* [Cd. 7273], p. 8.

[105] Emma Griffin, 'The emotions of motherhood: love culture, and poverty in Victorian Britain', *The American Historical Review*, 123:1 (2018), pp. 60–85 at 67.

reports and his own *How the Poor Live* published in 1904.[106] In that publication he classified those earning under 15s. a week as being very poor and estimated there were several thousand in that class. Dr John Lumsden, Chief Medical Officer (CMO) of Guinness's Brewery started a focused study in late 1903 and published it in 1905. Inspired by work conducted by Rowntree in York and Paton, Dunlop, and Inglis's study of working-class Edinburgh, he aimed to conduct 'a systematic investigation into the actual conditions under which the Brewery families live'.[107] Lumsden was appointed in 1894 in the general medical services of Guinness's brewery and became its CMO in 1899. From the outset, according to Dennison and MacDonagh, 'he became involved in preventive medicine' and he went to great lengths to ensure the well-being of the company's employees.[108] His resulting survey provides an impression of the everyday of what he termed 'average brewery families', the humblest of which were better off than most in Dublin City. For his informants, Dr Lumsden chose 'twenty women whose statements I could trust' from households where three regular meals were taken together daily and he tried to ensure that the families were of equal stature.[109] His selected families ranged in occupation and status from ordinary labourers to widows of pensioners (ten wives of ordinary labourers, four widows, three wives of foremen, two of tradesmen, and one pensioner's wife).[110] Lumsden did not include the calorific values of alcohol in his study and added in a footnote how carefully chosen the families were, those of 'particularly steady men, and of exemplary character both inside and outside the brewery'.[111]

Even with these selection criteria, some families emerged with economic vulnerabilities: Lumsden accounts for a Mrs Daniel G. (39), 27 Emerald Square, off Cork Street, wife of a charger (aged 40): they had eight children, girls aged 17, 14, 13, 11, 9, and 1, and two boys aged 7 and 5. They occupied a two-bedroomed dwelling but all the children slept in two beds contained in one room. In that instance Lumsden advised that the parlour be converted to a sleeping quarter:

The general appearance of the place is dirty, and the children, although healthy looking, are not kept as clean as they should be. This is a regular Irish family, living a hand-to-mouth existence, liking a little bit of show; and a filthy room to

---

[106] Charles A. Cameron, *How the Poor Live* (Dublin, 1904), pp. 4–5.

[107] Benjamin Seebohm Rowntree, *A Study of Town Life* (London, 1901); D. Noel Paton, James C. Dunlop, and Maud Inglis, *Studies of the Diet of the Labouring Classes in Edinburgh: Carried Out Under the Auspices of the Town Council of the City of Edinburgh* (Edinburgh, 1901).

[108] S.R. Dennison and Oliver MacDonagh, *Guinness 1886–1939; from Incorporation to the Second World War* (Cork, 1998), pp. 130–1.

[109] John Lumsden, *An Investigation into the Income and Expenditure of Seventeen Brewery Families and a Study of their Diets* (Dublin, 1905), p. 1.

[110] Lumsden, *An Investigation*, p. 1. According to the 1911 census returns the family retained occupancy of their two-bedroomed dwelling, but in 1904 all the children slept in two beds contained in one room (Lumsden, *An Investigation*, p. 35).

[111] Lumsden, *An Investigation*, p. 10.

entertain their friends in, is of more account than a healthy sleeping apartment for the children.[112]

Earning an aggregate sum of £24 10s. over fourteen weeks, their household was just 9d. over what Lumsden considered the poverty line. Despite their slender means, Lumsden remarked that 'a wise selection of foods was made'.[113] He noted twelve different animal proteins (milk, buttermilk, butter, mutton, pigs' legs, dripping, eggs, bacon, fish, beef, bones, and pigs' cheek) and ten vegetable sources (bread, sugar, potatoes, cocoa, flour, oatmeal, syrup, cabbage, turnips, and jam).[114] According to information received from Boland's Ltd and Johnston Mooney and O'Brien Ltd, two of the city's main bakeries, the average price of a 4lb loaf of bread delivered was 5¼d.[115] We have no way of knowing how food was apportioned within families, but greater portions and higher levels of protein were given to men. Mrs T.B. 'aged about 50' and her time-keeper husband (aged 55), lived with their five children at 28 Reginald Street which was a two-storey artisan cottage on the Meath estate; it had two bedrooms, a scullery, a concrete yard, and a WC. The couple shared their bedroom (1,989 cubic feet) with their two sons (17 and 15), while the three girls (24, 18, and 13) occupied the back bedroom (864 cubic feet). She shopped on Thomas Street on Tuesdays and Saturdays and paid for everything in cash. Lumsden informs us that B was a 'steady decent man' who only kept back 2s. a week for personal needs.[116]

Middle-class access to working class homes was as limited in Dublin as Hewitt found in Britain, but it was Lumsden's positioning as company doctor that gave him an advantage.[117] During the ten- to fourteen-week study, Dr Lumsden paid regular visits to the households involved; a few of the women revealed to him that their neighbours viewed the survey with great suspicion and as some form of a ruse to make the case for lowering wages and pensions. In overall terms Lumsden found the homes to be 'dangerously overcrowded' and a 'large number of our people reside in old tenement houses most of which places are dens of disease, and are both overcrowded and insanitary'.[118] Mrs P.S. 19 Usher's Island was the wife of a Guinness pensioner who kept a 'nurse-child (illegitimate)' for 14s. per month. When she lost the benefit of her son's income, after his employment at the Inchicore Railway Works ceased, she made up the shortfall in cash income by taking in a brewery widower and his 5-year-old son for 15s. a week.[119] This economic dexterity was replicated throughout the city and came at the great cost of limiting domestic space for family life even further. The S. family shared their

---

[112] Lumsden, *An Investigation*, p. 35.   [113] Lumsden, *An Investigation*, p. 36.
[114] Lumsden, *An Investigation*, pp. 38–9.   [115] ARRG, 1900, p. 21.
[116] Lumsden, *An Investigation*, p. 90.
[117] Hewitt, 'District visiting and the constitution of domestic space in the mid-nineteenth century', pp. 120–41.
[118] Lumsden, *An Investigation*, p. 132.   [119] Lumsden, *An Investigation*, p. 56.

front yard and water closet with twelve other families who lived in the two tenement houses at Nicolas Avenue at the back of the Four Courts, which Dr Lumsden
described as 'a dirty insanitary neighbourhood...with noisy neighbours of a low
class, and the signs of much poverty only too evident about'.[120] One of Lumsden's
suggestions for the improvement of living standards was the 'Encouragement of
healthy out-of-door sports, Athletic Exercise and Gymnastics amongst the men
and boys'.[121] These leisure-time activities were not that accessible to inner-city
dwellers. Further to Goodbody's Tobacco, Messrs Pim Clothing and Jacobs's biscuits factories were the primary sources of employment for children and youths
in Dublin, that is if they were lucky enough to get in.[122] The importance of child
and youth earnings to working-class household budgets has been reiterated by
several scholars, and the among the more notable are Sara Horrell and Jane
Humphries. Although they deal with an earlier period, rich data, and the very
different opportunities industrial Britain afforded, their time series analyses show
that some labouring households relied heavily on child income.[123] Guinness
brewery workers were fortunate to have job security and the cradle to grave care
of a paternalistically motivated employer. That Lumsden carefully selected 'good'
households and they exhibited vulnerabilities means that large swathes of the
inner-city population were in even more precarious circumstances with few safety
nets other than charity, the pawn, and, as a last resort, the 'Union'.

Working-class life was unpredictable—outside of 'jobs for life' in companies
with paternalistic values, few had security. Established companies had nepotistic
tendencies too and employed generations of the same families, which limited
opportunities for outsiders. For women married to precariously employed men,
reliance on the pawn was high.[124] Beverly Lemire has shown that, in England,
clothes were the most significant form of alternative currency with a recognisable
value; in Dublin it was the same.[125] In his study of the poor published in 1904,
Charles Cameron estimated that 2,866,084 pawn tickets were issued in one year,
and it was usually clothes and shoes that were pawned to buy necessities when
money ran out on a Monday or Tuesday—they were bought back the following

---

[120] Lumsden, *An Investigation*, p. 74.   [121] Lumsden, *An Investigation*, p. 142.
[122] Lumsden, *An Investigation*, p. 135.
[123] Sara Horrell and Jane Humphries, ' "The exploitation of little children": child labor and the family economy in the Industrial Revolution', *Explorations in Economic History*, 32:4 (1995), pp. 485–516;
Sara Horrell, Jane Humphries, and Jacob Weisdorf, 'Family standards of living over the long run,
England 1280–1850', *Past & Present*, 250: 1 (2021), pp. 87–134.
[124] Lumsden, *An Investigation*, pp. 24, 51. Mrs Catherine C. of 8 Cameron Street was a brewery
widow and her ex-soldier son, aged 26, managed to get a job in Guinness's and all four daughters were
employed by Goodbody's Tobacco Factory. Similarly, Mrs C. of 68 Manor Street was a brewery widow
and her son worked at the brewery too. Mrs J.L.'s 16-year-old son was a messenger at Guinness's earning 9s. a week while her husband was a foreman in the Forwarding Department: Lumsden, *An
Investigation*, p. 85.
[125] Beverly Lemire, *The Business of Everyday Life: Gender, Practice and Social Politics in England,
c.1600–1900* (Manchester, 2006), pp. 90–1.

Saturday if wages permitted.[126] Relative, absolute, and secondary poverty co-existed in tenement areas where credit, barter and the pawn were as significant as a wage to the local economy.

For older people without supporting relatives, life was full of uncertainties and potentially even greater hardships. Older women found ways of staying out of the workhouse by using a combination of charity and the pawn. The following three cases share similar survival strategies, Sarah Sheffield, aged 80, had been unwell. The week she died, she had asked her friend Bridget Leake to get a ticket for the SDU. She had been living on charity for ten years; she had a small sum of money in a post office savings account and was insured in the Liverpool Victoria Society Lord Edward Street. In this very poignant case, the retired silk-weaver (Messrs Pim Clothing) and spinster left her estate to the Hospice for the Dying in Harold's Cross, but her nephew who had not bothered with her for three years showed up. Sarah Jane Waterhouse, with whom she regularly took tea, made her posthumous wishes clear to the DMP. In order to make that bequest, Sheffield did without, and her lodgings at 41 Bride Street were described in the DMP report as being in a filthy condition.[127] Anne Grill, described as a pauper, was suffering from rheumatism and kidney disease, had 'no means of living', and had relied on co-religionist benevolence from 'charitable ladies belonging to the Protestant institution in Fishamble, Werburgh and Anglesea St' for a number of years.[128] Those without charitable inroads had to make do in other ways. Winifred Kelly, who was described occupationally as a widow and a pauper, had ten pawn tickets, 10s. 9d. in cash, and a purse on her person when she died of cardiac disease. Given that she was 65 and ailing in health, there was little hope of her earning the money to recover her pawned items—she had no addresses for her sons, one of whom was in America and another in England.[129]

Married Irish women did not enjoy the same property protection as in England. The agency of women was curtailed by statute; for example, the Divorce and Matrimonial Causes Act of 1857 did not apply to Ireland and the only recourse for women was the parliamentary process which, as Diane Urquhart states, was 'costlier, lengthier and more socially and gender biased'.[130] Both Urquhart and Sarah-Anne Buckley have argued that Irish society had its own way of dealing with marital disputes. In popular terms, resolution to unhappy unions particularly for the poorer classes was found in 'Irish-style' divorces; that is, informal separation outside official means.[131] There are a few such cases of emotionally,

---

[126] Cameron, *How the Poor Live*, p. 3.
[127] NAI/1900/18 Inquest on the body of Sarah Sheffield, 7 May 1900.
[128] NAI/1900/176 Inquest on the body of Anne Grill, 25 November 1900.
[129] NAI/1901/15 Inquest on the body of Winifred Kelly, 14 January 1901.
[130] Diane Urquhart, 'Irish divorce and domestic violence, 1857–1922', *Women's History Review*, 22:5 (2013), pp. 820–37 at 820.
[131] Sarah Anne Buckley, 'Men, women and the family, 1730–1880', in James Kelly (ed.), *The Cambridge History of Ireland: Volume 3, 1730–1880* (Cambridge, 2017), pp. 231–54.

economically, and, consequently, physically vulnerable spouses coming before the coronial court, such as the case of John Lane who lived in a lodging house at 4 Northumberland Square—he had been estranged from his wife and family for four years when he suffered a cardiac episode in a pub on Trinity Street.[132] Francis Moran, a 38-year-old 'married clerk' was also separated from his wife—he shared a room with two other men at 28 Cuffe Street. One of his co-lodgers was unknown to them (and refused to be named in the DMP report) but the other, Patrick O'Kane, stayed up with him the night before he died and 'gave him whiskey at intervals.'[133] Couples also parted temporarily for the purposes of seeking aid. Hayseed dealer John Campbell, aged 63, died in a hay loft at Beresford Terrace where he had been sleeping for the previous fortnight. The DMP report noted how his wife had been an 'inmate of NDU until a few days ago. She was sleeping with the deceased last night & she seems to be somewhat silly.' It transpired that his wife survived the bitter cold of the previous two weeks because she had spent some of that time at the NDU. He complained of a cough and had attended Coleraine Street dispensary three weeks prior.[134] Living in stables and outhouses caused other health problems: Edward Reilly's pneumonia cannot have been helped by his living conditions, a stable at the rear of 11 George's Hill. He was a single labourer and was not in care of a doctor. He was 44 when he died of cardiac failure, death consequent to pneumonia.[135]

Children were particularly vulnerable when resources were spread over two households and Chapter 2 discusses these cases in greater detail. There are several examples of how 'illegitimacy' was managed. Child protection legislation provided an instrument to collect maintenance but again had low numbers; for example, in 1900 there were ten applications to the courts and eight orders.[136] There were undoubtedly plenty of cases where men took responsibility for their extra-marital children, but only one in this sample, that of dairy proprietor, Peter Kavanagh, 19 East James Street, who paid for the lodgings of Margaret Scott at 31 Lower Liffey Street. At five weeks, her female infant was still unnamed, which should have prompted more DMP suspicion but acute colic was returned as cause of death. At that time, Scott was co-residing at 10 Tolka Cottages with Michael O'Sullivan.[137]

Childcare was a poorly regulated sector of the Irish economy, and it was in this context that evidence of a particular form of cruelty came before the coroner's court. Elsewhere I have described the sector and the loopholes that permitted this

---

[132] NAI/1901/296 Inquest on the body of John Lane, 25 November 1901.

[133] NAI/1901/289 Inquest on the body of Francis Morin, 13 November 1901.

[134] *Irish Daily Independent*, 22 February 1901; NAI/1901/49 Inquest on the body of John Campbell, 21 February 1901.

[135] NAI/1901/212 Inquest on the body of Edward Reilly dated 12 August 1901.

[136] *Judicial Statistics, Ireland, 1900* [Cd. 725, 682], p. 117.

[137] NAI/1901/283 Inquest on the body of Unnamed Scott, 6 November 1901. Kavanagh was 44 and unmarried: http://www.census.nationalarchives.ie/reels/nai003818065/ (accessed 10 November 2021).

informal economy to emerge but it warrants a brief summary here.[138] In what Margaret L. Arnott describes as a 'panic about baby-farming' and 'general framework of middle-class concern about working-class motherhood', the Infant Protection Act 1872 was introduced.[139] It was primarily intended to respond to criminal child neglect cases and made it mandatory for non-relatives caring for more than one child for over twenty-four hours to register with the local authority. This meant that women were permitted to care for one so-called 'nurse child' for payment without notifying the authorities and day care was excluded.[140] Those caring for more than one child for periods over twenty-four hours had to register with the local authorities. Another major milestone in the child protection movement was the foundation of the NSPCC in 1889, but it focused attention on what it regarded as unfit parents. The 1897 Infant Life Protection Act permitted local authorities to employ of female inspectors. Some other cosmetic amendments were made with respect to 'nurse-children'; for example, the notification period for the receipt of a child was increased from twenty-four to forty-eight hours.[141] In evidence taken before a Royal Commission in 1907, Miss Fitzgerald-Kenney, a Local Government Board inspector employed under the 1897 clauses, contended that the act missed the opportunity to alter the one-child exemption which, as Daniel Grey has argued, allowed plenty of room for bad actors to continue to ply their trade until the Children Act 1908 (Chapter 2 discusses child neglect and its links to household economics).[142] The nurse child sector was a legitimate way to supplement meagre incomes, but the payments demanded were beyond the means of low-paid and young single women.

Gendered Parameters

The poles of highly stylised working-class tropes make up a segment of the cases discussed here and the majority of the deaths were as a result of deep and systemic social inequalities. If we adopt a Judith Butler (Butlerian) lens then the construction of gender norms in Irish society was very much shaped by social class

---

[138] Ciara Breathnach, 'Infant life protection and medico-legal literacy in early twentieth-century Dublin', *Women's History Review*, 26:6 (2017), pp. 781–98.

[139] Margaret L. Arnott, 'Infant death, child care and the state: the baby-farming scandal and the first infant life protection legislation of 1872', *Continuity and Change*, 9:2 (1994), pp. 271–311.

[140] Buckley, *The Cruelty Man*, pp. 16–17; Infant Life Protection Act, 1872 (35 & 36 Vict.), c. 38.

[141] Infant Life Protection Act, 1897 (60 & 61 Vic.) c. 57.

[142] *Report from the Select Committee on Infant Life Protection. Together with the proceedings of the committee, minutes of evidence, and appendix. 1908 (99)*, p. 55. Daniel Grey '"More ignorant and stupid than wilfully cruel": homicide trials and 'Baby-Farming' in England and Wales in the wake of the Children Act 1908', *Crimes and Misdemeanours*, 3:2 (2009), pp. 60–77 at 65.

and religion.[143] Elite Anglo-Irish women, for instance, were expected to perform their identities in accordance with strict social norms of 'respectability' and, with the exception of tearooms and the relatively new concept of shopping in fashionable department stores, they were not factored as part of city life.[144] Patrick Joyce, using a photograph, or, what he terms a 'quotidian scene of Victorian life', of Deansgate in Manchester in the 1880s, argues that through 'dress, deportment, manners, action, all can be seen to perform urban life and social relations at the level of practice'.[145]

Photographs and accounts of streetscapes show that unless they were engaged in endeavours befitting of their social class, philanthropy for instance, then upper-class women rarely, if ever, frequented working-class areas of Dublin. None of the inquests discussed here includes voices of middle- or upper-class women.

Women and their needs were rarely taken into consideration by city authorities, and Flanagan uses the absence of public amenities to exemplify this deliberate exclusion.[146] Implicit in prevailing discourse was that respectable women would not dream of ever using a public toilet so it was a more pointed attack on the working classes who had fewer recourses, but not without options.[147] What it illustrates is that Dublin authorities were so ideologically patriarchal that the exclusion of women was normative and this permeated all aspects of urban planning. Working-class men were targeted too: while Dr Steevens' Hospital was constructing a new nurses' home in 1900 it petitioned the Public Health Committee to remove a urinal located adjacent to the new building on nuisance grounds and it was successful.[148]

In relative terms, gender performativity for poor women took on masculine attributes, and some forms of working-class masculinity were atavistic compared to their elite counterparts.

Gillian Rose argues that, with respect to 1930s London slum photography, 'the figured bodies in fictive spaces' were also gendered in spatial and corporeal terms. The popular representation of the maternalised body, with babe in arms, simply getting on with life in tough circumstances was to Rose a form of 'ordering' the 'spatial chaos' of the slum and a particular kind of femininity, which she juxtaposes with the predominantly white, male, and middle-class photographer.[149]

---

[143] Butler, 'Performative acts and gender constitution'.

[144] Stephanie Rains, *Commodity Culture and Social Class in Dublin 1850–1916* (Dublin, 2010).

[145] Joyce, *The Rule of Freedom*, pp. 6–7.

[146] Flanagan, *Constructing the Patriarchal City*, pp. 150–5. From the 1890s, Dublin Corporation was busy building public amenities for men, but the idea of doing the same for women was repugnant. It was mooted by Dublin Corporation on a few occasions but resisted by Sir Charles Cameron for years and flatly rejected by business owners who successfully sued the authorities in 1907 and managed to keep the city free of women's public toilets until the 1920s.

[147] Flanagan, *Constructing the Patriarchal City*, p. 155.

[148] *Dublin Corporation Report, Vol. 2, 1900*, pp. 629–30.

[149] Gillian Rose, 'Engendering the slum: photography in East London in the 1930s', *Gender, Place and Culture: A Journal of Feminist Geography*, 4:3 (1997), pp. 277–300.

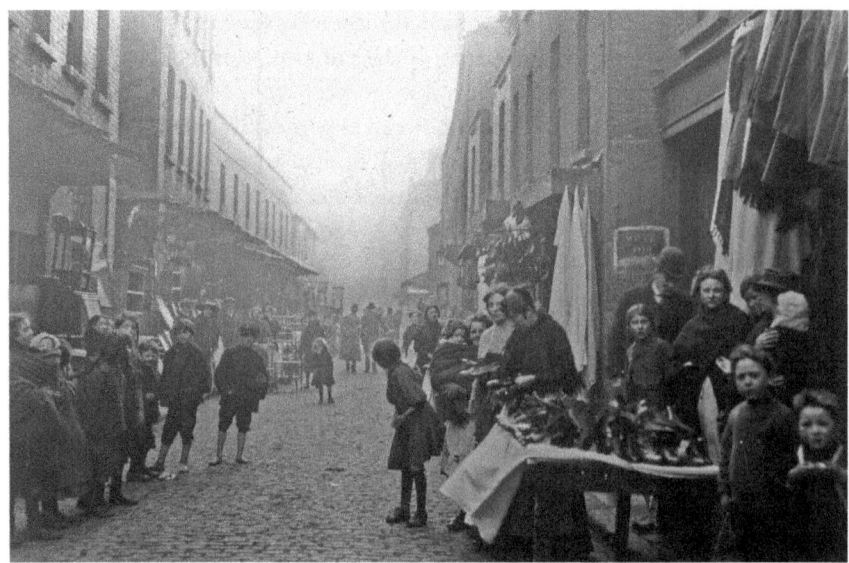

Figure 1.2 Street view, Coles Lane, Dublin City, Co. Dublin, Ireland

Note: I am grateful to Sarah Connaghan, Librarian, RSAI, for kind permission to reproduce here.

Source: Royal Society of Antiquities of Ireland, RSAI, BOX07_088. 'Street view, Coles Lane, Dublin City, Co. Dublin, Ireland', http://rsai.locloudhosting.net/items/show/24414 (accessed 10 February 2019).

Similar aspects of that composition are in evidence in Dublin streetscape photographs; for example, Figure 1.2 shows Cole's Lane off Henry Street on the city's north side. Captured in 1913 by NSPCC Inspector John Cooke when it was a busy market area, the photograph forms part of the 'Darkest Dublin' collection.[150] The eighteenth-century architecture was sadly, as Erika Hanna has documented, destroyed to build a shopping centre in the 1970s.[151] In this splendid photograph we can see the rough and tumble nature of a street occupied by, and commercially inclined more towards, the working classes. Another very striking element of this photograph is the number of children present—it is highly likely that some of them were engaged in paid work as messengers and other unpaid duties like care of younger siblings. There are two discernible, what Anna Davin calls, 'little mothers', that is, older daughters looking after younger siblings, in the frame.[152] Dangers to children working in the streetscape, as outlined in the 1902 commission on street trading, included keeping late hours, truancy, beggary, fighting, playing games that took up vehicular space, using bad language, going into licensed

---

[150] Buckley, *The Cruelty Man.*

[151] Erika Hanna, *Modern Dublin: Urban Change and the Irish Past, 1957–1973* (Oxford, 2013), p. 39.

[152] Anna Davin, *Growing Up Poor: Home, School and Street in London, 1870–1914* (London, 1996), p. 63.

premises to hawk goods, and smoking.[153] In her comprehensive analysis of the commission, Gillian McIntosh argues that from an urban middle-class perspective there was a very narrow margin between children trading and begging, and when things went awry it was mothers as opposed to parents who were blamed.[154]

Children and women were positioned and understood in relation to men. To better understand the positioning of poor women, then, it is important to consider the ways in which working-class Dublin City men were excluded from the dominant 'idealised' masculinity forms. Anglo-American hegemonic masculinity has been used by scholars since the 1980s to define what masculinity and manliness are, and what they mean in any given context, but its application in colonial settings is very problematic—more problematic still are instances where there are racialised differences.[155]

In her original thesis, Connell contended that the power and construction of hegemonic masculinities relied primarily on the subordination of women.[156] She defined hegemony as 'cultural dominance in the society as a whole. Within that overall framework there are specific gender relations of dominance and subordination between groups of men.'[157] Connell's original thesis, as Ben Griffin has asserted, offered no accommodation for intersectionality and the framework is certainly not a good fit for working-class Dublin where power operated in different ways to other cities in the United Kingdom.[158] In the first instance, the colonial setting has the added complexities of being held in comparison with the heteronormative behaviours of the coloniser, which makes few allowances for cultural factors and, in the case of Ireland, resulted mainly in the stereotypical colonised other. We must also be careful to consider how Irish masculinities were constructed from within and without.

John Tosh's definition of manliness as 'a cultural representation of masculinity rather than a description of actual life' is sensitive to local factors and Irish men

---

[153] *Street-Trading Children Committee (Ireland). Report of the Inter-Departmental Committee on the Employment of Children During School Age, especially in street trading in the large centres of population in Ireland, appointed by His Excellency the Lord Lieutenant of Ireland. Together with minutes of evidence and appendices (1902)* [Cd. 1144], p. vi: 'As regards street trading generally, the police returns show that in Dublin there are 214 boys under the age of 14, and 219 from 14 to 16, making a total of 433; and there are 32 girls under the age of 14, and 148 from 14 to 16, making a total of 180, following this occupation. In the case of the boys, the large majority, viz., 366, are engaged in selling newspapers; 180 of these are under 14, and 180 from 14 to 16. As regards girls—20 are employed in selling newspapers, 76 selling fruit, 48 selling fish.'

[154] Gillian McIntosh, 'Children, street trading and the representation of public space in Edwardian Ireland', in Maria Luddy and James Smith (eds), *Children, Childhood and Irish Society* (Dublin, 2014), pp. 46–64.

[155] Charlotte Hooper, *Manly States: Masculinities, International Relations, and Gender Politics* (New York, 2001), p. 5.

[156] R.W. Connell, *Masculinities* (Cambridge, 2005, 2nd edn), pp. 77–80; Ben Griffin, 'Hegemonic masculinity as a historical problem', *Gender & History*, 30 (2018), pp. 377–400 at 380.

[157] Connell, *Masculinities*, p. 78.

[158] Connell, *Masculinities*, p. 77.

occupied several liminalities during the long nineteenth century.[159] Connell's initial binary model, which was inherently linked to the 'legitimacy of patriarchy', or subordinacy was often too rigidly enforced but it formed the basis of men's studies. In light of the significant body of research the original thesis begot, in 2005 she reassessed with James Messerschmidt the problematic elements of the framework. Of particular relevance to this study was the acknowledgement of the plurality as well as the hierarchy of masculinities and the recommendation that hegemonic masculinity should not be used 'as a fixed, transhistorical model'.[160]

At a macro level, Ireland's loss of political autonomy in 1801 not only had an enormous impact on the economic climate, but it affected the national psyche deeply and caused a splintering of identity. Anglo-Irish elites were quick to take advantage of their status and the inherent privileges that it bestowed. Even if they were effectively outsiders in London, they were predominantly Protestant, which set them apart from Roman Catholics and the lower Irish orders as they could infiltrate English high society. In socio-economic terms, Ireland under the union can be crudely parsed into pre- and post-Famine eras, but with respect to political activism and masculinities, further divisions can be found. Griffin advises that 'active resistance' to the normative model is as important a consideration as 'Complicity, marginality and subordination'.[161] Internal and external perceptions of Irish masculinities differ greatly—they were constructed and broken repeatedly in the intervening period of the failed rebellions of 1798 and 1916. Resistance in Ireland gave rise to the repeal movement that sought to undo the union; the land question that began in the 1860s and culminated in the land acts of 1881, 1891, 1903, and 1909; and the overlapping national or home rule question that began in the 1870s and resulted in the slow partition of Ireland from 1920 to 1922. In the same timeframe a sharp urban/rural dichotomy emerged as each constituency engaged in its own socio-economic and cultural battles. Michael de Nie has shown that in the British press not only was Irish agrarian unrest written as cowardly in comparison with English manliness, but it was portrayed as monstrous.[162] More generally, the Irish in British newspapers and periodicals were

> shadowy man-monsters [who] stood in stark contrast to the upright British suitors and saviors... This unmanliness did not translate into effeminacy, as in cartoons of the French, but rather into inhumanity. The most degraded of the Irish were so unmanly, in fact, that they became less than human—they were drawn as Calibans and eventually as creatures with little or no human features at all.[163]

[159] John Tosh, 'What should historians do with masculinity? Reflections on nineteenth-century Britain', *History Workshop Journal*, 38 (1994), pp. 179–202 at 181.

[160] R.W. Connell and James W. Messerschmidt, 'Hegemonic masculinity: rethinking the concept', *Gender & Society*, 19:6 (2005), pp. 829–59 at 838.

[161] Griffin, 'Hegemonic masculinity as a historical problem', p. 382.

[162] Michael de Nie, *The Eternal Paddy: Irish Identity and the British Press, 1798–1882* (Madison, 2004), p. 161.

[163] de Nie, *The Eternal Paddy*, p. 264.

"Look on this picture, and then on that."—SHAKSPEARE.

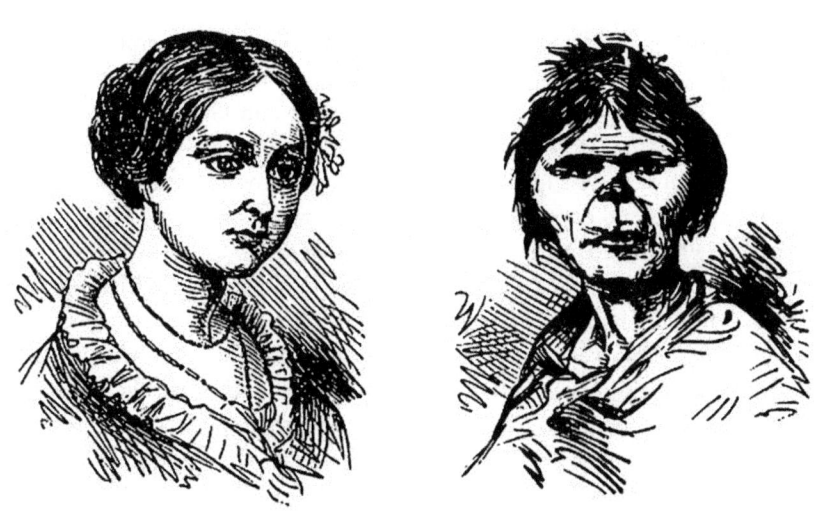

Figure 1.3   Contrasted faces: Florence Nightingale and Bridget McBruiser
Source: Samuel R. Wells, *New Physiognomy or signs of character, as manifested through temperament and external forms, and especially in the 'the human face divine'* (New York, 1886), p. 537.

Further to this, a drinking culture marred the Irish reputation at home and abroad even if, as Diarmaid Ferriter contends, per capita alcohol consumption data does not support the contrived view of shameful levels of excess.[164] Allegorical images of Ireland as a woman for several centuries were that of binaries too; in some instance, she was a beautiful young woman that needed protection, not from John Bull, but from brutish Irish men. Meanwhile, in the post-Famine era, popular print representations of poor Irish female migrants were made masculine, simianised, or both, as Figure 1.3 shows.

Inasmuch as illustrated newspapers played an important role in creating the simianised Irish man-monsters, they also played a critical role in its undoing. Sectarian fault lines in newspaper production were far more apparent in post-Famine Ireland, when Irish newspapers very definitely engaged in politics and more specifically identity politics.[165] By the late nineteenth century, the *Freeman's Journal* was solidly nationalist in its ownership and outlook, and the *Irish Times*,

[164] Diarmaid Ferriter, 'Drink and society in twentieth-century Ireland', *Proceedings of the Royal Irish Academy: Archaeology, Culture, History, Literature, Vol. 115C: Food and Drink in Ireland* (2015), pp. 349–69 at 352; Diarmaid Ferriter, *A Nation of Extremes: The Pioneers in Twentieth-Century Ireland* (Dublin, 1999).
[165] Marie Louise Legg, *Newspapers and Nationalism: The Irish Provincial Press, 1850–1892* (Dublin, 1999).

which was very definitely founded in 1857 on Tory principles, continued with its conservative, Protestant and unionist ethos.[166]

Men who were implicated in foul play at the coroner's court were viewed from the perspectives of social class, occupation, and religious sensibilities. Whether they were deemed to be without blame hinged to a large degree on the presentation of evidence showing that they were decent and God-fearing, which was mediated through their marital status, occupations, prior behaviours and/or their sobriety. Manliness, like Joanne Begiato found in early modern Britain, had universal attributes and expectations of full employment, marriage, and fatherhood, and those who did not achieve such markers were othered. Masculinity indicators equivalent to those Begiato identified can be found in urban Irish society but because unemployment, underemployment, and precariousness were more commonplace they were accepted in Dublin working-class communities as being factors beyond individual control.[167] Perceptions of Dublin working-class men in the coroner's court ranged from 'honest' family men, to under- and unemployed. Lower 'types' included drinkers and vagabonds unable to give good account of themselves, and then there were the criminal classes. Scholars of Irish masculinities are in agreement with Joe Valente's contention that the Irish were emasculated by virtue of being colonial subjects but had the 'double bind' of being agents of the imperial experiment at all levels of social class. A number of the cases discussed in Chapters 2 and 4 involved Irish soldiers in British regiments, whose representation in nationalist newspapers carried discernible biases—for example, the case of William 'Bill' Holmes, a soldier in the 10th Hussars, who was on furlough when he was involved in two separate and serious physical assaults on women. He came to the attention of the courts when one of his victims, Kate Anderson, subsequently died from her injuries. The *Irish Daily Independent* used the caption 'Soldier's Brutality' to describe the article accounting for his involvement in her demise and his later indictment.[168] Holmes belonged to a multiple masculinity model, subordinate in his urban working-class Irishness yet complicit with imperialism in his occupation. A few cases detail men who were clearly traumatised by their experience of the South–African wars, and while shell shock was not recognised until the First World War, there was a strong sense, and a broad understanding, that these were men troubled by what they had experienced.[169]

---

[166] James H. Murphy, *The Politics of Dublin Corporation 1840–1900* (Dublin, 2020), pp. 95, 105–6.

[167] Joanne Begiato, *Manliness in Britain, 1760–1900: Bodies, Emotion, and Material Culture* (Manchester, 2020), p. 7.

[168] *Irish Daily Independent*, 4 December 1900.

[169] Michael Robinson, *Shell-Shocked British Army Veterans in Ireland, 1918–39: A Difficult Homecoming* (Manchester, 2018); Brendan D. Kelly, '*He Lost Himself Completely*': Shell Shock and Its Treatment at Dublin's Richmond War Hospital, 1916–19 (Dublin, 2014); NAI/1901/161 Inquest on the body of Patrick O'Neill, 17 June 1901. '"He belonged to the army and was invalided home from South Africa some time ago, he was semi employed as a letter carrier in the GP Office" he was supposed to

Popular representations of urban masculinity differed greatly from their rural equivalents, and outside Dublin a new form of Catholic muscular identity emerged under the auspices of the Gaelic Athletic Association (GAA) founded in 1884. Ancient and rural Ireland was where it found the idealised male body and sports like hurling that set the Irish apart. Further to this the GAA invented its own version of football to implement what Aidan Beatty terms 'muscular visions of reborn Irishness', which was at the core of its mission.[170] In these muscular cultural nationalist terms, working-class men in Dublin City, where Association Football had taken a greater hold, were set apart again. Neal Garnham's work traces the first stronghold to Belfast in 1880 and he argues that, in the early days, outside Ulster few rural areas engaged in it. Following the foundation of the Dublin Association Football Club in 1883, some teams emerged but their composition, primarily soldiers and students, meant that tournaments were beset by the absences of furlough and inter-semester breaks, respectively.[171] In his analysis of the casualties arising from a fracas that occurred at a match in Belfast in 1912, Garnham surmises that the majority spectatorship was young, male, and working class.[172] Like elsewhere, Association Football in Dublin had the 'industrial patronage' of major employers like Guinness's Brewery and Jacobs's biscuit factory.[173]

Virtuosity, masculinity, and order were prized characteristics of Gaelic football and hurling, and the alignment with anti-colonial values was exemplified in exclusionary codes.[174] Through the introduction of the divisive 'Rule 21' in 1897 that banned members of the Royal Irish Constabulary (RIC), DMP, and British army, the GAA actively sought in its constitution to other those Irishmen who were complicit in the imperial project, 'thus further exacerbating the relationship between the Gaels and the garrison'.[175] A further motion was passed in 1902 that prohibited GAA members from attending, supporting, or participating in 'non-Gaelic games'.[176] Irish newspapers played an important role in communicating a recalibrated 'Gaelic' Irish masculinity, which was constructed in part to

---

present for a medical exam but did not.' The same was true of harness maker James Farrell: he was formerly a Dublin Fusilier and returned from South Africa last April owing to ill-health. He lived at 117 North King Street in a lodging house belonging to Mary Deegan. He was not under medical care, and he refused to go to a doctor. His breathing was laboured for previous few weeks prior to his death (NAI/1901/250 Inquest on the body of James Farrell, 23 September 1901).

[170] Aidan Beatty, *Masculinity and Power in Irish Nationalism, 1884–1938* (Basingstoke, 2016), p. 62.

[171] Neal Garnham, *Association Football and Society in Pre-Partition Ireland* (Belfast, 2004), pp. 5–6.

[172] Garnham, *Association Football*, pp. 116–17.

[173] Garnham, *Association Football*, pp. 48–9.

[174] Patrick F. McDevitt, 'Muscular Catholicism: Nationalism, Masculinity and Gaelic Team Sports, 1884–1916', *Gender & History*, 9:2 (1997), pp. 262–84 at 263.

[175] Aaron Ó Maonaigh, '"Who were the Shoneens?": Irish militant nationalists and association football, 1913–1923', *Soccer & Society*, 18:5–6 (2017), pp. 631–47 at 633.

[176] Ó Maonaigh, '"Who were the Shoneens?"', p. 641 note 11. Rule 21 remained in place until 2001 and Rule 27 until 1971.

counteract the competing narratives of the simianised, bigoted, and lazy stereotypes of Irishmen that were perpetuated in certain parts of the Anglo-American
illustrated press.

By eschewing foreign games and actively participating in Gaelic games, the
Irish, as McDevitt has argued, created a form of masculinity that was distinctive
and 'would stand apart from British or Imperial manhood'.[177] He argues that
between the fall of Parnell in 1891 and the Easter Rising of 1916 new forms of
muscular Catholicism were articulated in the flourishing of hurling and football
under the remit of the GAA. It acted as a very powerful unifying force in Irish
nationalism and a foil to the 'corporeal colonialism' of foreign games like the
kicking and passing games of Association Football and rugby. Urban attempts to
legitimise claims to Gaelic games and 'distance themselves from the taint of the
Anglicized city' were discredited, as McDevitt notes. Citing the GAA's observations, he argues that there was an implicit rural bias which went so far as to
clarify that the early successful urban teams were composed of internal migrants
from rural Ireland.[178] Indeed, Paul Rouse, quoting a newspaper article published
in 1882, contends that hurling 'was dead to Dublin' and it took some years before
it was properly revived.[179] Fatalities on playing fields were highly unusual but
there was one case in the coronial court sample I use here: Patrick Smyth of
Harristown died after playing a Gaelic football match for his club, Broughan, at a
pitch known as 'the Booth' in Piperstown near Swords on the northern outskirts
of the city. He collided with another player but in keeping with prevailing notions
of masculinity, he continued to play on—his death the following day was from
acute peritonitis.[180]

Cultural nationalism was also reinforced by the Gaelic League when it was
founded in 1893 to revive the Irish language, and together with the GAA it
formed a critical backbone to the revolutionary period and the muscular nationalism that emerged in the 1910s. In that iteration, Sikata Banerjee has found par-
allels with Indian nationalism, where the chaste female body represented
nationhood against the 'adult male body poised to sacrifice and kill for the nation',
which emerged periodically in the Irish context and more specifically during the
1912 to 1922 revolutionary period.[181] While social class dictated every element of
opportunity for men in Ireland, so too did religion and even if there was a rapidly

---

[177] McDevitt, 'Muscular Catholicism', p. 264.
[178] McDevitt, 'Muscular Catholicism', p. 270.
[179] Paul Rouse, *The Hurlers: The First All-Ireland Championship and the Making of Modern Hurling* (Dublin, 2018), p. 1.
[180] NAI/1901/147 Inquest on the body of Patrick Smyth, 29 May 1901; *Evening Herald*, 29 May 1901; *Skibbereen Eagle*, 1 June 1901; *Freeman's Journal*, 29 May 1901.
[181] Sikata Banerjee, *Muscular Nationalism: Gender, Violence, and Empire in India and Ireland, 1914-2004* (New York, 2012), p. 2. In Banerjee's account, 'Examples of muscular nationalism center an adult male body poised to sacrifice and kill for the nation.... This gendered binary remains stable as long as women do not act to challenge the expectations of chastity.'

rising Roman Catholic elite in Dublin, initially upward mobility was limited to a small minority of the so called 'Castle Catholics' of the upper middle class. By the late nineteenth century, these middle classes were amassing wealth and influence, and nationalist politicians were working actively towards achieving home rule constitutionally in local and national political structures. Irish Catholicism was also strengthened, and the role of the hierarchy was systematically entrenched in the provision of cheap health, welfare, and education systems from the 1860s onwards. Several factors coalesced to produce associational mechanisms for mobility. Muscular Christianity, the dominant narrative in the late nineteenth-century scramble for Africa, prompted a form of what Joseph Nugent termed 'Gaelo-Catholic' manliness.[182]

While women received little quarter in the early days of the GAA, they were invoked when it suited the agenda of the architects of a carefully crafted Irish masculinity. Furthermore, it was selective in the type of woman it championed. The GAA eschewed the corseted, made up urban dwellers aping their social betters and instead championed what Paul Rouse, citing Micheal Cusack, terms 'free and easy, full hearted, picture of health like daughters, mothers sisters and aunts'.[183] Implied in Cusack's binary model was that these rural-dwelling women, whose identities were mediated through familial ties invariably to male kin, were wholesome and those who lived in urban areas occupied dangerous spaces where tradition and morality could be corrupted.

If Dublin men were othered from these new forms of Irishness by imperial associations, then women were even more so, when they figured at all. They were viewed narrowly either in life cycle or in marital status terms: single women were presented as innocent domestics 'up from the country', morally suspect or spinsters, while married women were either good or neglectful mothers and housewives. The vast majority, as Lynn Abrams has cogently argued about the women of Shetland, occupied the middle ground of making do with very little. The hardships of urban living marked the lives of most women in this study but those who erred in their responsibilities for children were heavily scrutinised in coronial court inquiries.[184]

---

[182] Joseph Nugent, 'The sword and the prayerbook: ideals of authentic Irish manliness', *Victorian Studies*, 50:4 (2008), pp. 587–613 at 608. In his discussion of the clergy's attempts to mobilise St Columcille to reinvigorate a particular type of Irish masculinity, Nugent states that 'Out of the turn-of-the-century search for authentic Irishness, perhaps always doomed to failure, a distinctly Gaelo-Catholic ideal of manliness did emerge. The product of a contentious dialogue between the highly gendered discourses of Victorian imperialism, Roman Catholic praxis, and Irish racialized nostalgia, that ideal endured until at least the middle of the twentieth [century].'

[183] Paul Rouse, *The Hurlers: The First All-Ireland Championship and the Making of Modern Hurling* (Dublin, 2018), pp. 66–7. Rouse cites an account Michael Cusack made in the *Celtic Times* in October 1887 of a hurling match in County Louth where he describes the strong presence of rural women and their opposites as 'wasp-waisted, artificial-chested young ladies of the promenade'.

[184] Lynn Abrams, *Myth and Materiality in a Woman's World: Shetland, 1800–2000* (Manchester, 2005), p. 158.

Gender-Based Violence and Family Breakdown

Domestic abuse in Irish society has received very little systematic scholarly attention, but it has been argued by Elizabeth Steiner-Scott that culturally there was a
very high tolerance towards it.[185] Researching the topic is notoriously difficult
because first it relies on women to come forward with complaints and to perse-
vere with the fullness of the legal process. There are so many reasons why we
cannot use the judicial statistics as a barometer of domestic violence—much of it
was literally absorbed by the victims' bodies and was unreported. Some victims
relied on relatives (both male and female) to mete out their own forms of vernacular justice. Few women had the economic resources to bring cases to court
and unless the Crown prosecuted on their behalf, perpetrators could, and did,
escape notice. Sarah-Anne Buckley has uncovered evidence of female agency
whereby working-class women used the courts to bring their errant husbands
into line but stopped short of sending the breadwinner to jail. The judges in those
instances recognised the canny way in which women used the legal apparatus
available to them and were, in many respects, complicit.[186]

No specific legal provision for the protection of women in their homes existed;
for example, the 1853 Criminal Procedure Act that sought specifically to punish
perpetrators of aggravated assaults against women and children was not extended
to Ireland or Scotland.[187] Even if it were, and as Steiner-Scott contends, the
act was essentially toothless and did little to deter would-be perpetrators.
Paradoxically, the built environment of the tenements both facilitated and curbed
domestic violence. Fuelled by poverty, alcohol, and precarity, it always simmered
under the surface of Irish society but punishment for violent behaviour was not
always meted out in the courts. Vicky Holmes argues that when men beat their
wives in Victorian Britain they 'not only faced the opprobrium of their neighbours' but they were increasingly likely to find themselves before the courts.[188]
While the former might have been true in Ireland the latter was not, as relatively
few cases of domestic violence made it to the criminal courts.[189] What is quite
extraordinary in the cases discussed in Chapter 4 is that the perpetrators were
treated very leniently.

---

[185] Elizabeth Steiner-Scott, '"To Bounce a Boot Off Her Now and Then": domestic violence in post-
Famine Ireland', in Maryann Valiulis and Mary O'Dowd (eds), *Women in Irish History: Essays in
Honour of Margaret MacCurtain* (Dublin, 1997), pp. 125–43.

[186] Buckley, *The Cruelty Man*.

[187] An Act for the better Prevention and Punishment of aggravated Assaults upon Women and
Children, and for preventing Delay and Expense in the Administration of certain Parts of the Criminal
Law, 1853 (16 &17 Vic.), c. 30.

[188] Vicky Holmes, *In Bed with the Victorians: The Life-Cycle of Working-Class Marriage* (Basingstoke,
2017), p. 133.

[189] Annmarie Hughes, 'The "non-criminal" class: wife-beating in Scotland (c.1800–1949)', *Crime,
History and Societies*, 14:2 (2010), pp. 31–54.

Despite their presence as a very significant minority ethnic grouping in Britain, Shani D'Cruze, in her examination of sexual violence in her sample areas of Lancashire and Cheshire, found no Irish women bringing cases. D'Cruze surmised that this did not mean that they did not experience it; rather, she suggests that their absence in court records owed more to their distrust of the judicial system and 'alternative strategies to obtain redress or vindication within their own community'.[190] Extra-judicial means could include surveillance by neighbours; the close quarter living forced violent men and, to a much lesser extent, women to behave themselves and there are examples of interventions in the coronial court data. Joanne Bailey has advised against adopting linear narratives of domestic violence and suggests that a more fruitful approach might include 'analyses of contemporary understandings of "public" and "private" by demonstrating that, where wife beating was concerned, contemporaries equated "private" with secret or hidden abuse and "public" with open or witnessed abuse, rather than home and not-home'.[191] Her caution is well noted here. Other people's homes, particularly confidantes of the abused, complicated the narrative. Once women had reached their personal threshold of abuse and sought help outside their own walls, it instigated extra-judicial and, to a lesser extent, judicial processes. There were instances where, owing to the flimsy walls of some Dublin tenements, domestic disputes could never be private but among the working classes there was respect for individual and household agency. Even if physical violence was overheard by neighbours, wife-beating was considered a private matter and few would interfere. Concerned eavesdroppers in this sample only made interventions when beatings sounded too severe. When women had endured their threshold for abuse and went outside of their private lives to seek help, that made it public too, but much depended on who they told, and if that person had influence in the community. For legal actions to be taken against punitive husbands, charges had to be brought by victims or it had to burst outside and be witnessed by an agent of the law.

The absence of specific legal charges in the Irish records makes tracing cases of domestic abuse, in all its guises, difficult. If we turn to the annual judicial returns to parliament then efforts to find domestic abuse is frustrated by the aggregation of criminal statistics. With respect to serious crime, statistics were returned under six categories—offences against the person, against property with violence, against property without violence, malicious injuries to property, forgery and currency related crimes, and a catch all 'other offences not included in the above classes'. Of these categories the first is the one in which serious domestic abuse

---

[190] Shani D'Cruze, *Crimes of Outrage: Sex, Violence and Victorian Working Women* (London, 1998), p. 2.

[191] Joanne Bailey, '"I dye [*sic*] by inches": locating wife beating in the concept of a privatization of marriage and violence in eighteenth-century England', *Social History*, 31:3 (2006), pp. 273–94 at 274.

can be detected—in 1900 it accounted for 681 cases of which thirty-eight were of murder and fifty-four of manslaughter.[192] Unfortunately, the bulk of domestic abuse cases are buried in common assault and drunk and disorderly charges, and no breakdown is given. Desertion was dealt with in courts of summary jurisdiction and were so few as to be negligible—fifty-four applications resulting in fifty-two orders.[193] Richard MacMahon has posited that homicide rates were low and that when men assaulted their wives it was invariably with levels of non-lethal violence and they were unlikely to come to the direct attention of the coroner's court.[194] Of the thirty-eight murder cases in 1900, twenty concerned infants aged 1 and under.[195]

In Ireland only a fraction of domestic violence came before the courts and invariably it was because incidents occurred in public—if they caused disturbances the police were forced to deal with the matter. These cases came before the courts in the form of common assault and drunk and disorderly charges, of which the former comprised 19,994 in 1900 and the latter an enormous 97,457. The judicial statistics provide no breakdown of how these were gendered in terms of perpetrator or victim.[196] Furthermore, it would require a large-scale study of petty sessions and prison records to precisely ascertain the extent of domestic abuse cases, and with ambiguity in the classification of crimes (common assault, for instance, tells us nothing about longer term victimhood) coupled with patchy record survival it would be somewhat impressionistic unless some efforts were made to link various data and to re-categorise cases.

Overall, as Steiner-Scott contends, the law was inadequate, sentencing was erratic, and recidivism rates were high.[197] This demonstrates the patriarchal nature of Irish society and of the judiciary, coupled with Roman Catholic sensitivities and dictates surrounding the sanctity of the family. The depressing facts are that women had very little recourse when their own personal thresholds for abuse were met or exceeded. But that is another book. The women at the centre of the domestic violence cases here were, sadly, victims of homicide and only one proceeded to capital punishment. It was a particularly heinous case that repulsed Judge Kenny to such a degree that he flatly refused to alter his capital sentence. I have discussed that case in greater detail elsewhere and followed it through to hanging at Mountjoy, but such a judicial response was a rarity.[198]

---

[192] *Judicial Statistics, Ireland, 1900* [Cd. 725], 682, p. 13.

[193] Married Women (Maintenance in case of Desertion) Act, 1886 (49 & 50 Vic.), c. 52.

[194] Richard McMahon, *Homicide in Pre-Famine and Famine Ireland* (Liverpool, 2013), pp. 59–65; Steiner-Scott, '"To Bounce a Boot Off Her Now and Then"', pp. 125–43.

[195] *Judicial Statistics, Ireland, 1900. Part I.—Criminal Statistics* [Cd. 725], 682, p. 13.

[196] *Judicial Statistics, Ireland, 1900. Part I.—Criminal Statistics* [Cd. 725], 682, p. 14.

[197] Steiner-Scott, '"To Bounce a Boot Off Her Now and Then"', p. 131.

[198] Ciara Breathnach, 'Capital punishment in Irish prisons', *Health and History*, 22:1 (2020), pp. 1–22; NAI/CRF/1901/556-72 T-6-1901 John Toole Criminal Reference File; NAI/1901/70 Inquest on the body of John Toole, 7 March 1901.

Drinking Culture

Geographies of disadvantage are inextricably linked to patterns in addiction. For those who could afford it, drinking was a daily pursuit, and Dublin tolerated high levels of alcohol consumption. Patrick Joyce has argued that 'the language of character' imbued all aspects of Victorian political intellectualism and habit formation, and the control of habits was not only 'a particularly sensitive locus of governance' it was 'where desire and compulsion are mediated'.[199] Temperance was undoubtedly a lively topic of debate in late Victorian Dublin but it made little impact in a city where social drinking was deeply engrained. In fact, Guinness brewery's predominantly male workers were entitled to a daily allowance of two pints of porter (which was also widely advertised as Guinness's Stout[200] and colloquially known as a 'pint of plain'[201]), but for those who did not imbibe, they could cash these in for a 'scrip' valued at 2d. and total abstainers could recoup 1s. a week.[202] Effectively, drink formed part of payment for one of the most important employers in the city. For those who were precariously employed, drinking was intrinsic to getting work and getting paid. Greer and Nicholson use the example of dock workers in Dublin to exemplify the dynamics of exploitation—not only was their piecemeal work arranged in public houses, all too often they were paid by their gaffer/ganger in the pub so that they were obliged to buy rounds of drink as 'sweeteners' so they might be looked favourably upon for the next job.[203] Those who did not drink missed opportunities for paid work.

As I have established, there were multiple masculinities co-existing in Ireland and each was sensitive to location and class. In his study of fertility decline, Simon Sretrzer suggests the use of communication communities as a more appropriate way to view social class and Ben Griffin reiterates the importance of this framework with respect to masculinity studies.[204] In that regard it allows analysis 'by shared engagement in the mechanisms through which individuals were socialised into particular sets of norms, values and expectations'.[205] Whether teetotaller or not, drinking culture had a strong bearing on how working-class men fared in several aspects of Irish social life. Drinking was both a rite of passage for men and

---

[199] Patrick Joyce, *The State of Freedom: A Social History of the British State since 1800* (Cambridge, 2013), p. 253.

[200] *Mayo News*, 24 March 1900.

[201] NAI/1900/149: James Millar had taken a mouth full of 'a glass of plain' and fell on his way to lavatory down thirteen steps and hit his head at a house, 21 North Earl Street on 27 October 1900.

[202] Lumsden, *An Investigation*, pp. 30, 134.

[203] Desmond Greer and James W. Nicholson, *The Factory Acts in Ireland, 1802–1914* (Dublin, 2002), p. 237.

[204] Simon Szreter, 'Populations for studying the causes of Britain's fertility decline: communication communities', in P. Kreager, B. Winney, S. Uilaszek, and C. Capelli (eds), *Population in the Human Sciences: Concepts, Models, Evidence* (Oxford, 2015), pp. 172–95.

[205] Emma Griffin, *Bread Winner: An Intimate History of the Victorian Economy* (New Haven, 2020), p. 385.

an accepted coping mechanism for life's ups and downs, and the public house was much more than just a site of consumption.[206] In Ireland the association between the autonomous manly man and the ability to continue sociable drinking in the pub even when married with responsibilities was an intrinsic part of their working-class identity. Emma Griffin found the same pattern of behaviour in British cities, where

> The elevation of male labour as a marker of masculinity severed men from the comforts of home and thrust them into the masculine, alcohol-drenched world of the pub. We can see men turning away from the home as the source of human company and personal identity, and searching for these things in the public world of pubs and clubs instead.[207]

Another feature of Irish pub-going was the 'treating or the buying of rounds' which accelerated the pace of drinking and had undoubted consequences for individual finances and household budgets.[208] Nineteen-year-old John McLelland died from wounds he received in a fracas at Carroll's Public House, Christ Church Place, between 5 p.m. and 6 p.m. on 5 August 1901, from a man named Edward McDonagh. They had words over money; McDonagh struck the deceased who fell. Witnesses stated that the origin of the disagreement was that McLelland would not 'stand a pint of porter'. James McDowell, who had been drinking with him, stated that the victim was not that drunk and that he witnessed McLelland being dropped home. His mother put him to bed; she initially thought he was just very drunk but when he had not recovered the following day she called Dr Ashe who advised sending him to Cork Street Hospital where he died a few weeks later. The coroner's jury found that there was insufficient evidence to attach blame to Edward McDonough, but an arrest warrant was subsequently issued. He turned himself into Chancery Lane Station and was later sentenced to one calendar month for assault.[209]

Drinking was normative behaviour for working-class men—it was external observations of its consumption that othered these perceived 'anti-patriarchal' behaviours and made associations between them and the flawed masculinities Begiato describes in Britain.[210] Kevin C. Kearns spent decades gathering oral

---

[206] Ferriter, *A Nation of Extremes*, p. 47.
[207] Griffin, *Bread Winner*, p. 133.
[208] Ferriter, *A Nation of Extremes*, p. 48.
[209] NAI/1901/239 Inquest on the body of John McLelland, 9 September 1901; *Freeman's Journal*, 10 September 1901. The entire inquest was odd. Two men who were not summoned were in the jury box and were identified as frauds by another man present. Mr Chance the clerk stated that one man named Johnson purported to be a juror named John Carroll of 1 Christchurch Place. He claimed he was sent by Carroll who was subsequently fined. McDonagh served 1 calendar month:
NAI, PRIS 1/43/02 General register of convicted male prisoners, Mountjoy, no. 3249.
[210] Begiato, *Manliness in Britain*.

histories around inner-city Dublin and although he deals with a later era than this study his findings are relevant here and resonate in the coronial court records. He identified the prevalence of so-called 'hard men' who emanated from:

> A difficult urban environment of unemployment or irregular work, frustration, alcoholism, diminished self-esteem took a toll on many men. Most coped and behaved decently. But by all accounts, a good many degenerated into "hard men", the commonly used term for those miscreants who were controlling, bullying and tyrannical. Violent. Men who were a menace to their wife and children. The old, familiar boast heard around Dublin's tougher parts, "Ah me husband never took a hand to me" was in itself, suggestive of the prevalence of hard men.[211]

A raft of legislation was introduced between 1860 and 1906 to deal with the confusing licensing system and Sunday opening hours. Despite efforts to set the GAA apart in the script of bucolic imagery and ancient Irish traditions, Paul Rouse argues it was 'awash with drink':[212]

> Drinking was, from the beginning, a central element of the day's entertainment. Alcohol was sold on the sideline (under licence) at some GAA events, drawing occasional complaints that it was overpriced and pubs in the vicinity of pitches were thronged on match days.[213]

In 1878, a new law was introduced to prohibit the sale of alcohol on Sundays but Dublin, Belfast, Cork, Limerick, and Waterford were exempt from the blanket restrictions, and were required instead to close between the hours of 2 p.m. and 7 p.m.[214] Trains, away matches and willing publicans facilitated the mobilisation of the 'bona fide traveller' clause and their entitlement under the 1874 act, after a three-mile journey, to refreshments in a pub—the 1906 act changed the stipulation to five miles.[215] Many of the main stations of the Midland Railways company, like Broadstone Terminus and Mullingar Junction, had refreshment rooms which served 'wines, liqueurs and spirits'.[216] Association Football drinking culture was

---

[211] Kevin C. Kearns, *Working Class Heroines: The Extraordinary Women of Dublin's Tenements* (Dublin, 2018), p. 116.

[212] Paul Rouse, *The Hurlers: The First All-Ireland Championship and the Making of Modern Hurling* (Dublin, 2018), p. 70.

[213] Rouse, *The Hurlers*, p. 70.

[214] The Sale of Liquors on Sunday (Ireland) Act, 1878 (41 & 42 Vict.), c. 72.

[215] Licensing (Ireland) Act 1874 (37 & 38 Vict.), c. 69: section 28 defined a bona fide as a 'person for the purposes of this Act and the principal Act shall not be deemed to be a bona fide traveller unless the place where he lodged during the preceding night is at least three miles distant from the place where he demands to be supplied with liquor, such distance to be calculated by the nearest public thoroughfare'; Intoxicating Liquors (Ireland) Act 1906 (6 Edw. 7.), c. 39.

[216] *Freeman's Journal*, 5 December 1862; *Freeman's Journal*, 19 December 1862.

the same as the GAA, and the rise of leisure time and the extension of the railways further facilitated the growth of destination hotels, inns, and public houses
in coastal towns.

Proselytism was a continuous worry for Catholic and Protestant authorities
alike, but they put differences aside to advocate for the reverent observation of the
Lord's Day, to which Sunday leisure activities posed a real threat. The *Belfast
Newsletter* reported how, at a synod held in Glendalough, the Church of Ireland
Archbishop of Dublin bemoaned its secularisation. The same article discussed a
meeting of the Church of Ireland Temperance Society in Belfast in October 1902;
one delegate, Major Wellesley, described the system of 'bona fide' as 'a perfect
disgrace, and he was told that the state of some of the railway carriages on Sunday
evenings was quite scandalous'.[217] Although Dublin was exempted from the rules,
there are a few examples of Sunday outings ending in disaster, like that of William
Redmond's daytrip to Howth in September 1901. He took the train to the popular
seaside village on the north side of the city where he had a few pints. On his
return journey he got off at the wrong stop and proceeded to walk back along the
tracks—he was knocked down and all four of his limbs were fractured. He admitted that he was to blame and that he was under the influence of drink. The jury
found that he died from his injuries and, because he was a decent man with three
children, they recommended that his wife receive some compensation from the
rail company and glossed over his state of inebriation as follows in a rider: 'We
exonerate the motor man[;] we recommend the line be better lighted and some
further protection be put up'.[218] The temperance movement was driven by Roman
Catholic and Evangelical Protestantism at the close of the nineteenth century and
these forces were external to the close-knit working-class communities in Dublin
City. Ferriter argues that, during the nineteenth century, politicians were cautious
about affiliating with temperance and nor was the Catholic hierarchy universal
in its support of it. Instead, both took the easier option of advocating
moderation.[219]

Local authorities in Dublin had much to answer for, while judges of the higher
courts regularly expressed their dismay and personal disgust at the high levels of
drunkenness coming before their benches—licences for the sale of intoxicating
liquor were granted freely by the DMP divisional justices and magistrates presiding over the petty sessions dealt leniently with offending vendors.[220] A Royal
Commission was appointed to examine the licensing laws and trade in the United
Kingdom and it found, using 1896 data, that Dublin had 901 public houses and

[217] *Belfast Newsletter*, 22 October 1902.
[218] NAI/1901/242 Inquest on the body of William Redmond, 14 September 1901.
[219] Ferriter, *A Nation of Extremes*, p. 48 (see also pp. 12, 16–17).
[220] Royal Com. on Liquor Licensing Laws: Statistics relating to Number of Licensed Premises in
Great Britain and Ireland, 1898 [c. 8696], p. 7.

twenty-three refreshment house and wine licences with on-licences, that is, where intoxicating liquor could be bought and consumed on site, a ratio of one licensed premises to 275 people in 1896. There were 355 off-licences in Dublin according to the 1896 data.[221] Off-licences comprising 289 spirit grocers (200 sold retail beer and 77 wholesale and retail selling rights), 45 beer retailer licences, and 21 wholesale beer dealers also sold alcohol. Dublin vintners were a powerful political lobby—several by the mid-nineteenth century considered themselves middle class and respectable, and regarded themselves as a cut above the beer house and spirit grocers.[222] Elizabeth Malcolm traces their ascendency to the 1860s when they established further trade protection societies, which by the 1890s translated into harder political power in local authorities like Dublin Corporation.[223] Underscoring this newly won prowess, however, was the clout of the brewing and distilling industry and its enormous value to the Irish economy. The strong commitment to philanthropic endeavour (for example, by the Guinness family) preserved the industry from any real opposition or criticism and few politicians would speak out in favour of the temperance movement.

Ubiquitous in its availability, nearly every grocery shop sold alcohol, and further to licensed premises there were countless shebeens where illicit sale was conducted.[224] Public houses in the timeframe under review were permitted to sell alcohol between 7 a.m. and 11 p.m. save on Sunday, Good Friday, or Christmas Day where there was a requirement to close at 9 p.m.[225] When the Sunday opening debate arose again in the early 1900s, Ferriter argues that temperance reformers were not content with the proposed changes to Sunday opening and licensing laws that would restrict the renewals, and cites the argument made by Cardinal Logue that as long as grocers with mixed-trading capabilities were permitted to continue as normal the piecemeal actions were futile.[226]

Accounts of public houses and their patrons reflect what Stella Moss terms 'specific embodied practices and performative cultures; that is to say, particular practices and habits were considered as both constituting and reflecting manliness, and as such were widely practised.'[227] Public houses in Dublin were, in general terms, male-dominated spaces—there are very few references to couples

[221] Royal Com. on Liquor Licensing Laws, pp. 238, 248.

[222] Bradley Kadel, *Drink and Culture in Nineteenth-Century Ireland: The Alcohol Trade and the Politics of the Irish Public House* (London, 2015), p. 36.

[223] Elizabeth Malcolm, *Ireland Sober, Ireland Free: Drink and Temperance in Nineteenth-Century Ireland* (Dublin and Syracuse, 1986), p. 208.

[224] Royal Com. on Liquor Licensing Laws: Statistics relating to Number of Licensed Premises in Great Britain and Ireland, 1898 [c. 8696], p. 248.

[225] Refreshment Houses (Ireland) Act, 1860 (23 & 24 Vic.) c. 107, section 29.

[226] Ferriter, *A Nation of Extremes*, p. 53.

[227] Stella Moss, 'Manly drinkers : masculinity and material culture in the interwar public house', in Jane Hamlett, Hannah Greig, and Leonie Hannan (eds), *Gender and Material Culture in Britain since 1600* (Basingstoke, 2015), pp. 138–52 at 139.

drinking socially together. Holly Dunbar has argued that 'female drinkers entered cultural and physical spaces that were seen to be masculine, as opposed to the "feminine", domestic realm of the home and family life, and secondly, that being drunk or absent from the family home adversely affected their abilities to fulfil their perceived primary role of motherhood.'[228] From the perspective of the coroner's court, women who drank in pubs were of ill-repute. Apart from those who were accompanied by spouses, few stayed on site to consume their beverages. There is plenty of evidence in the court records and in the newspapers to provide a profile of the average female drinker and the locus of their drinking. Unfortunately, these are exceptional cases concerning criminality in some form or another so capturing an overall impression of the everyday of female alcohol consumption is next to impossible. Citing the high numbers of women arrested for drunkenness in 1907 (1,772 compared to 2,941 men), one contemporary observer lamented that 'I don't suppose there is any city in the world where there is so much drunkenness among women as there is in Dublin, except it be in Glasgow and Edinburgh...Women stagger from the doors of saloons along the sidewalks with dishevelled hair and disordered garments without attracting any attention whatsoever.'[229] If women were permitted to share public drinking spaces then the rules were overtly masculine and if the course of an evening's drinking took a terrible turn, then female alcohol consumption was subject to much closer scrutiny in the coroner's court and shown far less sympathy in the criminal courts. Despite legislation prohibiting the sale to minors under 13, under the 1886 act and section 14 under the 1901 act, in this sample and in criminal court records there are cases concerning deaths of small children where women used children to 'send for' glasses of porter and were accused of alcohol-related neglect. These 'sent for' glasses were freely sold and handed to young children, who acted as messengers and their errand-running received protracted attention in subsequent evidence given.[230] In cases of violent crime inquiries into the sale of alcohol to victims or perpetrators, volumes consumed and indeed into whether or not the sale of alcohol was illegal are consistent attributes.

Mauger argues that Irish nationalism found common cause with the Pioneers' Total Abstinence Association, and an ideology that created inextricable links between the social purity of temperance and political independence.[231] The Ennis

---

[228] Holly Dunbar, 'Women and alcohol during the First World War in Ireland', *Women's History Review*, 27:3 (2018), pp. 379–96 at 379.

[229] William Eleroy Curtis, *One Irish Summer* (New York, 1909), p. 360.

[230] The Intoxicating Liquors (Sale to Children) Act, 1886 (49 & 50 Vic.) c. 56; Intoxicating Liquors (Sale to Children) Act, 1901 (1 Edw. 7.) c. 27.

[231] Alice Mauger, '"The Holy War Against Alcohol": alcoholism, medicine and psychiatry in Ireland, c.1890–1921', in Steven J. Taylor and Alice Brumby (eds), *Healthy Minds in the Twentieth Century: Mental Health in Historical Perspective* (Basingstoke, 2020), pp. 17–51 at 29.

State Inebriate Reformatory was opened in 1899—it was, as Conor Reidy argues, an unprecedented government intervention aimed at tackling alcoholism.[232] Although problematic alcohol consumption was primarily a male-dominated problem, the efforts of the Inebriate Reformatory, focused disproportionately on women: in its first year it treated six male and ten female 'drunkards'.[233] That gendered trend continued: in 1907 it was reported in the House of Commons that 'thirty-eight men and sixty-nine women have been committed, of whom twenty-nine men and fifty-two women have been discharged'.[234]

Alcoholism was pathologised but not 'medicalised' by the turn of the nineteenth century—its management was moral and primarily through abstinence. There were three cases where high alcohol dependencies were implied by the identification of withdrawal symptoms in the cases of William Caruthers (already mentioned) and the following two cases. The first case was that of Joseph Boylan, whose landlady testified that he left his accommodation in Drumcondra at about 11 a.m. to go to mass on St Stephen's Day 1901. When he returned at 5 a.m. the following morning he was 'covered in Street mud', and it was surmised that he fell while drunk. Unable to go to work he stayed in bed for the day and was in such pain that night he got his co-lodger to bring him to the Mater Hospital—his arm was broken and very bruised. His cause of death identified alcohol withdrawal symptoms and delirium tremens, as well as cardiac failure and pneumonia.[235] A few days later, another heavy drinker, Cornelius Connelly, whom the DMP report documented as being of no fixed abode, died after suffering the adverse effects of alcohol withdrawal after he entered Mountjoy prison (he is counted among the institutional deaths). He was sentenced to two months for the ill-treatment of his children. Medical officer Dr Dowdall reported that he was very agitated and had assaulted other prisoners in Mountjoy, and that left him with no choice but to use a restraint jacket at 10.15 p.m. By 12.57 a.m. his condition had deteriorated—his pulse was weak and his breathing rapid; Dowdall sent for the chaplain. The jury found that he 'Died from sudden heart failure consequent on his condition from excessive drinking. And we are of the opinion this man should have been examined by a doctor in the police courts and that he should never have been sent to prison while in the condition he was in.'[236]

Female alcohol consumption was heavily scrutinised in the coroner's court and cases associated with the notorious brothels of 'Monto' (an area that included Montgomery Street) were regarded in moralistic terms by DMP officers and

[232] Conor Reidy, *Criminal Irish Drunkards: The Inebriate Reformatory System 1900–1920* (Dublin, 2014), p. 19.
[233] Anon., 'The Treatment of Inebriates', *Charity Organisation Review*, 10:57 (1901), pp. 151–4 at 153.
[234] House of Commons, Debate, 19 March 1907, vol. 171, cc. 648–9.
[235] NAI/1901/322 Inquest on the body of Joseph Boylan, 30 December 1901.
[236] NAI/1902/1 Inquest on the body of Cornelius Connelly, 1 January 1902.

jurors alike.[237] Some brothels around 'Monto', which Boyd describes as 'the British Isle's only sanctioned zone of iniquity', and O'Keefe and Ryan describe as one of 'the most notorious red-light districts in the world', doubled as 'shebeens' (from the Irish síbín) and were unlicenced premises. As O'Keefe and Ryan explain, 'Monto was allowed be an "other", an "othered" and an "othering" landscape within the city.'[238] By virtue of living in the area, poor single women were viewed with great suspicion and ran the reputational risk of moral ruin by association. In reality Monto was where cheap lodging could be found. The inclusion of the descriptor of prostitute in the coronial records was a deliberate act to distinguish between them and 'respectable' poor women, but was often used to cast aspersions on character and doubt over their word in witness statements. The Public Health Committee repeatedly brought the insanitary and dilapidated state of housing on Montgomery and Mabbot Streets to the attention of the corporation, but to little avail, although it did have powers to condemn certain buildings as uninhabitable.[239] Even when buildings were condemned by the Public Health Committee, it took time before those orders were fully executed—indeed, many orders were ignored.

Public opinion did not regard breaching licensing law or illicit drinking as serious offences and it is for such reasons that Elizabeth Malcolm argues that the clergy had no real control over drunkenness. She notes that the police were slow to arrest those involved in the illegal sale and consumption of alcohol.[240] It is hard to imagine how in a 'small town' like Dublin that shebeens could carry on business without the knowledge and complicity of the police. Shebeens were hidden in plain sight—only the problematic ones were reported and shut down.[241] For instance, Mary Sweeney's sudden death from respiratory problems in 1901 drew attention to the dire public health conditions of the notorious 'Monto'. She lodged at 61 Montgomery Street, which was described in the DMP report as 'a brothel and bad shebeen'.[242] There were several shebeens in the area—Mary Smith of 12 Mabbot Street and Margaret McDonagh of 28 Lower Tyrone Street (both streets were part of 'Monto') were sentenced to fourteen days for the unlicensed sale of porter, while Mary Traynor of Cumberland Street got ten months for

---

[237] Gary A. Boyd, *Dublin, 1745–1922: Hospitals, Spectacle and Vice* (Dublin, 2006), pp. 178–9: 'the area, known colloquially as Monto (or alternatively the "the Kips", "the Digs" or Macktown after Mrs Mack one of its more infamous denizens) was located just a few hundred yards to the east of Sackville Street... Towards the end of the century, however, the more visible aspects of prostitution had more or less been cleared from central areas to become almost exclusively concentrated in Monto.'

[238] Tadhg O'Keeffe and Patrick Ryan, 'At the world's end: the lost landscape of Monto, Dublin's notorious red-light district', *Landscapes*, 10:1 (2009), pp. 21–38 at 28.

[239] *Dublin Corporation Printed Reports* (Dublin City Library & Archive), Volume 1II, 1900, p. 501.

[240] Malcolm, *Ireland Sober, Ireland Free*, p. 214.

[241] Boyd, *Dublin, 1745–1922*, p. 178; O'Keeffe and Ryan, 'At the world's end', pp. 21–38.

[242] NAI/1901/58 Inquest on the body of Mary Sweeney, 25 February 1901.

'keeping porter for sale' in December 1901.[243] All three women had several aliases and were probably well known to the police. The area was generally very closely monitored; for example, Lizzie 'Bargess' Ryan of 56 Montgomery Street was occupationally described as a prostitute and convicted for the illegal sale of porter in 1901.[244] The national average of those summarily convicted for the illicit sale of drink from 1896 to 1900 was 1,151.6.[245] Of the 1,048 persons proceeded against in 1900, nine had charges withdrawn, 320 had the charges dismissed, and 719 were convicted, twenty-three of whom received prison sentences of one to three months, 116 of fourteen days to one month, and 55 under fourteen days; but the vast majority, or 523, received fines.[246] Almost a third, or 318 cases, occurred in the DMP area, and while some may have been repeat offenders it gives an idea of how superficial statistics with regard to legal sales of alcohol were. Actual consumption was much higher.[247]

Malcolm cautions against constructing an idea of sales from judicial statistics, which she rightly claims are a partial impression of police activity that cannot account for the scale of the illicit sales industry.[248] She also notes that there was a whole system of whistles and shrills to notify shebeen managers of potential DMP raids in the 1870s, and the early 1900s were no different.[249] Maria Luddy's work has argued that 'visibility and containment' were the primary concerns of vigilance societies and the general public in this timeframe.[250] This selectivity with respect to the application of the law forms part of what Joyce calls a system of 'subtle reciprocities' that maintained a certain status quo and permitted policing to operate in tandem with communities in a consensual manner.[251] Apart from loss of taxation revenues and rates, illicit sales created potential for the adulteration of drink. When Edward Dempsey died of carbolic poisoning, it was alleged that he had been drinking at a shebeen. He had fallen on the tram line. DMP Constable Thomas Grant took a statement from him at the hospital and he claimed that he was sold a bottle of porter by 'Rooney's of Boyne St and paid two pence hapenny for it'. On further investigation, Grant discovered three Rooney families living there: Anne Rooney of 16 Boyne Street, Mrs Bridget Kinsella and Elizabeth Rooney, both of 11 Boyne Street, and Anne Rooney of 2 Cottage Place

---

[243] NAI, PRIS 1/44/02, General register of convicted female prisoners, Mountjoy, nos. 5385–7. Mary Traynor was described as a domestic and cook in the 1901 census: http://www.census.national-archives.ie/reels/nai003683530/ (accessed 8 August 2020).

[244] NAI, PRIS 1/44/02 General register of convicted female prisoners, Mountjoy, no. 5369, Lizzie 'Bargess' Ryan.

[245] *Judicial Statistics, Ireland, 1900. Part I.—Criminal Statistics* [Cd. 725, 682], p. 51.

[246] *Judicial Statistics, Ireland, 1900. Part I.—Criminal Statistics* [Cd. 725, 682], p. 103.

[247] *Judicial Statistics, Ireland, 1900. Part I.—Criminal Statistics* [Cd. 725, 682], p. 108.

[248] Malcolm, *Ireland Sober, Ireland Free*, pp. 212–13.

[249] Malcolm, *Ireland Sober, Ireland Free*, p. 216.

[250] Maria Luddy, *Prostitution and Irish Society, 1800–1940* (Cambridge, 2007), p. 40.

[251] Joyce, *The Rule of Freedom*, p. 111.

off Boyne Street all deposed that they never sold a bottle of porter in their life and that they had never seen Dempsey before.[252]

Coronial court records provide incredibly detailed levels of insight into daily alcohol consumption and in the following chapters I aim to tease out the moralistic language used to describe, measure, and form judgements on inebriation and how it was gendered. Echoing elements of the deserving and undeserving poor discourse that was so prevalent in the context of the Poor Law, evidence of alcohol abuse was an automatic slur on the character of those presenting at the coronial courts, especially when the slender means of most households is taken into consideration. It is equally interesting to note high levels of medico-legal awareness among publicans and their patrons, which is why this book and the final section on violent deaths in particular takes note of the contemporary knowledge of what is now termed alcohol by volume (ABV). Either people lied and erred on the side of conservatism when discussing the number of drinks taken in the coronial courts, or the ABV they were consuming was extremely high. Guinness's brewery controlled a large part of the domestic market and sold its products under the brand names of Porter and Extra Stout, which had ABVs of 6 per cent and 7.5 per cent, respectively.[253] These so called 'gravities' were not reduced until after the First World War, but quality control mechanisms in brewing and distilling were not uniform.[254] The final chapter will take advantage of Ordnance Survey maps and GIS (Geographic Information Systems) to map the centrality of public houses and the availability of alcohol, and to visualise the scenarios in a sample of graphically described murders that went from the coroner's to the criminal courts.

Conclusion

In this chapter I have provided an overview of how biopower functioned in Dublin City at the turn of the century to firstly position the coroner's court within the architecture of medico-legal frameworks and secondly to show how its smooth operation hinged on close collaboration with hospitals, individual doctors, the DMP, the judiciary, and, to a lesser extent, the DFB. In order to fully understand the cases that form the basis of the next three chapters, I have presented a spatial reading of city life. I believe it is important to consider the parameters of ordinary lives from the size of homes to the spaces available to them 'outside' during the day. Intangible boundaries of gender and class governed

---

[252] NAI/1901/183 Inquest on the body of Edward Dempsey, 10 June 1901.
[253] Patrick Lynch and John Vaisey, *Guinness's Brewery in the Irish Economy 1759–1876* (London, 1960).
[254] I am grateful to Eibhlin Colgan, Archive Manager, Guinness Archive for this information.

public space and is why I have presented an overview of Dublin City from these perspectives. Women and children were positioned in proximity to male kin in all classes, and for the working classes respectability could be achieved if the male head of household was 'a good man'. Urban working-class men faced employment difficulties and, as we shall see, many had perilous and precarious jobs, so achieving middle-class notions of manliness was complicated by factors that were beyond their control. This broad sketch of the limitations of the patriarchal city is necessary to help unravel the primary causes of death in the coroner's court, which were inextricably linked to social class.

2

Sudden and Accidental Deaths in Domestic Settings

Sudden deaths were most likely to occur in the home and they usually pertained to people who were not under any form of medical care—they account for just over half or 307 of the 611 cases in the dataset used for this study. In this tally are deaths of people who were living rough, and those who managed their final illnesses in domestic contexts but died on their way to hospital. It is no surprise that the home should be so strongly represented in these data, but it is important to consider why. The domestic deaths investigated by the coroner's court represent the lower levels of the working-class poor—many were living in poverty and some of whom were destitute. The circumstances had a very broad range of causation, and in most cases the coroner deemed an investigation necessary because the deceased had not been under medical supervision prior to their deaths. As discussed in the previous chapters, the instruments of biopower were neither inviting nor approachable for those who feared its reach. For older people, fear of death in the workhouse and the social stigma of the pauper burial was very real. Engagement with the Poor Law for impoverished parents was always a calculated risk that brought child custody into the equation.

The purpose of an inquest was to rule out foul play, even in cases with clear evidence of death by natural causes. Some came to the attention of the authorities because they occurred in suspicious circumstances but for most cases the cause was more mundane. Low living standards and poor living quarters had a profound impact on health and gave rise to serious medical problems. Others occurred because of defective domestic architecture, for example poor ventilation and overcrowding. Combined deaths from burns and scalds accounted for sixty-eight domestic deaths (including five smoke inhalation cases), accidents owing to the decrepitude of housing was another but less prominent cause of death in sixteen cases. Many of the deaths associated with fires and scalding were preventable, as were falls owing to damaged fixtures. Families eked a hand to mouth existence, and relative poverty coexisted alongside absolute poverty, which was characterised by rough living, neglect, and malnutrition. As living arrangements were often very fluid, in this chapter I include cases that occurred in domestic settings even if it was not the deceased's residence. The first part of this chapter directs attention towards living conditions and standards, and the range of socio-economic

Ordinary Lives, Death, and Social Class: Dublin City Coroner's Court, 1876–1902. Ciara Breathnach, Oxford University Press. © Ciara Breathnach 2022. DOI: 10.1093/oso/9780198865780.003.0003

conditions we can discern from the dataset. It then provides a flavour of the medical cause of deaths occurring in domestic settings, for example from cardiac syncope and lung disease. The second part examines accidental, or indeed, preventable deaths. It concludes with a section on child neglect in domestic settings.

Cold Comforts

By the 1840s, the grand Georgian houses of one-family households in Dublin had begun to transition into tenements or a hotchpotch of lodging houses with anything up to seventy occupants (see Figure 2.1). Social change did not occur quickly enough in London or Dublin and as Drew Gray found in Victorian London these lodging houses were of enormous importance to the poor who

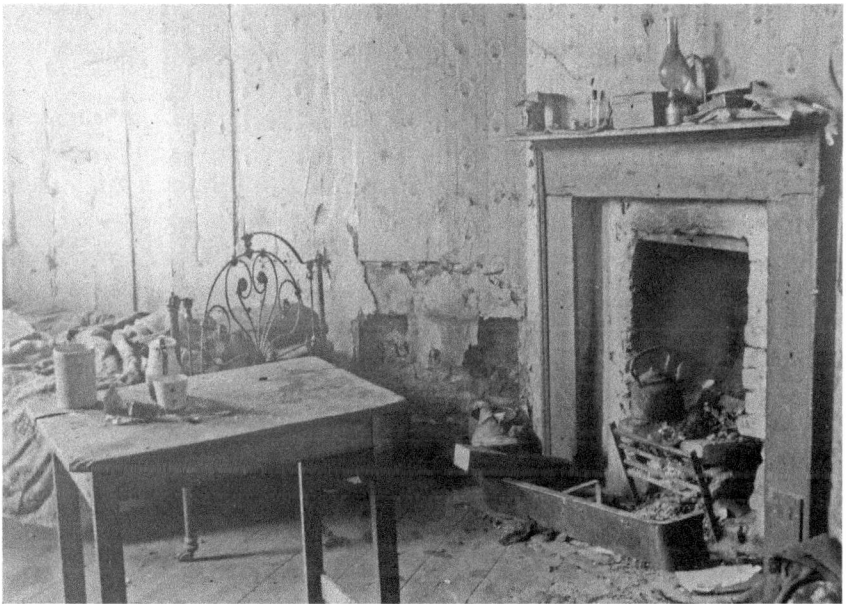

Figure 2.1 Tenement room

Note: I am grateful to Sarah Connaghan, Librarian, RSAI, for kind permission to reproduce here.

Source: Royal Society of Antiquaries of Ireland, RSAI, BOX07_083. Georgina McMahon, 'Tenement interior, The Coombe, Co. Dublin, Ireland', http://rsai.locloudhosting.net/items/show/24409 (captioned '33 Coombe – Tenement Furnished 4/1' and 'T. Mason, 5, Dame Street, Dublin') (accessed 3 February 2019).

could find a cheap bed or part of one on a nightly basis.[1] Ruth McManus's research has shown Dublin's tenements had a similarly messy pattern of rental.[2] Among the worst kind of accommodation I have found in this sample was a shakedown of straw on the floor, which was, of course, common in rural Ireland but less so in urban areas.[3] The inquest into the death of Michael Kennedy illustrates how strangers were thrown together in lodging-house arrangements. The 68-year-old, married handyman, took his last meal at 8 p.m. and retired to a room he shared at 168 Church Street with four other lodgers, Joseph Doyle, Joseph Burke, Michael Kavanagh, and a man unknown. Kavanagh shared the same bed with Kennedy, and he gave deceased some water between 11 p.m. and 12 p.m. on the night he died of 'aortic disease'.[4] Daniel Paderischi/Pedreschi was a single plumber who lived in what was described as 'a closet off the front parlour' of a tenement house on Shaw Street. He took his meals with his family at 8 Wentworth Place and when he missed dinner one evening and breakfast the following morning they went to check on him. He died of 'cardiac syncope consequent on tubercular disease of his lungs'. Recorded as Pedereskye in the 1901 census, he was living at 10.3 with fellow plumber James Monks. Monks occupied the main compartment of the room and stated Pedreschi's 'closet' was partitioned from his domestic space. From Monks's account we can surmise that the closet had a door and it is highly likely that his sleeping accommodation was poorly ventilated, which cannot have helped his chronic respiratory condition.[5]

Taken together, all forms of death from tuberculosis in Dublin amounted to 1,951 cases of the 9,976 deaths in 1900 and while they are not broken down by age or location, it is worth noting that 228 were from *tabes mesenterica*, a form of tuberculosis that predominantly affected children.[6] I have argued elsewhere that its prevalence is indicative of serious public health problems and how virulent forms of tuberculosis were in constant transmission in Dublin City. Very often tuberculosis was only discovered in post-mortem contexts and in death registrations it was often referred to obliquely to spare 'respectable poor' families the associated shame. This type of compassionate reframing of socially stigmatising diseases was not afforded to those perceived as the undeserving poor.[7]

[1] Drew Gray, *London's Shadows: The Dark Side of the Victorian City* (London, 2010), p. 130.

[2] Ruth McManus, 'Dublin's lodger phenomenon in the early twentieth century', *Irish Economic and Social History*, 45:1 (2018), pp. 23–46.

[3] Ciara Breathnach, 'Capital punishment in Irish prisons', *Health and History*, 22:1 (2020), pp. 104–25.

[4] NAI/1901/297 Inquest on the body of Michael Kennedy, 26 November 1901.

[5] NAI/1901/143 Inquest on the body of Daniel Paderischi, 20 May 1901; census return, http://www.census.nationalarchives.ie/reels/nai003733223/ (accessed 20 July 2021).

[6] ARRG, 1900, p. 166.

[7] NAI/1900/89 Inquest on the body of Jane Gaffney, 6 August 1900, https://civilrecords.irishgenealogy.ie/churchrecords/images/deaths_returns/deaths_1900/05753/4625098.pdf (accessed 3 January 2021).

Chief among the primary causes of these deaths were cardiac problems in older cohorts. Of the 143 cardiac cases in this sample, 136 were of adults—in six adult cases the age was not given, and the average age was 49. Pulmonary diseases were mentioned in sixty-eight deaths located in domestic settings, and of these forty-two were coupled with heart disease. Many of those who died from cardiac and lung diseases were either unaware of their underlying condition or were managing their illnesses privately and outside of physicians' care. With respect to respiratory health there was a high tolerance of chronic conditions and ailing health in the community. Elizabeth Ormsby's death from pulmonary haemorrhage must have been a frightful affair. She was a married 39-year-old shirt maker living at 1 Portobello Square, Clanbrassil Street, living with chronic lung disease. Her sister Bridget Bright of 2 Winnfield Cottages stated that she had been ailing for two years and suffered regular nose bleeds, but was never treated by a doctor. At 8 a.m. on the morning she died, she knocked on her neighbour's door to seek help in getting her sister a few doors away. Catherine Ryan opened her door to find Ormsby standing by a pool of blood and vomiting blood. She lost no time and a few minutes after she returned with her sister Mrs Neill, from number 5, and Catherine Hegarty, number 6, Ormsby died. Fr Hickey was sent for too, but she was dead by the time he got there.[8] The house, being a tenement, was considered unfit for an inquest. Post-mortem found 'old standing disease of both lungs'.[9]

'Pensioner's sudden death: Another case of Refusing to See the Doctor'

Thus ran a headline in the *Evening Herald* in 1901, and with good cause: neglect of personal health problems or indeed a lack of awareness of underlying health conditions are threaded throughout the coronial court cases. The brief newspaper article was referring specifically to the case of James Molloy who lodged at 25 Upper Mercer Street with Mary Reilly—she noticed his failing health and had tried to get him to see a doctor but he declined. In her defence she argued that the army pensioner had not been complaining the night he died, but with pneumonia as cause of death it is unlikely that he was asymptomatic prior to his death. When he became critically unwell, a priest was called and he was tended to by Fr Flanagan of St Michael and John's Chapel. Dr Bryne, the *Evening Herald* reported, made a point of impressing the importance of having medical men attend the ill,

---

[8] NAI/1902/19 Inquest on the body of Elizabeth Ormsby, 5 February 1902; *Freeman's Journal*, 6 February 1902.
[9] Her marriage to William Ormsby in 1879 was registered—they had no census entry for 1901 and were long-term residents of Portobello Square: https://civilrecords.irishgenealogy.ie/churchrecords/images/marriage_returns/marriages_1879/11082/8055666.pdf (accessed 7 November 2021).

irrespective of their own personal agency.[10] At a granular level there is strong evidence of fear of, and aversion towards, medical care, which may have to do with the extent to which it was associated with Poor Law administration and the loss of personal agency, particularly for older cohorts. Robert Floyd was 11 years old when he noticed his mother, Francis (*sic*), ailing in the chair where she worked at 11 p.m. making matchboxes. He alerted his father who was sleeping by shouting 'My Ma is dying'—her condition was undoubtedly grave. It was revealed in the DMP report that Mr Floyd's first recourse was to go to the Bridwell Lane police station as he was unable to pay for a doctor for her. Sergeant Gilmore 23D went with him to the relieving officer Mr Kidney, who issued him with a 'red ticket' entitling health care in the home. While he responded immediately, by the time Dr John P. Garland arrived, she was dead from 'apoplexy'.[11] Mr Floyd was not admonished for ignoring his wife's health needs but a month later, Edward Byrne of 16 Werburgh Street was subject to Dr Byrne's opprobrium for permitting his brother to die without medical assistance for pneumonia. James Byrne refused to allow a doctor to be called, and his brother, who visited him every day at 102 Upper Dorset Street in his final week, respected his wishes. The coroner 'thought the conduct of the brother was certainly open to censure' and that the deceased could not have known his own mind in the delirium of illness.[12] When Elizabeth Ledwidge died in March 1901 she had not been attended to by a doctor, but a priest was sent for when she was found unconscious. Dr Byrne made the point at her inquest that there was an onus on lodging house keepers to ensure that their residents were medically attended to even if it was against their express wishes.[13]

Calling a priest as opposed to a doctor was a common reaction to medical emergencies—a good death, last oils, and an act of contrition were deemed important in the Roman Catholic tradition. It is also indicative of fear, or of the perception that going to a doctor was an exercise in futility. Francis McCabe's health slowly deteriorated over a period of three years. He did not attend a doctor and self-medicated with cod liver oil. On the night of his death at 3 Fingal Street, off Cork Street, he had a violent fit of coughing, which worried his brother John to the extent that he went for a priest. Fr McSweeny anointed him and he died shortly thereafter. It was only at this point that his sister Maggie went to Dr Stritch of Harrington Street, who could do nothing except advise her to go to the DMP to report the death.[14] Sadly, medical services were not the primary recourse for the very poor: doctors were only called or mentioned in twenty-one cases in the overall sample of 611, priests were called in eighteen cases and, in three instances,

---

[10] *Evening Herald*, 12 February 1901.

[11] NAI/1900/27 Inquest on the body of Frances Floyd, 24 May 1900.

[12] *Evening Herald*, 25 June 1900; NAI/1900/48 Inquest on the body of James Byrne, 25 June 1900.

[13] *Evening Herald*, 4 March 1901; NAI/1901/66 Inquest on the body of Elizabeth Ledwidge, 4 March 1901.

[14] NAI/1902/22 Inquest on the body of Francis McCabe, 11 February1902.

the doctor and priest were called simultaneously. Medical officers were perceived as agents of local surveillance and in vulnerable communities there were high degrees of resistance towards them. While some of this reticence was certainly associated with reconciling physical decline and illness with masculinity, it may be partially explained by popular beliefs about seeing a doctor as portending doom. In a cruel twist of fate, those who expressly refused to engage with medical care were subject to the post-mortem scalpel. Patrick Brennan's family observed his aversion to medical science even after his death. The former soldier, who had served 'in the Militia' in South Africa had been complaining about pains in his limbs for three months. When he died his family refused to allow his remains to be brought to the morgue, but their resistance was futile. It was later found that the 42-year-old died from 'Fatty degeneration of the heart following Bright's disease'. Particulars of his death escaped the notice of media attention.[15]

Despite the fact that Dublin was very well served by maternity hospitals, the Rotunda Lying-in to the north and the Coombe and the National Maternity Hospital to the south of the Liffey all operating comprehensive dispensary services and domiciliary services for women who chose to birth children at home, some women managed pregnancies and childbirth unaided. On the night before Mary Darley of 51 Ballybough Road died she complained of a severe headache— her husband went to the Rotunda Lying-in (hereafter the Rotunda) to seek assistance, but because she was not in her confinement they stated she was not a case for them. That the Rotunda was his first port of call indicates that she may have been pregnant, which would explain why her husband went there as opposed to the four other nearby dispensaries or the Mater Misericordiae Hospital. Pregnancies were rarely cited in cause of death data unless a woman was in childbirth or she died from haemorrhage or puerperal fever post-partum. Further to that, the Rotunda dealt with cases strictly—unless women were in labour they were turned away. One of the two doctors that Darley dealt with at the Rotunda accompanied him to Dr Crinion in Amiens Street, who did not arrive until 8.40 a.m. at which point it only remained for him to pronounce life extinct.[16] Harriet Ferguson, whom I have written about in greater detail elsewhere, was heavily pregnant but was denied care because she 'was not in her confinement'.[17] Dr Crinion, who was derelict in duties on a few occasions, also featured in that tragic story where a mother died of chronic respiratory disease owing to lack of medical attention. Her husband set out in the early hours of the morning and traipsed to the Rotunda followed by four dispensaries to find medical help and by the time he got home from his unsuccessful endeavours she had expired. All of the doctors

---

[15] NAI/1902/31 Inquest on the body of Patrick Brennan, 25 February 1902.

[16] NAI/1900/117 Inquest on the body of Mary Darley, 22 September 1900; Dr Sexton at the Rotunda is named.

[17] Ciara Breathnach, 'Respiratory disease and death registration, Dublin 1900–1902', *Annales de Démographie Historique,* 142:1 (2022), pp. 39–72.

involved were exonerated.[18] In a rare instance in 1902, Dr Crinion was taken to task by a coroner's jury for not having adequate cover for urgent night cases.[19]

While it is unlikely that any late stage medical intervention would have helped Darley or Ferguson, the case of Anne McEveney was one that would definitely have benefitted from more skilled help. She died from haemorrhage at Shovehouse Lane Chapelizod after she had a stillborn male child under a certified and local midwife, Maryanne Clark. Efforts to procure medical assistance were hampered by the fact that the doctor would not attend without a note from the midwife—these delays proved fatal. By the time he arrived she was dead. He too was exonerated in the rider, although his concern for bureaucratic probity was clearly a factor.[20] Sarah Phibbs died of heart failure following septicaemia after the birth of her child at 36 Arklow Street. She had the baby on 7 December and died a week later—during that time she was attended to by a Nurse Morris. Public health nursing and community midwifery was important for women who did not meet the criteria or have the wherewithal to gain access to the maternity hospitals. The jury added a rider: 'we consider she did not get proper skilled treatment…and a Doctor should have been called in'.[21]

Accidental Death

Occupants of 'top back rooms' were most likely to perish in fires and to suffer fatal falls from windows or by falling down stairs. It stands to reason that they would have been the most inaccessible for the fire brigade and highest in terms of falls, which accounted for sixteen accidental deaths in domestic settings, half of which involved children under 12. Although Maurice Joseph Carroll and Gerald Barry occupied opposite ends of the social spectrum, the circumstances of their deaths were precisely the same. Occurring while momentarily out of adult supervision, both children fell through open upper-floor windows. The *Weekly Irish Times* reported how the coroner's court cited Carroll's mother's absence but it stopped short of calling her negligent—the Lad Lane Station Sergeant Thomas Cullen's report noted that there was an old bed nearby from which it was easy to

---

[18] NAI/1901/113 Inquest on the body of Harriet Ferguson, 18 April 1901.

[19] Mrs Doyle sought medical assistance for her husband but failed owing to absences. NAI/1902/18 Inquest on the body of John Doyle, 29 January 1902: 'Died from apoplectic seizure and we wish to add that we consider it a serious matter that Dr Crinion who is a dispensary doctor has no arrangements made for answering urgent night calls. And we also consider that Dr O'Brien showed a want of Professional feeling and kindness towards this poor woman in not going with her in her distress.'

[20] NAI/1901/241 Inquest on the body of Anne McEveney, 12 September 1901.

[21] NAI/1901/310 Inquest on the body of Sarah Phipps, 16 December 1901: her death was recorded (https://civilrecords.irishgenealogy.ie/churchrecords/images/deaths_returns/deaths_1901/05712/4611404.pdf) and Sarah, her daughter's birth was registered on 2 January 1902.

reach the window sill, but stated it 'was wholly accidental'.[22] Domestic chores were the root cause of 10-year-old Anne Flynn's death: she fell while taking a jacket off the clothes line that led out from the lobby window at 79 Chancery Street. She suffered a fractured skull from the impact of her fall from a height of 14 ft to a concrete yard and was rushed to Jervis Street Hospital where she died later that day.[23]

Clearly, all three falls from windows were tragic accidents but some of the other cases were owing to the appalling state of repair of the tenement buildings and, because the home was so central to child's play, there were inevitable consequences. Stairs and common areas were where younger children played. Permitting children to play on the landing outside their room doors offered them the company of others and their mothers the chance to get on with daily chores. It was as normal at the close of the nineteenth century as it is now to allow children 'out to play' but none of the accident prevention measures of modern life were in place; for example, gates on stairways. Even if they were in place they would not have prevented the death of Edward McQuaid, who was 5 years and 8 months when he accidentally fell through bannisters at the tenement house 54 Jervis Street—the coroner's court was told that they were not in proper condition.[24] It was found that Jane Murtagh, aged 5, died from 'coma following laceration of the brain' when she fell over the bannisters at her home, 5 Upper Tyrone Street. She lived in the top back room and was playing with two other children on the top landing. Her mother had gone to empty water on the ground floor, and she had the horrific experience of watching her child fall through the space at the centre of the spiral staircase—from a height of 35 ft. The jury added an insipid rider that aimed to encourage rather than shame slum landlords into taking more responsibility for the safety of children. It stated: 'And we consider that in every tenement house a grating should be placed at each landing over the open space outside the bannisters to prevent a similar occurrence in future.'[25] In what might have been a childcare arrangement, Richard Boyle was visiting the home of Mrs Margaret Stynes at 27 Arran Quay when he fell down the stairs and four stories. Stynes occupied the top front room. The 8-year-old from 53 Smithfield was playing in the early afternoon with Stynes's 3-year-old son when the accident occurred. Dr Garland, who was located next door, was called immediately, but he could do little for the child's fractured skull and he died a few hours later. No suspicion was attached to anyone.[26] John McVeigh was only 8 years of age when he fell while

[22] NAI/1900/105 Inquest on the body of Maurice Joseph Carroll, 3 September 1900; NAI/1901/141 Inquest on the body of Gerald Barry, 18 May 1901; *Weekly Irish Times*, 8 September 1900.
[23] NAI/1901/252 Inquest on the body of Anne Flynn, 21 September 1901.
[24] *Dublin Daily Nation*, 25 August 1900.
[25] NAI/1902/71 Inquest on the body of Jane Murtagh, 19 April 1902.
[26] NAI/1901/220 Inquest on the body of Richard Boyle, 26 August 1901; *Freeman's Journal*, 27 August 1901.

sliding down the bannister—although it was a genuine accident it points to the unsuitability of such environs for child's play.[27]

Anna Davin notes children's preferences for being 'outside' as it was where they were 'freer'.[28] Catherine McMahon, aged 7, went out to play between 9 p.m. and 10 p.m. Her parents thought nothing much of it, as it was summertime, but when she had not returned by 11 p.m. a search was initiated, according to the DMP report. Her father testified that at 10.45 p.m. he went out to search for her. At 2 a.m. he found her in the yard of their house and took her at once to the Meath Hospital. The family occupied the 'top back room' at 50 Francis Street. There were no witnesses, but it was presumed that she fell from the top of the ten stone steps at the back of the house 'rising a height of about 9 feet'. There was a wall on one side of the steps but the iron rail on the other side was detached leaving a gap between the building and the stairs, and it seems that she fell through the opening onto the flagged ground below.[29] Her injuries—serious head wounds, several broken ribs, a broken arm and wrist—were so severe as to be more consistent with a fall from a greater height but there were no witnesses and the line of questioning at the inquest was understandably sympathetic. By the time she was admitted to hospital, House Surgeon Dr Charles Kendall Bushe estimated she had been dead two or three hours.

Another element of cramped living environs was the lack of places to put dangerous substances out of child's reach. That was how Winifred Lambert, aged 4, died of alcoholic poisoning caused by drinking whiskey out of a naggin bottle at the residence of her parents at 1.1 Coles Lane, which was a mixed shop and tenement building. Her father stated that he had obtained the bottle for his younger daughter's teething. It was purchased at Messrs Williams and Company on Henry Street and one of its employees testified that it was '18 degrees under proof'.[30] Winifred drank from it and her father stopped her; he replaced it on the mantle but the child got up again and drank again from it—this time it was their 'servant Mary Dowd' who happened upon the incident as her father was sleeping. The child began to sweat; her father 'applied vinegar' and her mother brought her to Jervis Street Hospital, where she died later that night, on 21 July 1901.[31]

---

[27] He was sliding down the bannister—'he over balanced himself and fell to the ground a distance of about 30 ft thereby sustaining a serious injury to the head'. He was immediately conveyed to Jervis Street Hospital by his father. NAI/1901/157 Inquest on the body of John Brennan, 10 June 1901: 'Died from coma the result of fracture of the skull caused by accidentally falling over the bannisters of the staircase of the house 9 Upper Buckinghamshire St on 8th inst said death taking place at JS Hospital on the 9th inst.'

[28] Anna Davin, *Growing Up Poor: Home, School and Street in London, 1870–1914* (London, 1996), p. 63.

[29] NAI/1901/159 Inquest on the body of Catherine McMahon, 14 June 1901; *Freeman's Journal*, 15 June 1901.

[30] *Evening Herald*, 23 July 1901.

[31] NAI/1901/195 Inquest on the body of Winifred Lambert, 23 July 1901; census return, http://www.census.nationalarchives.ie/reels/nai003772256/ (accessed 20 July 2021).

Poor health, infirmity, and the mobility issues posed by stairs claimed at least three lives. John Bolger, aged 58, had been suffering from bronchitis for about a year, and Charles Howard, aged 75, had been delicate for some time. Both died as a result of falls in their homes but, as they were ailing in health, neither case raised much by way of newspaper interest.[32] Bolger's death received no attention, as it was overshadowed by two drownings in the River Liffey that came before the court on 17 June and, as implied suicides, they received more coverage (discussed in Chapter 4). He had not received medical attention for a year prior to his death, and after his accident a priest was called, but no doctor. The verdict in his case was 'coma caused by fracture at the base of skull, the result of a fall down nine steps at 34 Bride Street'. The post-mortem was conducted by Dr Frank Sharpe Porter Newell from 18 Upper Baggott Street, and the brief report was somewhat superficial. It amounted to a sentence on the identity of the deceased followed by the verdict—his chronic lung condition was not mentioned at all. One witness, Rose Cleary, told DMP constable Sergeant Daly 124A that he 'was somewhat under the influence of drink', and, while no other witnesses corroborated her statement, there were several mentions of 'being out', the deceased 'who had been out', and both his son and daughter 'were out at the time of the occurrence'. Given that the accident took place at 11 p.m. on 15 June it is likely that they had all been at public houses or shebeens. Charles Howard's age was incorrectly reported and, as his inquest occurred amid two other cases that day, a tragic drowning of a 9-year-old boy and the death of a man who fell on the street, his case received bare mention.[33] The final case of limited mobility was that of Michael Hendrick who was only 35 years of age when he fell downstairs at 14 Glencullen Terrace. He had been in receipt of medical attention for 'weak action of the heart' when he fell down twelve steps at his new lodgings. He had just moved there from 6 Upper Gloucester Street, and was showing his nephew Patrick Hendrick around the new place when the accident occurred between 11 p.m. and 12 p.m. He died at 3 a.m.[34]

The power of the coroner's court was limited to inquiry, but strongly worded riders tended to find greater traction in the newspapers and that could have a bearing on whether action was taken by urban sanitary officers of the Dublin Corporation or the DMP. The remit of the Sanitary Act of 1866 and the Public Health Acts 1874–8 also extended to safety. Property owners were responsible for structural defects.[35] The extent to which sanctions were taken against landlords arising from such riders is deserving of more thorough investigation, but is

---

[32] NAI/1901/165 Inquest on the body of John Bolger, 18 June 1901; NAI/1901/208 Inquest on the body of Charles Howard, 8 August 1901.

[33] *Evening Herald*, 8 August 1901.

[34] NAI/1902/30 Inquest on the body of Michael Hendrick, 23 February 1902; the *Irish Times*, 25 February 1902, called him Michael Henry; as did *Belfast Newsletter*, 26 February 1902.

[35] First report of Her Majesty's commissioners for inquiring into the housing of the working classes [C402 C402-I C402-II], p. 4.

beyond the scope of this study. Dublin Corporation had powers to sanction landlords who neglected their water and sanitation obligations, and to condemn housing as being unsuitable for habitation. Landlords were responsible for the state of repair of communal areas like stairwells and hallways, but the emphasis was more on matters of public hygiene and in the cubic feet of air per individual housed. Sanitary sub-officers operating under the Infectious Disease (Notification) Acts 1889 were empowered by a Local Government Board circular in 1900 to issue sanctions against slum landlords for matters of overcrowding owing to the threat of bubonic plague as an outbreak had occurred in Glasgow.[36] The problem with follow through was, of course, resourcing; it was expensive to conduct inspections and Dublin had very few sanitary inspectors. Their attention was primarily focused on public health rather than public safety. The powers emanated from by-laws associated with the sanitary and public health acts which viewed overcrowding narrowly and simply as an impetus for the spread of communicable diseases. The dangers posed by additional wear and tear from over-occupancy and its impact on stairs, bannisters, and fittings hardly registered as a problem. With the prospect of little to no sanction, tenements deteriorated further and the often appalling state of repair caused a number of preventable deaths.[37]

Crumbling interiors were the direct cause of a few adult deaths, but nearly all were linked to alcohol consumption, so this added another layer of complexity to causation and the dispersion of blame. James Robertson stayed the night at 101 Francis Street after having a few drinks—there was no door to the room and he fractured his cervical vertebrae when he fell down the stairs in this house. The jury recommended that a door be placed on the room.[38] The absence of a bannister and handrail was a primary factor in the death of 30-year-old labourer John Doody, but he had been out on Christmas Eve 1900 and had taken a few drinks. It is interesting to note how his drinking was not problematised by the court, which marvelled so frequently at female alcohol consumption to the point of obsession. He stumbled and fell down the stairs of number 20 Gardiner Street and the resulting fracture at the base of his skull proved fatal. DMP inspector Thomas Lenehan, Store Street, found the stairs in 'a dangerous condition' with no bannister or handrail and deemed it the cause of death.[39]

Deaths from falls within tenement buildings were recurrent: James Kelly, a vanman, fell on the stairs while inebriated at 35 William Street and he crashed his head on a flagged floor below.[40] His fall was reported as being from a mere five

---

[36] Circular No. 174 M/1900, Twenty-ninth Annual Report of the Local Government Board for Ireland, for the year ending 31st March 1901 [Cd. 1259] p. 74.

[37] Thomas Rogers Forbes, 'Crowner's quest', Transactions of the American Philosophical Society, 68:1 (1978), pp. 1–52 at 26 mentions darkness as a factor in domestic and streetscape accidents.

[38] NAI/1900/76 Inquest on the body of William Robertson, 25 July 1900; Irish Daily Independent, 26 July 1900.

[39] NAI/1900/203 Inquest on the body of John Doody, 26 December 1900.

[40] Evening Herald, 2 March 1901.

feet but the effects of coma and brain abscess were immediate—he spent almost three weeks at Mercer's Hospital where he died on 1 March.[41] Thomas Quinn, aged 37, had drink taken when he called to his friend's house at 39 Upper Mercer Street on 25 May 1901. He was leaning over the bannister and fell down into the cellar; he was conscious but refused initially to get medical attention. He died four days later at Mercer's Hospital from a fractured vertebra, which had caused breathing difficulties.[42] Richard Sullivan's fall over the bannisters at 17 Great Longford Street caused ruptures to his kidney and spleen; he died in the Adelaide Hospital on 6 October 1901. He had been drinking in Murphy's public house on Stephen Street with his brother and sister-in-law, who testified that he only had a pint and a half or two pints of porter.[43] Three weeks later a similar case, that of Catherine Sweeney, aged 64, came before the coroner. She was visiting a friend when she fell in the dimly lit abode at 4 Talbot Lane—it transpired that she had lived there in the past and would have known the layout of the building; there were no witnesses to her fall.[44] Although questions about her sobriety were raised at the inquest, there was no evidence to say she had taken any drink. She fell in a communal area, 'it was evening and lighting was not great'. Further to that, a DMP inspector deemed the staircase to be 'in a dangerous condition'—a verdict of accidental death was returned and it is unlikely that anyone profiteering from these tenements were prosecuted or taken to task in any way.[45]

Living Rough and Alcoholism

There are a number of cases in this dataset of people who were living rough or had no fixed abode. Nearly all involved alcohol abuse and separation from family, or both. I classify them as domestic cases because their deaths occurred in the locations where they slept ordinarily even if they were of no fixed abode. For example, Patrick Kenny lived in a cottage with no roof on Weaver's Lane in Phibsboro, and took his meals at Margaret Hughes's house, 3 Weaver's Lane. Worried that he had not been taking care of himself, Hughes went round to check on him and found him dead. His place was described as a 'dilapidated thatched cottage where deceased slept at night, but which was not inhabited by any other human being'.[46] Rough living took its toll on the 36-year-old who died from

---

[41] NAI/1901/65 Inquest on the body of James Kelly, 2 March 1901.

[42] NAI/1901/149 Inquest on the body of Thomas Quinn, 30 May 1901; *Belfast Newsletter*, 31 May 1901.

[43] NAI/1901/257 Inquest on the body of Richard Sullivan, 7 October 1901; http://www.census.nationalarchives.ie/reels/nai003727536/ indicates that he was unmarried at the time of the March 1901 census but the inquest states he was married (accessed 2 December 2020).

[44] NAI/1901/274 Inquest on the body of Catherine Sweeney, 28 October 1901.

[45] *Evening Herald*, 29 October 1901.

[46] NAI/1900/158 Inquest on the body of Patrick Kenny, 8 November 1900.

'cardiac failure secondary to disease of lung, liver and kidney'—he was not attended by any doctor.[47] Stephen Kennedy, aged about 50, was considered by the *Evening Herald* to be a case of 'Destitution and death'.[48] He was found in the top back room at 20 Great Longford Street, where he died from natural causes and tubercular disease. Mary Vesey of the same address noticed that he regularly came in to the building and squatted in the top back room which was empty—she gave him water two days before he died. Another woman in the building named Kate Mahon had given him tea and bread in the days leading up to his death. The DMP report noted how the house was 'condemned by the Corporation and the room was dis-used'; he slept on the bare floor which was described as 'in a wretched state of filth and vermin'. In that case there was no mention of alcohol consumption.[49] Charles Hackett was just above the point of rough sleeping and 'lived from one lodging house to another'; he died at 23 Stafford Street, a tenement house. It was thought that he had been a draper's assistant at one point but was addicted to drink and lived in very poor circumstances. He had been in the care of Dr Walter Leonards who was not surprised to learn that he had died of respiratory and cardiac complications.[50]

Grief may have pushed Sarah Perry into a spiral of heavy drinking after her husband died of phthisis on 14 August 1899.[51] She had secured a place in the newly constructed and much sought after Guinness Buildings; she had eleven children living but was clearly very unwell. On the day she died, her daughter saw her getting sick into a bucket and fall backwards on the floor—she ran to get help from a neighbour.[52] Mrs Connor testified that Kathleen Perry came to her in a panic saying, 'my mother is fainting'; she went at once to assist and gave her some water. Sarah Perry died within seconds from 'cardiac failure as a [sequelae] to tubercular disease of the lungs' and it was registered accordingly.[53] Her brother-in-law John Toole, a former DMP Superintendent, living at 63 Summerhill, identified the body. Rather unusually for a widow of her social class, her funeral notice was placed in the *Freeman's Journal*.[54] Toole took her two children to his residence. When both parents died, families invariably disintegrated, and it seems that some of Sarah Perry's children were taken in by close relatives in Dublin and

---

[47] *Freeman's Journal*, 9 November 1900.
[48] NAI/1900/154 Inquest on the body of Stephen Kennedy, 7 November 1900; *Evening Herald*, 7 November 1900.
[49] NAI/1901/154, report dated 7 November 1900.
[50] NAI/1901/230 Inquest on the body of Charles Hackett, 2 September 1901.
[51] See https://civilrecords.irishgenealogy.ie/churchrecords/images/deaths_returns/deaths_1899/05788/4636906.pdf (accessed 27 November 2021).
[52] NAI/1900/24 Inquest on the body of Sarah Perry, 20 May 1900; evidence of Kathleen Perry 30B Block Guinness' Buildings, 20 May 1900.
[53] See https://civilrecords.irishgenealogy.ie/churchrecords/images/deaths_returns/deaths_1900/05762/4628121.pdf (accessed 3 January 2021).
[54] *Freeman's Journal*, 22 May 1900.

County Kildare, and her youngest daughter was boarded out and living with four other boarded out children in Swords, according to the 1901 census.[55]

Eliza Murphy who was 'addicted to drink' lived at 4 Ayres Court—she went to bed between 4 p.m. and 5 p.m. and between 6 p.m. and 7 p.m. she complained of pains in her head. For reasons unknown she was living under her maiden name Martin. The DMP found a pawn ticket on her person from Mrs Crinion's—she was using her possessions for liquidity despite the fact that her husband was a soldier in the 1st Leinster Regiment serving in South Africa and she held a separation allowance of £3 4s. 7d. from the Military Office. She apparently left it there for safe keeping.[56] It is unlikely that her death would have piqued much interest from the newspapers but as it happened it was overshadowed by what the newspapers described as the 'Horrible Fatality' and workplace accident of miles man (railway worker) John Doyle at Serpentine Avenue. It was held by the county coroner Christopher Friery, who was legally qualified.[57] The following day, the death of Evelyn Flood commanded the headlines as a middle-class 'inferred suicide' case.[58]

Heavy alcohol consumption in domestic settings was common to a few female cases. Thirty-nine-year-old Norah St Laurence Burke's death in a better class of lodging house at 12 Lower Mount Street was alcoholism-related. She came to lodge there with her husband, Mr Walker Burke, a bank clerk out of employment about nine months prior to her death. In that time Sebina Sloper the landlady noticed her physical decline. The DMP report documented how she 'lived principally on drink ["for past week" was struck out], which was brought into her by her husband, and a servant in the house'.[59] Sloper was concerned about the impact of the recent heavy drinking and sent for a nurse, Clare Shee from the Mater Hospital, who advised that she be admitted. While she was away making the necessary arrangements Norah expired; her husband was comatose alongside her following a heavy drinking session and had not noticed anything awry. Dr John Burgess found evidence of her excessive alcohol consumption which corresponded with liver damage and how it was 'enormously enlarged' but the adherent clot he found in the right ventricle was deemed to be the primary cause of death thus sparing her the association with liver disease and the inferences of alcohol abuse in the verdict and her subsequent death registration.[60]

[55] See http://www.census.nationalarchives.ie/pages/1901/Dublin/Swords/North_Street/1267221/ (accessed 7 February 2021). I am grateful to Dr Rachel Murphy for her assistance in tracking down the Perry family.

[56] NAI/1901/307 Inquest on the body of Eliza Murphy, 11 December 1901.

[57] Irish Daily Independent, 11 December 1901; Evening Herald, 12 December 1901.

[58] NAI/1901/308 Inquest on the body of Evelyn Flood, 12 December 1901.

[59] NAI/1901/39 Inquest on the body of Norah St Laurence Burke, 7 February 1901.

[60] NAI/1901/39 DMP report dated 7 February 1901. The addresses of the jurors were not recorded on the inquisition form. See https://civilrecords.irishgenealogy.ie/churchrecords/images/deaths_returns/deaths_1901/05738/4619908.pdf (accessed 24 November 2021).

Informal 'inebriates' were in operation in Dublin. Chronic alcoholism caused Isabella Ford to lodge at 17 Lower Gloucester Street. She was identified as being 'addicted to drink for past 15 years and living apart from her husband for 18 months, who allowed her 10s. a week to live on'. She complained to her landlady Mrs Flanagan of pains in her chest but she would not see a doctor or go to hospital. The DMP report accounted for the fact that she was a regular problem for the Summerhill Station because of her heavy drinking over the previous two years and the fact that she 'frequently drank methylated spirits'.[61] Her post-mortem found extensive kidney inflammation, an enlarged liver, and her right lung 'was consolidated + in the pneumonic state'. Death was from 'cardiac failure due to pneumonia'.[62] Her landlady's daughter Kate Flanagan 'noticed her very bad' on 10 February and encouraged her mother (unnamed) to seek help. The landlady knew the whereabouts of her husband and went to seek his assistance—on her return she found her dead.[63] In another informal arrangement to contain and conceal female alcoholism, Anne Wilson came from Glasgow to stay with her sister Norah Roberts and while in Dublin she began to drink excessively and refused medical aid. The post-mortem report noted congested lungs and enlarged liver and heart disease—the jury added 'resulting from excessive use of alcohol'. Although not what we could categorise as a rider, as the opinion was based on medical testimony, it was an adjudication and one the jury elected to emphasise, where in other cases like Norah St Laurence Burke's it was quietly elided. What differentiated her case was that when she could not get drink herself early in the morning she would send her 4-year-old grandson to a public house to purchase it for her. One of the jurors said that the publican deserved censure but Dr Byrne did not permit it to enter the record as he was not there to defend himself. Although her liver was very much enlarged, and her lungs were 'much congested', death was considered to have been from cardiac failure accelerated by the heavy drinking. Her death registration qualified the fact that her cardiac failure was 'from excessive use of alcohol'.[64] Another rather unusual case was that of Elitia Kearney whose inquest was held on 31 July 1901—the verdict was that she died of inflammation of the lungs and cirrhosis of liver. The jury received an anonymous letter stating that she was not the legal wife of Mr Kearney and that there was foul play afoot as it would save him £1 a week in maintenance. They had been living separately for three years and it was also stated that she bedded another man the

[61] NAI/1901/41 Inquest on the body of Isabella Ford, 11 February 1901.
[62] NAI/1901/41 Inquest dated 11 February 1901.
[63] NAI/1901/41 DMP report dated 10 February 1901.
[64] NAI/1900/58 Inquest on the body of Anne Wilson, report dated 6 July 1900; *Irish Times*, 7 July 1900; https://civilrecords.irishgenealogy.ie/churchrecords/images/deaths_returns/deaths_1900/05753/4625061.pdf (accessed 24 November 2021).

night she died. In that instance, the jury added the rider: 'we consider that the writer of the anonymous letter deserves censure'.[65]

Living Quarters: Burns and Scalds

Life in overcrowded one-roomed tenements weighed heavily on small children. Apart from accidents like falling from windows or down stairs that could occur in any household, there were a number of preventable deaths like burning and scalding that were a particular feature of the tenements. The architecture of the home and limited cooking facilities (see Figure 2.1) gave rise to these burns' cases. Between candles, oil lamps, and the reliance on open fires for heat and cooking, burns and scalds were omnipresent dangers—the injuries were both horrific and life limiting.

Few households had fireguards for the shallow hearths, initially intended solely for heating purposes in bedrooms and never supposed to function as cooking places. Charles Cameron noted how meat was boiled or fried in tenement houses as there were no facilities for roasting—he omitted the fact that fuel necessary for ovens and longer cooking times was prohibitively expensive for the households in question.[66] Susan Galavan's work on the architectural drawings for semi-detached Victorian suburbs coupled with the images from the 'Darkest Dublin' photographic collection provide an impression of the dimensions of the fireplaces in the upper floors of these erstwhile one-family dwellings. Usually only the kitchen fireplace, located in basements or lower floors, was purpose built with flagstone floors and properly recessed for cooking. While there are several mentions of households living in 'back kitchens', those living in upper floor bedrooms often had dangerously shallow fireplaces that could hardly accommodate fuel let alone precariously poised pots or kettles (see Figure 2.1).[67] The 1914 report on the condition of working-class housing stated that these small fireplaces were unsuitable for general use.[68] Deaths from fire, scalding, and asphyxia from smoke and carbon monoxide were all preventable. They occurred with such regularity that Dr Byrne was exacerbated by them, both as a clinician and as coroner. The *Irish Times* rarely carried reports from the coroner's court, but Dr Byrne's fatigue from the high number of fire-related deaths carried some currency. A 1908 article cited his efforts from 1905 using 'any little influence he possessed with the members of the Corporation'. His proposal that cheap fireguards be provided to the poor came

---

[65] NAI/1901/198 Inquest on the body of Elitia Kearney, report dated 31 July 1901.

[66] Cameron, *How the Poor Live*, p. 11.

[67] Susan Galavan, *Dublin's Bourgeois Homes: Building the Victorian Suburbs, 1850–1901* (London, 2017), pp. 61, 72.

[68] Report of the departmental committee appointed by the Local Government Board for Ireland to inquire into the housing conditions of the working classes in the city of Dublin [Cd. 7273], p. 4.

before the Public Health Committee, but it amounted to nothing.[69] As Tarr and Tebeau found in America, in Ireland the primary concern in the late nineteenth century was workplace risk management and the home safety movement, which was more firmly linked to the hazards of electrification, occurred much later.[70]

The perennial problems of deaths by burns and, to a lesser extent, scalds were a source of particular concern to the Dublin Sanitary Association, which documented that in the ten years from 1871 to 1880, 4,376 deaths were returned under this category and children under 5 accounted for 63 per cent of them.[71] These statistics were irregularly collated and, unfortunately, it is not possible to do an international comparative analysis. By and large the burns' cases concerning children were ones where clothing caught fire and was quickly extinguished. The medical history of fire and burns has received very little scholarly attention, yet their occurrence in the context of coroner's records is indicative of several socio-economic problems.[72] Of the fifty-nine fire-related cases (excluding five cases of smoke inhalation) fifteen cases involved adults and thirty-nine concerned children aged 12 and under. The locus of fire-related deaths in all but three of the fifty-nine fire-related cases discussed here was the home. This places Dublin at odds with the occurrences of fires in more industrially developed cities of the United Kingdom where people, as Shane Ewen argues, had an 'exploitative relationship' with it, and encountered it more frequently 'in the factory, the mill, the foundry', as well, of course, as the domestic hearth.[73] Reflecting the lower level of industrialisation in Ireland, fire-related deaths rarely occurred in the workplace; in fact, there were only two in these data: the first was that of Peter Eustace, a white deal worker/white wood worker, who sustained severe burns at his workshop at 2 Rotunda Market. It was late, and he was working by paraffin lamp—it overturned and when he went to pick it up his clothing caught fire. He went immediately to Jervis Street Hospital to have his wounds dressed; he returned two days later to have fresh dressings applied and, as his condition had deteriorated, he was detained as a patient. He died two days after admission.[74] The second occurred when a fire broke out during the night at the American Bar and despite

---

[69] *Weekly Irish Times*, 11 January 1908.

[70] Joel A. Tarr and Mark Tebeau, 'Housewives as home safety managers: the changing perception of the home as a place of hazard and risk, 1870–1940', in Roger Cooter and Bill Luckin (eds), *Accidents in History: Injuries, Fatalities and Social Relations* (Amsterdam, 1997), pp. 196–233.

[71] The Dublin Sanitary Association, *The British Medical Journal*, 1:1363 (1887), p. 349.

[72] The history of fire and burns in Ireland has received very little scholarly attention to date, with the exception of Tom Geraghty and Trevor Whitehead, *The Dublin Fire Brigade: A History of the Brigade, the Fires and the Emergencies* (Dublin, 2004); Gemma Clark, 'Arson in modern Ireland: fire and protest before the Famine', in D.M. MacRaild and K. Hughes (eds), *Crime, Violence and the Irish in the Nineteenth Century* (Liverpool, 2017), pp. 211–26; Shane Ewen, *Fighting Fires: Creating the British Fire Service, 1800–1978* (Basingstoke, 2010).

[73] Ewen, *Fighting Fires*, p. 2.

[74] NAI/1901/114 Inquest on the body of Peter Eustace, 13 September 1900.

DFB efforts, the live-in cook Mary Malone died from smoke inhalation.[75] The third non-domestic case involved a child named Mary Gargan who stopped to warm her hands at a fire lit by Alliance Gas Company workers near her home in Inchicore. She was one of a few children who had stopped to do the same thing and her dress caught fire; Mrs Stanley heard the child cry and ran out to assist. She took off the burning clothes and sent for her father, who brought the child straight to Dr Steevens' Hospital, where she died sixteen days later.[76] There were eleven cases of scalding, only one of which involved an adult, who was a psychiatric hospital patient. While she was being bathed her attendant momentarily turned her back—the patient turned on the hot tap and suffered scalds in the process; the jury rider recommended that two attendants should have been present.[77]

For nosographical purposes, coroners were instructed to record whether or not the death was due to burns or scalds and how long they lived after the wounds occurred. Death from either cause was usually owing to extensive skin trauma which left victims prone to sepsis and dehydration.[78] Scalding caused eleven deaths and limited cooking space was the primary issue in most cases. Some fires warranted the attention of the DFB. These included cases of asphyxia from smoke inhalation and carbon monoxide poisoning. Often the terms burns and scalds are used interchangeably but inaccurately. Taken together, my analysis shows that over a tenth of the overall dataset occurred from both; five deaths were as a result of smoke inhalation (Figure 2.2). Further to these, there were four instances of carbon monoxide poisoning occurring in domestic settings, which illustrates the

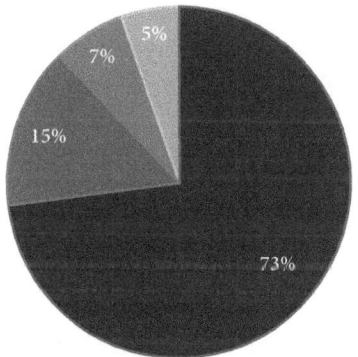

Figure 2.2 Burns, scalds, smoke, and carbon monoxide deaths
Note: Total of seventy-four cases.

---

[75] NAI/1901/298 Inquest on the body of Mary Malone, 26 November 1901. It was also where she lived so it straddles both domestic and workplace deaths.

[76] NAI/1902/25 Inquest on the body of Mary Gargan, 13 February 1902.

[77] NAI/1900/10 Inquest on the body of Annie Meehan, 30 April 1900.

[78] *Statistical Nosology*, 1864, pp. 56, 61.

impact of modernity and its uncomfortable layering beneath and on top of the existing city architecture.

Deaths of children caused by fires in the home followed a repetitious pattern. On 9 May 1901, Bridget Walsh was going about her daily chores at 25 Lower Stephen Street when she was alerted by her 3-year-old son that 'Katie is lighting'.[79] She ran into the next room and found her 4-year-old niece Catherine McLoughlin in the centre of the room in flames. Walsh immediately wrapped the bedclothes around her to smother the fire and the child was then conveyed by a neighbouring woman to the nearby Mercer's Hospital where she was detained as a patient.[80] The DMP report noted how despite best efforts she died before morning and it described her remains as 'shockingly burned'. The circumstances surrounding the incident have many shared characteristics with other child deaths coming before Dr Byrne's court. Katie was left in a room with a fire while her mother, Mary Connor, a fish dealer, went out to get some groceries; 'a half ounce of tea and some sugar' to be precise. Unlike the thrifty housewives of the Guinness Brewery who had reliable weekly wages, this household depended on fluctuating incomes, shopping locally (not in the markets), and in small quantities. According to the police report her mother had 'told Kate to mind the fire and not get burned. Mary Connor had only gone as far as the hall when she heard the fuss upstairs and went back'. The child's stepfather John Connor, a builder's labourer, was also out. In most cases where women left their children alone in tenement settings there was usually another mother or adult female nearby keeping a communal eye on all the children in the building—nearly all doors were left open or unlocked as there was a sense of community and, invariably, little to steal (see Figure 2.1). Families of Dublin City origin, as was the case with the Connor and Walsh households, tended to neo-locate and create a sense of community among kin; this permitted women to extend their watch over children from other households, within buildings and usually on the same floor.[81]

Number 25 Lower Stephen Street had six households and twenty-eight inhabitants, but Katie, who was a child born out of wedlock, was not accounted for in the census a few weeks prior (in any county, with all variations on her name and age) and it is also possible that the number recorded as resident on census night is not

---

[79] The census transcription states her son Patrick was 8 years old—this is an error. See http://census.nationalarchives.ie/reels/nai003727769/ (accessed 21 August 2021).

[80] NAI/1901/130 Inquest on the body of Catherine McLoughlin, 10 May 1901; report and evidence of Bridget Walsh dated 10 May 1901, 25 Lower Stephen Street.

[81] Prior to their marriage in July 1899, John Connor and Mary MacLoughlin both lived within a stone's throw of their marital home, at 39 Lower Stephen Street and 1 Dawson Court, off Lower Stephen Street, respectively. See https://civilrecords.irishgenealogy.ie/churchrecords/images/marriage_returns/marriages_1899/10390/5783131.pdf (accessed 5 November 2020).

a true reflection of total occupancy either.[82] Katie's death was registered on 11 May from 'information received'.[83]

Burns' cases were not just confined to tenement life in the inner city—they could be found in poor households in the more affluent suburbs, which were perceived and depicted as more wholesome. This is where biopower and the uneasy relationship poor people had with its instruments and agents become more apparent and Laurence Stone's ideas surrounding prosopography and its ability to elucidate social structure are most relevant.[84] By grouping these burns' cases together it is possible to examine them in the round and to see how a similar set of medical and social circumstances produced a uniformity in verdicts but a variance in jury riders, which reveal much about the prejudices of jurors towards the inner-city poor and, more specifically, towards those they believed to be morally transgressive.

The following three cases involve instances of mothers leaving their small children unattended or in the care of older children. Three-year-old Mary Josephine Smith was staying with her grandmother at 14 Weir View in Lucan in March/April 1900. When her grandmother went shopping in Dublin, a distance of some 8–11 kilometres or 5–7 miles, she left her grandchild in the charge of Bridget Kilmorey of 13 Weir View, who subsequently went out locally to get some essentials and left Mary Josephine Smith in the care of 7-year-old Mary Kilmorey/Kilmurey/Kilmuray (all derivatives are used in the records). It was in this absence that 3-year-old Mary Josephine Smith stood in front of an open fire and her clothes 'became ignited'. Seven-year-old Mary Kilmurray tried immediately to extinguish the flames but failed and brought the child to number 16. It was a neighbour, Frank Murray of 15 Weir View that cut the child's clothes off, wrapped her in a blanket and brought her to the Lucan Dispensary. The doctor 'applied some remedies' and advised sending her to Dr Steevens' Hospital, which her aunt Margaret duly did. Her head, face, and extremities were so severely burned that she died the following day, 31 March. The verdict was 'shock resulting from burns accidentally received'.[85] John Brien, aged 5, suffered burns when he was left in the care of his 10-year-old brother in a cottage at the Grange, Rathfarnam (a suburb south of the city), on 4 January 1901. His mother left them for a period of two

[82] See http://census.nationalarchives.ie/reels/nai003727771/ occupants of number 25, Connor family (accessed 5 November 2020).

[83] See https://civilrecords.irishgenealogy.ie/churchrecords/images/deaths_returns/deaths_1901/05729/4616824.pdf (accessed 5 November 2020). She may be the child registered by Holles Street Hospital but it is not possible to verify that in the absence of the full maternity records as her mother's address is not recorded. In any event the institution registered her birth, not her mother. See https://civilrecords.irishgenealogy.ie/churchrecords/images/birth_returns/births_1897/02140/1812859.pdf (I am grateful to Rachel Murphy for her assistance here).

[84] Lawrence Stone, 'Prosopography', *Daedalus*, 100:1; *Historical Studies Today* (Winter, 1971), pp. 46–79 at 46.

[85] NAI/1901/94 Inquest on the body of Mary Smith, 1 April 1901.

hours and on her return, she found a neighbouring woman applying oil to John's injuries. Mrs Brien brought the child to the local dispensary doctor, Dr Croly, who dressed the wounds and advised sending him to Harcourt Street Hospital. Mrs Brien did as the doctor instructed, but such were the extent of the injuries that the child died in hospital a week later on 12 January at 10.30 p.m. Although it was clearly a case of burning, the DMP report used the term scald and burn interchangeably. It was noted that his father Matthew was a labourer, and the verdict was that the child died from 'exhaustion following burns accidentally received'.[86] Mary Balfe, The Quarries, Terenure (another suburb to the south of the city), was 9 years old when her clothes became ignited while she was putting coal in the fire on 31 January 1901. She ran out into the street where neighbours clambered to save her. Two men, both with addresses on the nearby Saint Ignatius Road, used their coats to extinguish the flames. They then took off her clothes and were careful in their testimony to add that they immediately 'gave her over to Mrs Collins'. A Mrs Essie Murphy (no address given), travelled by cab with Mrs Bridget Collins to the Meath Hospital between 5 p.m. and 6 p.m. It transpired that Mary Balfe was in charge of her sister Daisy, aged 5, and brother John, aged 3, while their mother, also Mary, a widow, was out working. Her eldest child James, aged 12, was 'temporarily absent' when the incident occurred. It was decreed that Mary Balfe died from burns accidentally received at her residence and her death took place in the Meath Hospital later that day.[87]

A fairly consistent trope in fourteen of the thirty-nine child cases was the absence of adult supervision or that a child, aged 12 or under, was in the charge of a child. There is a sharp contrast between the straightforward verdicts in these suburban cases and those coming from the inner city. As Vicky Holmes has astutely observed in her Ipswich case study, the distance from shops and amenities posed risks to children. In the Dublin records there is evidence of how women often went an additional distance to access cheaper produce.[88] That was the underlying cause in the death of 5-year-old Mary Rourke who died at 11 p.m. on 3 February 1901. Her mother (also Mary) left their room at 7 Lower Gardiner at 1 p.m. to do her shopping on Britain Street, which was a distance of over a kilometre (about three quarters of a mile) away. She left the deceased and her brother Richard, aged 3, in a room where there was a lit fire; when she returned at 1.40 p.m. she found her daughter had been taken to hospital. The alarm was raised when a neighbour, Theresa Lynch, heard a noise from the back kitchen and went downstairs. Together with Mrs Jennette and Bridget Rice, another tenant, she pulled the burning clothes off the child and sent for the constable. The women

---

[86]   NAI/1901/13 Inquest on the body of John Brien, 14 January 1901; DMP report dated 12 January.
[87]   NAI/1901/29 Inquest on the body of Mary Balfe, 31 January 1901: death took place at the Meath Hospital.
[88]   Vicky Holmes, 'Home cultures', p. 319.

then entered the kitchen and found the bed on fire; they threw some buckets of water on it to quench the flames. It was thought that the children were lighting bits of paper, or, literally playing with fire. Dr John Begley conducted the post-mortem. Although the police report states that there was no suspicion of foul play, the verdict was 'Shock the result of burns accidentally received at her residence' the 'back kitchen' at 7 Lower Gardiner Street and her death occurred at Jervis Street Hospital. DMP constable Matthew O'Brien 171C, Store Street, who took the child by cab to the hospital, stated that 'The mother was not there when I arrived.'[89] Unlike the previous three cases, where children aged 12 and under were left *in loco parentis*, in the case of Mary Rourke the jury added the rider 'And we consider the mother guilty of gross neglect in leaving the children without any one to care for them in a room with a fire.'[90] All of these cases were tragic accidents but Mrs Mary Rourke, the inner-city dweller, whose husband was notable by absence in the DMP report and the witness statements, was brought before Mr Mahony at the Northern Police Court a fortnight later partly on the strength of the jury's rider. Mr Mahony showed compassion and dismissed the case stating that she had suffered enough already.[91] By then the newspapers reported that Mary Rourke was living at 3 Terrace Place, Bella Street, and by the time the census was taken on 31 March 1901, it seems the already 'weak family' had disintegrated altogether, and a 3-year-old Richard Rourke (the only one fitting his age and general profile in the Dublin area) was residing with the five-strong Matthews Family at 31.3 Grenville Street.[92]

Couples who left their children unattended stood a better chance of withstanding the pressure authorities could subsequently bring to bear if burns cases proved fatal. When Emily Murray decided to get oil for the lamp as her husband returned from work on Christmas Eve, she left their two small children Mary and Nellie, aged 3½ and 1½, respectively, in their top back room at number 24 Great Britain Street. Thinking that she would only be a few minutes away, she did not ask anyone to mind the children, but there was a lit fire in the room. James, her husband, went with her to get the oil at 194 Great Britain Street[93] and convinced her to stop for a quick drink while there. In evidence she stated that it was his fault that one became two whiskeys and she was anxious the whole time. On their return they met a neighbour who told them their room was on fire—James Murray ran in and rescued both children but Mary Murray died later that day from her injuries. The jury added the rider 'And we consider the parents guilty of gross carelessness in

---

[89] NAI/1901/37 Inquest on the body of Mary Rourke, 7 February 1901.

[90] NAI/1901/37 Report and evidence dated 6 and 7 February 1901.

[91] *Irish Examiner*, 22 February 1901.

[92] See http://www.census.nationalarchives.ie/pages/1901/Dublin/Mountjoy/Grenville_Street/1325765/ (there was no trace of him in the 1911 returns) (accessed 7 January 2019).

[93] See http://www.census.nationalarchives.ie/reels/nai003692079/ (accessed 17 November 2021); James Byrne, spirit grocers (*Thom's Directory*, 1894), p. 1363.

leaving the two children in a room in which a fire was lighting without someone to mind them.'[94] It seems they were not brought before the police courts, which were exceptionally busy with drunk and disorderly cases during the festive season, and three months later they were living with Ellen (Nellie in the coroner's report), at 12.6 Moore Street.[95]

Inflections of social class and perceptions of respectability characterised the case of Elizabeth Elliot, who was an 'illegitimate child' living with her late father's wife. Her guardian Mrs Rathborne went out 'on business' and left Elizabeth in charge of her two children Ruby and Anne Rodbourne/Rathborne, aged 5 and 3 years, respectively, at 35 Emorville Avenue at 9.30 a.m.[96] About an hour and a half after she left, John W. Kavanagh, a grocers' assistant, called on business to the same address and heard a child screaming inside. He knocked, and the door was opened by the child, whose clothes were in flames around her—Kavanagh at once tore the burning clothes off the child and then wrapped her in a rug. She was brought to the Meath Hospital by a DMP constable where she died shortly thereafter. Rathborne, whose defence was that she was 'delayed in several places', did not return until 3.30 p.m. She stated that Elizabeth was 11 years old, 'was very sensible' and she had left her in charge on 'many previous occasions'. The DMP report stated that Elizabeth was 8 years old. Her death registration stated she was 'about 11'.[97] Rathborne was a young and propertied widow, whose late husband's estate, valued at almost £505 in 1898, left her in a very comfortable position and her case of neglect of Elizabeth Elliot was permitted to fade from public view without jury censure.[98]

Dr Byrne was very concerned with propriety and, where permitted, he took negligence in all its hues to task. When Edith Ferns died at Jervis Street Hospital from 'Shock the result of burns accidentally received on Saturday the 8th March 1902 at her residence 18 Upper Dominick St', it transpired that her mother

[94] NAI/1900/202 Inquest on the body of Mary Murray, 26 December 1900; *Freeman's Journal*, 27 December 1900.

[95] See http://www.census.nationalarchives.ie/pages/1901/Dublin/North_City/Moore_Street/1333274/ (accessed 7 November 2021).

[96] According to Ruby's birth registration Henry Talbot Rathborne was a land holder and proprietor from Ballymore, County Meath, married to Jane Fanning (see https://civilrecords.irishgenealogy.ie/churchrecords/images/cert_amends/cert_1896/1826845a.pdf). They married in 1895 (see https://civilrecords.irishgenealogy.ie/churchrecords/images/marriage_returns/marriages_1895/10527/5834386.pdf) and he died aged 85 in 1898 (see https://civilrecords.irishgenealogy.ie/churchrecords/images/deaths_returns/deaths_1898/05841/4654608.pdf) (all links accessed 24 November 2021).

[97] NAI/1901/7 Inquest on the body of Elizabeth Elliot, 7 January 1901: death registration at https://civilrecords.irishgenealogy.ie/churchrecords/images/deaths_returns/deaths_1901/05738/4619866.pdf (accessed 24 November 2021); *Evening Herald*, 7 January 1901. I failed to find her civil birth registration.

[98] When she died in 1940, aged 65, she lived at Belgrave Square—her daughter Ruby was present at death: see https://civilrecords.irishgenealogy.ie/churchrecords/images/marriage_returns/marriages_1895/10527/5834386.pdf; for Rathborne's estate, see http://www.willcalendars.nationalarchives.ie/reels/cwa/005014910/005014910_00481.pdf (both links accessed 24 November 2021).

Margaret Ferns had initially been refused care at the Richmond Hospital.[99] The accident followed the same pattern as the other cases—her mother was doing housework and the child was standing at the fire in their room when her clothes ignited. Margaret immediately wrapped Edith in a sack and ran to the Richmond Hospital accompanied by Charles Canavan of the same address, but there was no vacancy. They then went to Jervis Street Hospital, and the time lost undoubtedly further aggravated the child's injuries. All else was in order—she was not insured, her father was employed as an engine driver, and her mother was present when the accident occurred. Dr Byrne asked if the jury wished to add a rider concerning the actions of the Richmond Hospital but it was declined.[100] Patrick Palmer was 'illegitimate' and living at 50 Goldsmith Street—his mother Annie 'Irene' Palmer was a domestic servant who had him 'out to nurse' with Mary Anne Parkes who kept the lodging house and had four other nurse children, who were all were registered with the local authority. The child appeared well cared for and Mrs Parkes burned herself while trying to extinguish the child's burning night shirt. She had vacated the room momentarily to get a cup at 9 a.m. on 21 February—she was dressing all children opposite the fire. No suspicion was attached to Mrs Parkes who, according to the 1901 census, had six nurse children and an adopted daughter listed as living with her; Irene Palmer was listed as a visitor.[101] The case received no newspaper coverage, whereas another inquest conducted on the same day did, that of Christopher McCullough's death following a scalding accident.[102] He had pulled a pot of boiling tea over his face and breast—his mouth, throat, and chest were scalded, and he was immediately brought to hospital. He was noted as having died at the Children's Hospital Temple Street, from 'shock the result of burns accidentally received' at his parents residence, 2 Church Avenue, Drumcondra.[103]

In contrast with burns, cases of scalding elicited a sympathetic reaction from the coroner's court; there was a sense of inevitability and an automatic absolution of blame. The careful scrutiny of maternal actions in the DMP or coroner's inquiry was not as prevalent as in the burns' cases—for example, the case of Ellen Reilly aged 3 years and 7 months that came before the court on 15 April 1901. She had been in the care of older siblings Mary, aged 17, and William, aged 6, at 7 Cross Kevin Street while her mother Bridget went out, and contrary to the burns' cases, the purpose of her absence was neither stated nor scrutinised. Shortly after her mother left, Mary took a pot of boiling water off the fire (see Figure 2.1) and

[99] NAI/1902/41 Inquest on the body of Edith Ferns, 10 March 1902.
[100] *Weekly Irish Times*, 15 March 1902.
[101] NAI/1901/53 Inquest on the body of Patrick Palmer, 23 February 1901, http://www.census.nationalarchives.ie/pages/1901/Dublin/Inns_Quay/Goldsmith_Street/1324536/ (accessed 8 February 2021).
[102] *Irish Daily Independent*, 25 February 1901.
[103] *Irish Daily Independent*, 25 February 1901; NAI/1901/52 Inquest on the body of Christopher McCullagh, 23 February 1901.

placed it on the floor where her younger sister had been playing. Ellen fell into the pot and was badly scalded. Mary ran immediately with the child to her neighbour, Mrs Celia Mould's room. Mrs Mould had the good sense to remove the clothes. It was at that moment her mother returned about 12 p.m. to 1 p.m. and she took the child straight to the Meath Hospital. Despite the best efforts of medical attendants, significant scalds about the back, abdomen, and thighs caused her death within twenty-four hours. The DMP report scripted by Peter Holohan, Station Sergeant at Chancery Lane, was careful to document the fact that this was a respectable poor family: 'James Reilly labourer father of the deceased was at work when accident happened.'[104]

Devices like marital status, occupational data, and children's ages were critical and, I contend, deliberately placed respectability indicators in the DMP reports. Their inclusion provided cues to the coroner as to the necessity for holding an inquest in the first instance and a professional opinion to the court as to whether or not there was suspicion of foul play. With scalds, the incident usually occurred in split seconds: Thomas Doyle 'died from shock the result of scalds accidentally received' when his mother Bridget Doyle momentarily turned her back on the saucepan of water she was boiling on the fireplace. She had gone to shut the door when her son aged 2 years and 6 months climbed up on a chair and pulled the handle, spilling the contents over his face and body. He was rushed to hospital but died within twenty-four hours.[105] The case of Patrick Power was slightly different—like others he was playing on floor when he hit a saucepan of potatoes his mother was lifting off the fire and was scalded about the neck and shoulders. While she sent for Dr Whelan of Synott Place and he came immediately to dress the wounds, she refused to follow his advice that the child be sent to the National Children's Hospital at Harcourt Street. When Dr Whelan visited the following day the child's temperature was 102.4. On the third day he was summoned again, but this time the child was dead. There was no suspicion of foul play.[106] Immediately preceding all scalding cases were the actions of a responsible adult—burns were different in that regard.

Domestic arrangements in the tenements afforded families very little privacy but in some cases this grassroots social surveillance was an important interlocutor to instruments of biopower. It was not only critical in terms of quick reaction times to accidents—it also forced violent or abusive people, in Foucauldian terms, to 'self govern' and behave themselves in a civil manner.[107] When Mrs Woodcock

---

[104] NAI/1901/111 Inquest on the body of Ellen Reilly, 15 April 1901; evidence dated 13–15 April 1901.

[105] NAI/1900/54 Inquest on the body of Thomas Doyle, 3 July 1900; DMP report is not appended.

[106] NAI/1900/180 Inquest on the body of Patrick Power, 30 November 1900.

[107] Michel Foucault, 'Technologies of the self', in L.H. Martin, H. Gutman, and P.H. Hutton (eds), *Technologies of the Self* (London, 1988), p. 18. Foucault identified self-government as a fundamental element of governmentality: 'technologies of the self, which permit individuals to effect by their own means or with the help of others a certain number of operations on their own bodies and souls,

went out for five minutes on 20 February 1901 to a nearby shop to purchase soap, she left her son aged 3 and her daughter, 9-month-old Isabella, at their abode at 16 Heytesbury Place. On her return, she found her infant daughter's clothing on fire. She immediately extinguished the flames and ran with her child to the Meath Hospital, but poor Isabella died two hours after admission. The jury found that she 'died from shock the result of burns accidentally received' and added the rider 'we consider the mother guilty of gross neglect'. What this verdict made little of, and what was reported in the newspapers (Figure 2.3), was that while she was out, her husband, a sorter at the General Post Office was working night shifts and was asleep in the next room. The DMP report intimated how he slept right through what must have been pandemonium and when the police returned with Mrs Woodcock to the house he finally got up 'and asked for his wife'. Sergeant Patrick Finn 76A punctuated his report with his observations of what he perceived as an air of menace; for instance, how an unnamed neighbouring woman was present but was 'afraid to come in'. Sergeant Finn noted how Mr Woodcock 'came out with me to the room where the accident occurred and then I called in his wife. He got into a terrible rage[;] she asked him to let her reason with him and explain'. It was at that point that Mr Woodcock levied allegations of past neglect against her to shift blame away from himself and place it firmly on to his wife. While no other witnesses corroborated it, Mr Woodcock's statement that 'the mother is in the habit of leaving the children alone while she remains for hours away drinking with other women in public houses and that he repeatedly asked her to bring the children with her', was entered into evidence. Sergeant Patrick Finn 76A documented the only words of comfort offered to his distraught wife as follows: 'now he says you have done it what will I do. You better go and I have a sleep and give

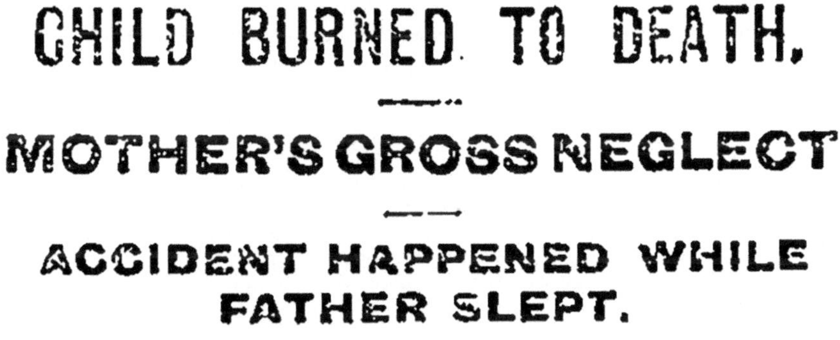

CHILD BURNED TO DEATH.

MOTHER'S GROSS NEGLECT

ACCIDENT HAPPENED WHILE FATHER SLEPT.

Figure 2.3 Sensationalised newspaper headline: burns and neglect
Source: Evening Herald, 20 February 1901.

thoughts, conduct, and way of being, so as to transform themselves in order to attain a certain state of happiness, purity, wisdom, perfection, or immortality.'

up your crying.'[108] If Sergeant Finn's inference of an unhappy home was too subtly put, then other coroner's inquests provide ample and overt evidence of domestic abuse and violence and will be discussed in greater detail in Chapter 4. The family had moved to 107 Church Street Upper in the six-week period between the accident and the census.[109]

Captain Purcell's annual reports to the Waterworks and Fire Brigade Committee, Dublin Corporation, usually conveyed the positive stories about the amount of insured property saved as a result of DFB operations, but in 1901 he had the grim task of reporting eight fire-related deaths.[110] All came before the coroner's court. There were two episodes of fires concerning multiple victims: three members of the Lynch family[111] died from burns when an oil lamp fell on their bed and four Doyle children perished because, despite gallant efforts in saving their mother, baby sibling, and other building occupants, the DFB officers could not reach them in time.[112] Prior to her death, Mary Lynch deposed that she had the oil lamp lit as she waited for her husband to return from work at 2 Willet Place, which was a two-roomed house according to the 1901 census.[113] Prompt actions by her father, Christopher McCabe, who also resided in the same house, served to save one of her sons. On his return to save his other grandson, reinforcements had arrived and the boy was gone, apparently rescued by another neighbour.[114] Mary Ellen Tully of 2 Moore's Cottages deposed that she saw a woman with a burned child in her arms at Willet Place between 11 p.m. and 12 p.m. Tully stated that 'I told her to bring it to the hospital, she said she would not. I then took the deceased from her and ran to Jervis Street Hospital with it and it was detained.'[115] The child was Mary Lynch, aged 2 years and 6 months. Constable Martin Touhy 64C was on the beat near Glorney's Buildings at about 11 p.m. and he responded immediately to Mary Lynch senior's calls for help. The DFB was on the scene immediately after that. Despite best efforts, Mary and her daughter Annie were burned extensively and succumbed to their injuries shortly thereafter, and young Mary Lynch died a day later.[116] The *Kerry News* reported that the accident was as a result of an exploding lamp.[117]

[108] NAI/1901/48 Inquest on the body of James Byrne, 20 February 1901.
[109] See http://www.census.nationalarchives.ie/reels/nai003686182/ (accessed 17 November 2021).
[110] *The Thirty Ninth Annual Report from the Chief of the Dublin Corporation Fire Brigade Department for the year ending 31st December, 1901* (Dublin, 1902), p. 5.
[111] NAI/1900/155/156/157 Inquest on the bodies of Mary, Annie, and Mary Lynch, 8 November 1900.
[112] NAI/1901/132/133/134/135 Inquest on the bodies of Sarah, Bartholomew, Joseph, and Peter Doyle, 13 May 1901.
[113] See http://www.census.nationalarchives.ie/reels/nai003760015/ (accessed 19 November 2020).
[114] *Irish Daily Independent*, 9 November 1900; *Evening Herald*, 8 November 1900.
[115] NAI/1900/155 Inquest on the body of Mary Lynch, 9 November 1900.
[116] See http://www.census.nationalarchives.ie/pages/1901/Dublin/Mountjoy/Willatt_Place/1327145/ (accessed 12 December 2021). Pat Lynch, widower, and his two sons Christy and Michal (*sic*) lived in the same house when the census was taken—they were classified as visitors; presumably they were living with Christopher McCabe.
[117] *Kerry News*, 13 November 1900.

Five months after the Lynch family tragedy, Peter, Sarah, Joseph, and Bartle (Bartholomew) Doyle, who ranged in age from 12 down to 6, were asleep when a fire broke out in the basement of 9 Green Street shortly after 4 a.m.[118] Mr and Mrs Joseph Doyle lay in a critical condition in the wards as the inquests on four of their five children proceeded in the morgue of Jervis Street Hospital. It was decided not to inform them of the deaths until 'they were in a stronger position to bear the shock'.[119] After hearing the evidence of a medical expert and several lay witnesses, the coroner's jury gave the verdict that the children were overcome by smoke and died of asphyxia.

According to the 1901 census conducted on the night of 31 March 1901, three families lived in the three-storey over basement building. Reflecting the fragmented nature of the Dublin rental market, Bridget Breen, a 62-year-old widow, was the contracted tenant, who sublet rooms to two other households.[120] Collar and harness maker, James Curran, his wife, and two children occupied the three rooms on the ground floor, one of which he had converted into a saddler's shop. Curran's apprentice, James Devine was also returned as a member of his household. Together with her adult daughter, son, and niece, Breen lived in the two rooms on the second floor, while seven members of the Doyle family occupied two rooms at the top of the house.[121]

DMP Constable Joseph Kelly 73D was on duty near the adjacent Green Street Station on the ill-fated night when he noticed smoke billowing from a broken window in the ground-floor shop. He immediately alerted his superiors and ran to assist. Kelly barged through the front door shouting 'fire' and that roused some of the occupants from their slumber; he then proceeded to carry the bed-bound invalid Bridget Breen out the front door and place her in the care of neighbours. An immediate response from the DFB at the nearby Bolton Street Station was critical to saving four of the top floor occupants by means of its 'fire escape' ladder.[122]

James Devine was asleep in the top back room, and when asked if he was smoking or had ignited a match he testified at the inquests that he went to bed about 10 p.m. and woke at 4 a.m. 'owing to smoke', which impeded his attempted escape through the front door. Despite the poor visibility and his semi-conscious state, Devine managed to find the Doyles' baby and hand it to fire officer Dunphy,

[118] NAI/1901/132–135 cases of Sarah, Bartholomew, Joseph, and Peter Doyle, respectively. I published this section on the Doyle family as a guest blog in July 2020. https://forgedbyfiresite.wordpress.com/2020/07/06/fire-hazards-and-housing-in-early-twentieth-century-dublin/ (accessed 12 December 2021). I am grateful to Dr Rebecca Wynter for the invitation and her feedback. Parts of the blog are reproduced here.
[119] *Evening Herald*, 13 May 1901.
[120] Ruth McManus, 'Dublin's lodger phenomenon in the early twentieth century', *Irish Economic and Social History*, 45:1 (2018), pp. 23–46.
[121] See http://www.census.nationalarchives.ie/pages/1901/Dublin/Inns_Quay/Green_Street/ (accessed 12 December 2021).
[122] *Freeman's Journal*, 13 May 1901.

who was on the fire escape affixed to the top window at the front of the building. Once Devine and the infant had been delivered to safety, Dunphy re-entered the building via the upper-floor window and sustained burns to his face and hands in his efforts to rescue the rest of the Doyle children. Such was the intensity of the smoke and the flames on the lower levels that the escape ladder caught fire. Reinforcement fire brigades from Chatham and Winetavern Streets had to take over from their Bolton Street colleagues to douse the flames and carry out the rest of the rescues. The latter brigades used a 'smoke helmet', which was an American invention that provided oxygen to the wearer. Both Mr and Mrs Doyle were unconscious throughout the rescue operation. Asphyxia from toxic smoke was not a common cause of death in domestic house fires, which usually yielded verdicts of 'shock following burns received'. Dublin Corporation was well aware of the problems and the fire hazards posed by mixed-use premises but with low-to-no surveillance of housing quality and weak enforcement of nuisance laws, saddler James Curran could conduct his business from his home, and store a half-ton of highly flammable and tightly packed straw in the basement. The straw acted as both cause and accelerant of what was deemed to have been a case of 'spontaneous combustion'. The burning straw combined with smouldering leather from the shop to emit a thick black smoke, which complicated an already challenging rescue environment. Arson was ruled out as the house, belonging to Mr Reid of 4 Dawson Street, was not insured and the personal effects and business property of all inhabitants was lost.[123]

Evoking the sense of a city on the pivot of modernity, accounts of this house fire provide sharp contrasts between the poor housing stock of the nineteenth century and the twentieth-century professionalisation of emergency responders. The technical effectiveness and swift cooperation of police and fire officers meant that eleven lives were saved. The Dublin City coroner's court relied heavily on the support of the DMP and the DFB for the smooth running of its service and it wasted no time in praising officers when appropriate. The coroner's jury added a rider to commend the bravery of the rescuers; it singled out Constable Kelly's 'plucky manner in which he entered the house and rescued Mrs Breen & roused the inhabitants' and also acknowledged the bravery of fire officers Dunphy and Gildea—all were recommended 'to the favourable consideration' of their employers. That year the DFB 'granted chevrons' to Inspector Guildey and firemen William Byrne, Thomas Dunphy, and Michael Fox. Their bravery was also recognised in monetary terms and they received an additional shilling per week in their salaries.[124]

---

[123] *Freeman's Journal*, 14 May 1901.
[124] *The Thirty Ninth Annual Report from the Chief of the Dublin Corporation Fire Brigade Department for the year ending 31st December, 1901* (Dublin, 1902), p. 5.

The adult burns cases differed in tenor from the child cases; the physical infirmity of some victims meant that the burns were far more severe. For example, Henry O'Grady, aged 70, was estranged from his family who were living at 18 Halston Street. When the shed he stabled his donkey, and lived in, caught fire at 1.25 a.m., he stood little chance of escape or rescue with his inflammable surrounds.[125] By the time police arrived at the scene at 15 May Lane the blaze was too advanced and the post-mortem described how his limbs were reduced to charcoal. The 'elderly' Henry O'Grady died on 30 April 1901— he was so badly burned that even the highly experienced assistant coroner, Dr John Burgess found it difficult to determine cause of death. His head and part of his neck were completely ravaged, and his limbs and trunk were charred. It prompted Dr Byrne to comment that he had never seen a body so extensively burned that it was beyond identification.[126] The case received very little newspaper attention which was more apt to report on the railway disaster in Tralee that claimed three lives.[127]

Within weeks of one another, two rag-pickers, Elizabeth Keating and Mary Walsh, both burned to death in their homes.[128] Fires occurring at night only came to prompt attention perchance—the former case happened at about 3 a.m. at Cole's Lane near Henry Street, and the latter was at 36 North Cumberland Street. Walsh's forename was unknown at that point, and she was deemed to be around 55 years of age. The jury added the rider 'And we consider that rags and inflammatory materials should not be allowed to be stored in rooms of dwelling houses as they are such a great danger to the inhabitants.'[129] Neighbours deposed that they had seen her about 8 p.m. and that she was drunk. She had a terrible death— owing to the delayed alarm her body was extensively charred and both legs were burned off.[130] Keating was a widow, and her case caused quite a stir only because the dramatic efforts of neighbours and the DFB involvement. A neighbour, Elizabeth Kennedy, first noticed the fire and sent her son to the fire escape at Nelson's Pillar. Brave actions of Peter Lynch who on hearing 'the alarm of fire' between 2 a.m. and 3 a.m. on 12 October selflessly ran up the stairs, broke down her door, and found her unconscious on the floor. He was in the process of carrying her out when he met the DFB and DMP officers. The fire was contained to one room; the DFB was prompt in its arrival and in extinguishing the flames. In both cases it was the heaps of rags and pickings that acted as an obstacle to escape and as fuel to the fire. Captain Purcell gave evidence at the Walsh inquest to the effect that such occupational hazards should not be permitted to accumulate in tenements.[131]

---

[125] NAI/1901/123 Inquest on the body of Henry O'Grady, 30 April 1901.
[126] *Freeman's Journal,* 1 May 1901.
[127] *Kerry Sentinel,* 8 May 1901; *Irish Examiner,* 6 May 1901.
[128] NAI/1900/136 Inquest on the body of Elizabeth Keating, 12 October 1900; *Skibbereen Eagle,* 20 October 1900; *Mayo News,* 13 October 1900.
[129] NAI/1900/151 Inquest on the body of Mary Walsh, 2 November 1900.
[130] *Irish Times,* 3 November 1900.   [131] *Irish Times,* 3 November 1900.

The jury added a rider in support of Purcell's recommendation. Dramatic rescue attempts nearly always received newspaper attention, even if the details were relatively mundane, if tragic, like the case of Mary Collins who was drying a mattress by the fire at 35 Jervis Street, when it ignited. She died from the effects of smoke inhalation. The DFB came quickly to the scene. Her son John identified her body and confirmed that she was 57 years of age.[132]

Anne Allen's death had some unusual features and some heroic actions, so it raised some attention from the newspapers. She was at her home at 22 Lower Mount Pleasant and her neighbours upstairs noticed smoke coming through the floorboards. Allen, aged 75, died from 'Shock the result of burns accidentally received' after her clothing caught fire. The jury praised 'the conduct of Sergt Rouse commendable in getting a priest and a doctor for the deceased'.[133] It is difficult to ascertain patterns in newspaper reporting terms apart from slow news days necessitating additional content. Bodies of lesser consequence in terms of newspaper interest included older people and prostitutes: for example, Sarah Nolan did not register any interest from the newspapers, details of her age were not given in the coroner's inquiry and neither was her occupation.[134] James Healy, aged 66, was under the influence of drink on the night it was suspected that either his pipe reignited in his shirt pocket or in an attempt to light a candle his shirt which 'was burned off him' caught fire. His neighbours found him drunk in the hallway of 71 Great Britain Street and had to carry him upstairs to his room.[135] Not all cases of burns came to full inquiry. A week prior to Healy's death another older man, Denis Doyle, aged 60, suffered significant burns at his home at 17 Mary's Lane—he was treated at Jervis Street Hospital but refused to remain. On 31 October, he was admitted to the NDU hospital where he remained until he died on 7 November 1900. Dr Byrne did not consider that the case merited an inquest, but it was reported in the newspaper on what was probably a slow news day.[136] Bessie Lambe was identified as a prostitute in her inquiry. She was heating cold meat on the evening of 30 March 1902 following a drinking session with Catherine Rourke when her dress got caught in the cooking apparatus and the contents spilled on top of her. Rourke later told Sergeant Devoy 10C that she informed Bridget Cullen who also lived at 57 Montgomery Street and they both brought her by cab to Jervis Street Hospital about 10 a.m. the following day. She died at 4 a.m. on 7 April. She had been under treatment for a number of years by Dr Oulton at the Summerhill Dispensary for chest and lung disease. Her cause of

---

[132] NAI/1901/302 Inquest, dated 6 December 1901; *Evening Herald*, 6 December 1901 (23 Jervis in newspaper).
[133] NAI/1901/256 Inquest on the body of Anne Allen, 7 October 1901; *Evening Herald*, 7 October 1901.
[134] NAI/1900/36 Inquest on the body of Sarah Nolan, 4 June 1900.
[135] NAI/1900/169 Inquest on the body of James Healy, 15 November 1900.
[136] *Evening Herald*, 9 November 1900.

death was registered as being from burns but it was in fact from scalds. Another aspect of newsworthiness was the competition factor—Lambe's was one of three inquests held on 8 April 1902,[137] none of which received attention from newspapers. The day before, two cases, that of a fatal cycling accident and a case of severe child neglect captured the headlines, and the day after Lambe died of her injuries her story coincided with an awful family tragedy caused by carbon monoxide poisoning, which was an important matter of public interest.[138] Parts of Ellen Lee's body were completely charred by the time her neighbour John Bowden responded to the cries of her 2-year-old grandson who was shaking the door in an attempt to get out. Hers was the only case that may have been as a result of smoking tobacco. She was 80 years old and was supported by her daughter Mrs McDonnell who was a cook at Mr Kennedy, Solicitor, Blackrock. The DMP report noted that she 'may have been lighting her pipe' when her clothes ignited.[139]

Some fire and asphyxia cases occurred as a result of defective equipment. Reflecting the extent of the problem across the four nations, a select committee was appointed in 1896 to consider the state of the petroleum industry and the use, sale, and storage of inflammable liquids. It deliberated the quality and variance in safety standards between mineral oils of high and low 'flashing' points.[140] Vicky Holmes argues that the phenomenon of exploding lamps was sensationalised by the British press to combat the flooding of the market with cheaper and 'inferior' American lamps.[141] There is nothing to suggest similar vested interests in Ireland—in cases where explosions are mentioned there was evidence. An oil lamp explosion was the root of Patrick Levy's death at his home at 24 Shepard Avenue on 11 October 1900. When his wife retired to bed she left Levy, a coachbuilder, reading in the kitchen—after about twenty minutes she heard the explosion.[142] Ordinary users were probably unaware of the dangers posed by inconsistencies in oil quality and the necessity for extra vigilance. The dangers associated with using paraffin oil were not clear to Mary Barret, a 21-year-old prostitute who threw it on a fire at her home at 28 Lower Tyrone Street and her clothes were set alight. William Harrison came to her aid and brought her to Jervis Street Hospital, where she later died.[143] Similarly, Margaret Maguire's clothing caught fire at her home at 119 Saint Stephen's Green when she was lighting a paraffin lamp. Her sister in law Miss McGuire/Maguire called for help and a Mr Parkes ran

---

[137] NAI/1902/62 Inquest on the body of Bessie Lambe, 8 April 1902; *Evening Herald*, 8 April 1902.
[138] 'Fatal accident to a cyclist', *Irish Times*, 8 April 1902; 'Alleged neglect of a child', *Irish Times*, 8 April 1902.
[139] NAI/1901/292 Inquest on the body of Ellen Lee, 18 November 1901.
[140] Report from the Select Committee on petroleum; together with the proceedings of the committee, minutes of evidence, appendix, and index, 1896 [xii.i].
[141] Vicky Holmes, 'Penny death traps: the press, the poor, parliament, and the "perilous" penny paraffin lamp', *Victorian Review*, 40:2 (2014), pp. 125–42.
[142] NAI/1900/135 Inquest on the body of Patrick Levy, 11 October 1900; *Irish Times*, 12 October 1900.
[143] NAI/1901/81 Inquest on the body of Mary Barrett, 21 May 1901.

in to help—he put his coat and a rug around her and had her conveyed by cab to Mercer's Hospital. The jury found that she died from 'Collapse caused by septic absorption the result of burns of back abdomen and arms. And we wish to put on record our estimation of the very manly and humane conduct of Mr Benjamin Parkes'.[144] Single father John Reilly fell asleep with an oil lamp lit and when his 13-month-old daughter Josephine pulled the cloth from underneath the lamp it fell into her cradle. Children were fascinated by fire and flames, and in that instance, the jury added how it 'attach[ed] no blame to the child's father'.[145]

Carbon monoxide poisoning was another lesser known chemical threat. There were two separate instances of carbon monoxide poisoning and four resulting deaths: James Clarke died because of defective mains piping under his house at 9 Eccles Street—he was found by his daughter naked and acting in a very strange manner. She called the local priest, Fr Byrne. In fact, the entire household was in a stupor, but the others were saved because of prompt action by neighbours.[146] The gas company had legal representation at the inquest and the depth of the mains was discussed. In that instance the jury recommended that such pipes should not be laid so close to the surface—there was no recommendation to compensate relatives of the deceased.[147]

A few months later, Augustine O'Neill, a fitter at the Railway Works, Inchicore, his wife Margaret, and their child Joseph, aged 5, died at 115 Rialto Cottages, which was part of a development built by the DADC and included the latest in modern conveniences (Figure 2.4). All succumbed to the noxious fumes when the sluice pipe was disconnected from the gas meter in the house.[148] Legal counsel for the gas company, Gerald Byrne, alleged that the deceased had tampered with the meter but Dr Byrne did not permit the besmirching of his character to proceed. Professor of Public Health, Dr Anthony Roche wrote to the *Freeman's Journal* and the *Irish Daily Independent* to raise awareness about the nefarious actions of the Alliance Gas Company, which was more concerned with profit than safety. He pointed to the potency of the particular type of gas supplied (containing water gas), which he argued, had an 8 per cent higher content of carbon monoxide than 'coal gas'. He cited the ten-fold increase in carbon monoxide poisoning deaths in New York, Brooklyn, and Baltimore because of this type of mixture.[149] Dublin's embrace of modernity did not extend to public safety campaigns, and the risks associated with new conveniences like piped gas supply were poorly understood.

---

[144] NAI/1901/222 Inquest on the body of Margaret Maguire, 27 August 1901.
[145] NAI/1901/62 Inquest on the body of Josephine Reilly, 26 February 1901.
[146] NAI/1901/293 Inquest on the body of Ellen Lee, 18 November 1901.
[147] *Freeman's Journal*, 19 November 1901.
[148] NAI/1902/65–67 Inquest on the bodies of Augustine, Margaret, and Joseph O'Neill, 9 April 1902; *Evening Herald*, 9 April 1902.
[149] *Freeman's Journal*, 10 April 1902; *Irish Daily Independent*, 10 April 1902; professor at the Catholic Medical School: *Belfast Newsletter*, 10 April 1902.

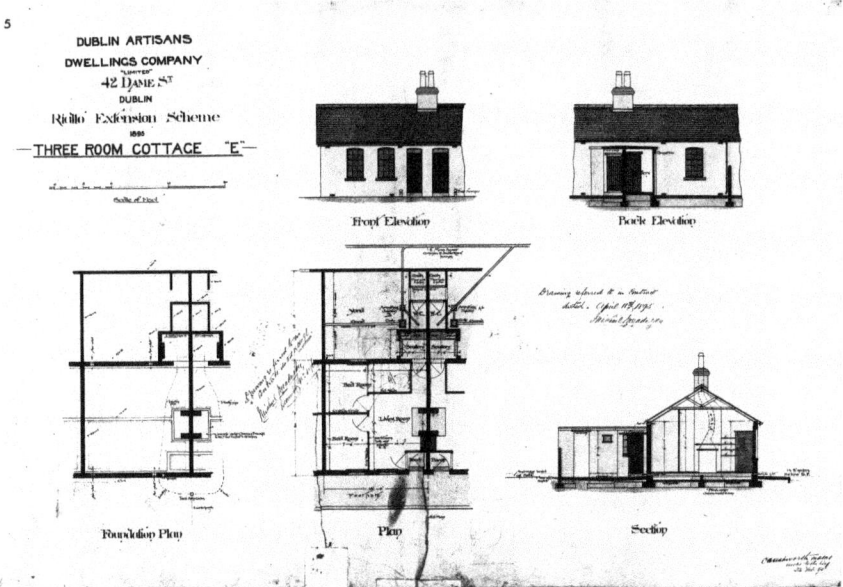

Figure 2.4 Architectural drawing of Rialto Cottages

Note: I am very grateful to Colum O'Riordan at the Irish Architectural Archive for this image.

Source: Irish Architectural Archive, 79/26.12/77R6. Type E cottage, E Cottage, Rialto Scheme Extension, 1895.

Treatments

A striking element of all these burns and scalding cases is the high levels of ver-nacular knowledge of what to do in these emergency situations where immediate actions of ordinary people could make extraordinary differences. Dampening flames with clothing was quickly followed by the removal of the victim's clothing which was a major factor in reducing the risk of further skin and tissue damage. There are no mentions of quenching flaming clothes or using cold water therapy to calm angry skin reactions in either burns or scalding episodes. Instead, bicar-bonate of soda, oil, and petroleum jelly were applied in a few cases. Dermatology was not an established medical specialty in 1900 but even in poor communities where fear of medico-legal dictates were heightened there was a clear understand-ing that burns and scalds necessitated immediate professional medical interven-tion. Clinical care of wound management primarily involved infection control through clean environments, careful dressings and observation.[150] According to Naylor et al.'s English translations of Fabry's 1607 treatise *De combustionibus*, the first book to delineate the classification system of burns into first, second, and

---

[150] Ian MacDonald, 'Picric acid in superficial burns', *The British Medical Journal*, 1:2002 (13 May 1899), p. 1152.

third degrees, was in circulation as early as 1643.[151] By 1900, a few treatments were in use. For the treatment of superficial burns and scalds Dr R. Chalders Miller advised the use of pleric acid in a letter to the *British Medical Journal* in 1897. He also advised keeping the wounded skin wet with Hazeline (a cream made from hazel extract) and its cheaper non-proprietory version (hamamelidis liquid distillatum) and not to remove any 'adherent portions of clothing' until such a time that the skin underneath had healed, for which he encouraged the use of zinc ointment.[152]

In America, cognate treatments had been in use for decades—Dr G.F. Waters of Boston Massachusetts provided cursory dermatological advice of wetting dry matter and drying wetter wounds—he recommended ointment and bicarbonate of soda, or potash if the former was not to hand.[153] In a comparative analysis of soda treatment versus carron-oil, Dr J. Johnston of Bolton described how in the case of an 18-month-old boy whose neck, chest, and abdomen were scalded by a cup of tea, and that of a 5-year-old boy who had scalded his lower arm to his elbow with water from a kettle, that the efficacy of the soda treatment was more apparent than the case of an 8-year-old boy who was treated for 'severe scald' using carron oil after he put his foot into a boiler. He concluded that the soda and camphorated water treatment was cheaper, better, reduced pain, and was far less of a mess than the oil. In the case of the infant he found him 'screaming in agony, and swathed in rags soaked in a sticky slimy compound of treacle, flour, etc'.[154] Because of its ability to 'exclude atmospheric air' and purported astringent properties, the use of treacle for burns and scalds had been popular among physicians in earlier decades of the nineteenth century and is probably how it came into common household usage.[155] It was discredited as a remedy when products like Hazeline became available. In 1936–7, when the Irish Folklore Commission collated the Schools' Collection, it found that a mixture of these cures were still in circulation in Dublin: James Corrigan collected the following cure from his 'Granny' Mrs A. Corrigan who lived in Mill Street, Ballbriggan: for burns and scalds she advised to 'dissolve a little bread-soda and hot water in a cup, soak a bandage in it and put it on the injured part, olive oil may also be used'.[156] Another variation was provided by Peter Gill, North Commons, Lusk to P. Brogan: 'Equal

---

[151] I.L. Naylor, B. Curtis, and J.J.R. Kirkpatrick, 'Treatment of bum scars and contractures in the early seventeenth century: Wilhelm Fabry's approach', *Medical History*, 40 (1966), 472–86 at 472.

[152] R. Shalders Miller, 'Treatment of superficial burns and scalds', *The British Medical Journal*, 2:1868 (17 October 1896), p. 1168.

[153] Anon., 'Burns and scalds', *Scientific American*, 38:25 (22 June 1878), p. 387.

[154] J. Johnston, 'Soda treatment of burns and scalds', *British Medical Journal*, 2:922 (31 August 1878), p. 313.

[155] A. Markwick, 'Treacle, a remedy for burns and scalds', *Provincial Medical & Surgical Journal (1844–1852)*, 11:26 (29 December 1847), p. 710.

[156] *The Schools' Collection*, Volume 0783, p. 309: https://www.duchas.ie/en/cbes/4498200/4383310/4507389 (accessed 25 November 2020).

parts of fresh lime water and linseed oil make an excellent cure for scalds or burns. It is called Carron oil.'[157]

Child Neglect in the Home

Section 12.1 of the 1908 Children Act permitted sanctions to be brought against those who did not seek medical assistance for sick children. Even if there was a moral expectation that parents and guardians would at least try to ensure children were kept out of harm's way until 1908, they were not compelled under the infant life protection or the offences against the person acts to attend to medical needs.[158] There were few public health visits for preventive purposes at the beginning of the twentieth century and children were at high risk behind closed doors. Neglect was often inadvertent and some mothers, and indeed their doctors, were reconciled to the idea that certain children were 'delicate from birth' and would never thrive, and thus their health was permitted to decline. Elsewhere I describe cases of children and youths whose deaths were described as 'rather sudden' yet their post-mortem examinations showed extensive evidence of deep-seated and old-standing pulmonary tuberculosis.[159] In these cases the mothers had not come to the attention of the authorities even though they had been neglectful of their children's health care needs. William Kenny's death at six weeks was deemed to have been as a result of 'asthenia', a vague term used to describe general weakness and failure to thrive and his mother made no effort to seek medical aid. She was recorded as being ignorant of its cause and the jury attached no blame to her. What worked in her favour was that she was married, and she had made efforts to safeguard her pregnancy. The child was born at 24 Great Clarence Street under the supervision of Nurse D'arcy from Holles Street Hospital and was not insured. It only came to the attention of the police because Dr Taylor at Sir Patrick Dun's Hospital thought the child was so emaciated as to constitute deliberate neglect.[160] It was not reported in the newspapers but it is worth pointing out that two women were gruesomely murdered in December 1900 and run-of-the-mill infant deaths paled into insignificance as a result.[161] Although the DMP report was clear in its assertion that there was 'no suspicion of foul play', 4-week-old Michael Francis

---

[157] *The Schools' Collection*, Volume 0786, p. 181: https://www.duchas.ie/en/cbes/4498381/4384161 (accessed 25 November 2020).

[158] An Act for the Prevention of Cruelty to, and better Protection of, Children, 1889, c. 44.

[159] Breathnach, 'Respiratory disease and death registration, Dublin 1900–1902'; NAI/1900/25 Inquest on the body of Hugh Malone, 28 May 1900; NAI/1900/138 Inquest on the body of Thomas Storey, 15 October 1900.

[160] NAI/1900/184 Inquest on the body of William Kenny, 5 December 1900. See https://civilrecords. irishgenealogy.ie/churchrecords/images/deaths_returns/deaths_1900/05746/4622699.pdf (accessed 27 January 2020).

[161] NAI/1900/184 Inquest on the body of William Kenny, 5 December 1900.

Cruise's case proceeded to inquest.[162] Parents Jane and Michael, a hall porter, lived at the DADC Crampton Buildings and had four other children—they took immediate actions to fetch a doctor when they noticed at 5.15 a.m. that the infant 'looked somewhat convulsed.'[163] Jane and Micheal Cruise were good, decent and respectable people but low-income families always came under scrutiny.

Sick children were even more vulnerable when their parents separated and the following three cases have definite links to the economic ramifications of trying to split limited resources between two households. While he died 'outside' and is not included as a domestic death, it is worth considering the case of Joseph Wall here. He had been subject to fits and his delicate health could not have been helped by his parent's 'Irish-style divorce' arrangements. Along with his mother and his 9-year-old sister Margaret, he stayed at the night asylum in Bow Street and they got food daily in the Mendicity Institute, Victoria Quay. On the day he died he had 'stirabout & new milk for breakfast and bacon & cabbage for dinner in the mendicity' but he had not received any medical care for the full year prior to his death. His mother was adept at negotiating the instruments of charity and must have known that the child was entitled to receive free medical care, but it seems she avoided the 'Union'. As I have argued elsewhere, engagement with the Poor Law embodied risks of losing child custody with increasing powers of guardianship granted to local authorities in successive legislation from 1862.[164] This might offer an explanation for her and other poor parents' decisions. Instead she opted for 'a powder in the chemist shop of Mr Murphy 48 Nth King Street'—it was only when he had a severe attack that she brought him to hospital. She stated in evidence that her husband had a job at Kennan's engineering works at Fishamble Street and lodged in Church Street.[165] Mr Wall was tracked down for the purposes of the inquest and he stated that he had given her 7s. on 8 September.[166] At the time that Joseph Wall's inquest occurred the newspapers were consumed with the highly unusual case of Bridget Gannon, whose body was exhumed for a second inquest at the county coroner's court as it appeared she had drowned in mysterious circumstances involving a serving policeman, and his case was not covered.[167]

Teresa Smith's parents were separated for the four months prior to her death and she lived at 54 Francis Street with her mother and grandmother. Tubercular disease had wasted the 26-month-old child to 11.5 lbs, and although visibly

---

[162] NAI/1900/109 Inquest on the body of Michael Francis Cruise, 8 September 1900.

[163] See http://www.census.nationalarchives.ie/reels/nai003723112/ (accessed 31 October 2021).

[164] Ciara Breathnach, 'Infant life protection and medico-legal literacy in early twentieth-century Dublin', *Women's History Review* 26:6 (2017), pp. 781–98; Guardianship of Infants Act 1886 (49 & 50 Vic.) c. 27, 28; Pauper Children (Ireland) Act, 1876, (39 & 40 Vic.) c. 8. s. 2; Orphan and Deserted Children (Ireland) Act, 1869 (32 & 33 Vic.) c. 25, s. 2.

[165] *Thom's Irish Almanac & Official Directory*, 1884, p. 1397.

[166] NAI/1900/112 Inquest on the body of Joseph Wall, 10 September 1900.

[167] *Irish Daily Independent*, 11 September 1900.

unwell she was not attended to by a doctor. Even the child's face bore the stigmata of neglect: she had two large ulcerous sores on her face and another on the back of her head—they were all so deep-seated that they must have been there a good while. Dr Byrne cautioned the mother not to say anything that might be later used against her in a criminal court.[168] The court was sympathetic and added the rider 'we consider the mother is not guilty of neglect'—it is no coincidence that her mother was sober.[169] By contrast, when Christina Reel died from bronchopneumonia, the jury added a rider to 'severely censure' her mother (also Christina), who was described in the newspapers as 'drunken', for not bringing the child to the 'Union' when she deposited another of her children there on 10 September 1901.[170] Instead, the following day, Eliza Cleary of 33 Beresford Street brought the sick child to the NDU on her behalf, and she died there three days later. Christina Reel senior used the NDU on a regular basis to manage her way out of cyclical addiction, homelessness, and poverty.[171]

Drunken behaviour, or allegations to that effect, sent inquiries along different lines, and evidence gathered in the coroner's court was used verbatim in the judicial proceedings that followed. Edward Caffrey, news vendor of 10 Golden Lane, reported that at 7 a.m. on the morning of 27 December his wife found their infant daughter dead in the bed. Perhaps in a fit of grief, Edward Caffrey directed his anger at his wife. In the short statement that was to identify the cause he indicated that the child had 'the whooping cough since it was a fortnight old' and he proceeded to then blame his wife.[172] He recounted how he had been drinking the day before and went to bed at about 10 p.m. with his children Kate, 5 years old, and James, aged 1 year and 8 months. In his retelling of the series of events leading up to the tragedy he claimed that he saw his wife at about 1 p.m. drunk and how she had been drinking for a few days. She denied being drunk, and her husband claimed he did not hear her going to bed on Saint Stephen's night. All slept in the same room and bed—the deceased 6-week-old infant was placed outside its mother.[173] For practical reasons, associated with night feeding, mothers slept on the outside—it also protected small children from being overlain by fathers or

---

[168] NAI/1901/294 Inquest on the body of Teresa Smyth, 22 November 1901; *Irish Daily Independent*, 23 November 1901.

[169] NAI/1901/294 reports, dated 22 November 1901.

[170] *Evening Herald*, 17 September 1901: headline: 'Dying child – drunken mother'; NAI/1901/247 Inquest on the body of Christina Reel, 17 September 1901.

[171] She was of no fixed abode when she entered on 6 September (NAI, BG 78/G 76, nos. 3317–3310) and from 1 to 30 October 1898 (NAI, BG 78/G 76, nos. 4302–4) with her daughters Mary Anne, aged 5, and Juliana, 14 months.

[172] NAI/1900/205 Inquest on the body of Ellen Caffrey, 28 December 1900—Samuel Ryder was the foreman.

[173] Vicky Holmes, *In Bed with the Victorians: The Life-Cycle of Working-Class Marriage*, pp. 43–4, notes that the purpose of the positioning of infants on the outside was likely to ensure the male breadwinner had quality sleep.

suffocating in between adults.[174] Mary Caffrey said that the child had whooping cough for a month but had not been seen by a doctor. Parents with meagre means often took calculated risks—Mrs Caffrey stated that 'When the kink would come on she would be seized with convulsions' but perhaps based on prior experience it caused her no worries. Assistant coroner Dr John Burgess conducted the post-mortem and found evidence of congestion in the lungs commensurate with what a mother of three would have recognised as whooping cough. But the imputation of licentiousness coupled with a life insurance policy cast Mary Caffrey into the neglectful category in the eyes of the jury. Infant Ellen weighed a mere 5.5 lbs according to Dr John Burgess's post-mortem report. Her husband stated that she was drinking the night that the child died. Byrne questioned her: 'Is it a fact that you were drunk that night, as your husband has made the charge against you at the police station?' When she responded in the affirmative, Byrne replied 'You ought to be ashamed of yourself.'[175] Other than Caffrey's naming and shaming in the evening newspaper (Figure 2.5), no further charges were made against her.

That afternoon another case of infant death arising from emaciation came before Byrne's court, but the mother had at least visited the doctor. The same jury was used in the case of 9-week-old Mary Anne Everard who weighed 7.5 lbs. This could also have been viewed as a case of neglect but the jury accepted the

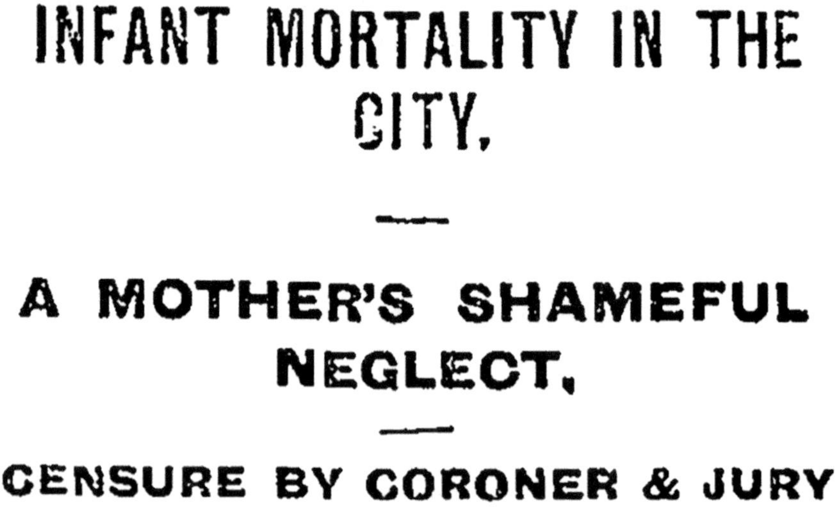

INFANT MORTALITY IN THE CITY,

—

A MOTHER'S SHAMEFUL NEGLECT,

—

CENSURE BY CORONER & JURY

Figure 2.5 Sensational newspaper headline: mother's censure
Source: *Evening Herald*, 28 December 1900.

[174] Overlaying is what Forbes explains as a 'suffocation of an infant by an older person lying on it': T.R. Forbes, *Surgeons at the Bailey: English Forensic Medicine to 1878* (London: Yale University Press, 1985), p. 114.
[175] *Evening Herald*, 28 December 1900.

convincing medical evidence of the child's failure to thrive since birth coupled with the presence of bronchopneumonia.[176] That her mother had sought medical attention is a moot point because she could not afford the 1s. 6d. for the treatment prescribed by Dr McWalter at the Leonard's Medical Hall on 15 December. Instead, she purchased 2d. worth of squills, which she administered until its death on 25 December.[177] A more comparable set of circumstances might be the case of Peter Gibbons who was 2 months old when he died of convulsions in February 1901 owing to acute disease of the lungs—his mother Teresa had not sought medical attention until the morning of his death. She sent for her husband who arranged for a 'red' relief ticket at the Castle Street Dispensary; by the time Dr Porter Newell arrived the child was deceased. Like the Caffrey case the child was insured for 1d. a week at the Scottish Legal Assurance Society but in the absence of a reference to alcohol there was no imputation of neglect.[178]

When mothers came to the attention of the police, their children came under scrutiny too. The involvement of the NSPCC was not necessarily a positive thing for children either, since it mainly targeted the conduct of mothers. If cases led to prosecutions and prison sentences, they ironically deprived children of their primary caregivers, as happened in the case of Bridget Connor, who was 1 year and 10 months old when she died of pulmonary and mesentery tuberculosis in October 1900. When her father Thomas reported her mother Mary to the NSPCC for 'intemperate and dirty habits', Bridget subsequently spent from 11 June to 29 August 1900 at the Dublin Auxiliary Union in Cabra while her mother served three months at Mountjoy prison for child cruelty.[179] After her release from Mountjoy, Mary Connor retrieved her child from the NDU. It seems that she, like Christina Reel, periodically used the NDU throughout 1899 to subsidise her family's meagre income.[180] On 25 October 1900, she entered again, with Bridget, and they gave their address as 53 Mabbot Street.[181] The Resident Medical Officer at NDU, Dr Bernard Burke Kennedy, testified that at that point the child 'appeared in a very dirty and wasted condition had sores on the head and was swathed around the body with wadding and oil'. But her decline and death in late October was a matter of weeks after she left institutional care—it is unclear if she was living with her entire family in the interim. Her post-mortem examination found 'her weight to be eleven and a quarter pounds, absence of fatty tissue throughout

[176] NAI/1900/206 Inquest on the body of Mary Anne Everard, 28 December 1900; *Evening Herald*, 28 December 1900.

[177] NAI/1900/206 Inquest on the body of Mary Anne Everard, 28 December 1900.

[178] NAI/1901/61 Inquest on the body of Peter Gibbons, 27 February 1901.

[179] NDU, admission and discharge records, NAI, BG 78/G 81 no. 2862, her father was listed as living at 53 Mabbott Street, she entered 11 June 1900 and was released to her mother 29 August 1900.

[180] For example, in 1899 Mary Connor and her two youngest daughters (Catherine and Bridget) spent the night of 26 May 1899 in the NDU—their address was 28 Marlboro Street and her husband was described as a coal labourer: NAI, BG 78/G 78, nos. 3847–9.

[181] NAI, BG 78/G 82 nos. 2750–1. Bridget died 26 October, her mother stayed until 29 October.

the body the lungs and mesentery tuberculosis and abscess of the left lung. In my opinion she died of acute tuberculosis.' No blame was attached to anyone, but the child had spent a considerable amount of time at Cabra. It is highly likely that it was there she contracted the disease and was definitely where her health deteriorated from it. In the same week that Bridget Connor died, the NDU was under scrutiny for its high infant mortality rates following allegations made by two Protestant clergymen, Rev. Canon Scott of Mountjoy Square and Rev. J.O. Gage Doherty.[182] With undoubted sectarian undertones, the newspapers reported that the Children's Department was run by the Sisters of Charity and, as if to refute the implied allegations of incompetency against 'nursing nuns', it also reported that there were two competent and trained lay sisters. In the inquest it was stated that Mary Connor had two other children who were aged 5 and 10 and were described as being 'clean and healthy and living with Father, a labourer, Thomas Connor 53 Mabbot St'.[183] Mary Ellen Connor, aged 11, and her sister Kate, aged 3, entered the NDU on 27 October 1900 and remained under Poor Law guardian care, it seems, until 2 May 1907.[184]

Cycles of addiction, scrapes with the law, imprisonment and general disadvantage characterised the lives of several mothers, who were directly implicated in the deaths of their children and/or swiftly blamed by their husbands for alleged neglect. For example, Thomas Conroy of 57 Montgomery Street accused his wife of overlaying their daughter, 6-month-old Mary. He woke between 3 a.m. and 4 a.m. to find his infant lifeless beside his wife Kate and rushed her to Jervis Street Hospital. The police report documented his swift rush to judge and blame his wife, whom he claimed was addicted to drink. In fact, both of them had a poor track record of parenthood. Childcare to his mind was women's work and he noted, without a hint of irony or duty, that while he was on his way to Connell's pub at 22 Mabbot Street the previous evening at 6.15 p.m., he saw his wife at the corner of Purdon and Mabbot Streets (Monto) under the influence of drink with the deceased infant in her arms. Thomas Conway proceeded to Connell's pub regardless—he claimed he had only one pint but he was there for over two hours. Prostitutes Polly Walsh and Lillie Cassidy who lived at 57 Montogomery said that both parents were drinking at 11.45 p.m.—all of the reported times contradicted.[185] His allegations of overlaying were not borne out in the post-mortem examination. The jury returned an open verdict following the evidence presented by Dr Edmund Glenny, who found bread in the child's airways and considered that

[182] *Freeman's Journal*, 26 October 1900; *Irish Daily Independent*, 27 October 1900; *Evening Herald*, 25 October 1900.

[183] NAI/1900/145, report dated 27 October 1900; *Freeman's Journal*, 29 October 1900.

[184] South Dublin Poor Law Union, workhouse admission and discharge records, NAI, BG 78/G 82, no. 2808; NAI, BG 78/G 80, no. 801; NAI, BG 78/G 84, no. 3560.

[185] NAI/1902/35 Inquest on the body of Mary Conroy, 3 March 1902. Walsh and Cassidy are returned as domestic servants in the 1901 census: http://www.census.nationalarchives.ie/reels/nai003684151/ (accessed 6 February 2021).

the child was too young for such solids. The *Freeman's Journal* reported it under the headline of 'An Error in Dietary' which was something Dr Glenny stated was a common problem and 'was a source of great trouble'.[186] By then, Kate Conroy was, and subsequently became, well known to the NSPCC. On 26 May 1900, her son Matthew died at 7 weeks from 'probably convulsions' with no medical attendant at 70 Montgomery Street—it was not investigated as a suspicious death.[187] Shortly after that she served six months for neglecting her children, aged 11 and 7, according to the *Freeman's Journal*. In January 1901, she was described in the Northern Police Court as a 'helpless drunkard' who had pawned clothes to buy drink while her husband was serving a month's jail sentence for a child neglect charge, and she was twice convicted for drunkenness in the month he was away.[188] Records pertaining to this family are inconsistent—although criminal records and newspaper accounts place them living on Montgomery Street before and after the 1901 census, there are no returns for them living there, or elsewhere in Dublin for that matter. They were truly on the margins of society, living hand to mouth, and the cycle of deprivation continued. In 1904, Kate Conroy was arrested and brought before Mr Mahony at the Northern Police Court for drunkenness and cruel ill-treatment of her then 9-month-old infant Christopher. At that stage, NSPCC Inspector McCloy stated that he knew her for the past five years. Abandoned and poor, she was living in an unfurnished room at 2 Ralph Place where she slept on the floor with her infant—it is unclear where her older children were at that stage. The court had issued a warrant for Thomas Conroy's arrest, presumably for desertion.[189]

Alcohol abuse precipitated the death of Delia Kelly who was 15 months old when she fell into a bucket of water. The child's mother, Jane Kelly, had been drinking with her own mother, Elizabeth Coughlan, and Mary Harrison from 1 p.m. at Hayes's public house in the company of other women, who were described as fish dealers. Harrison deposed that at about 5 p.m. Coughlan became 'the worse of liquor' and she helped Kelly to bring her home. It is unclear who was minding the infant or indeed her siblings, Mary, aged 7, Thomas, aged 5, and Elizabeth, aged 3 all this while, but Harrison advised taking the infant Delia with her as they went back to Hayes's public house.[190] At about 7 p.m. or 8 p.m., 11-year-old Patrick McDonagh saw Mrs Kelly vomiting and dropping the child outside the pub—he brought the child back to its home at 20 Charles Street and placed it in a bed with

---

[186] *Freeman's Journal*, 4 March 1902. Glenny, misspelt Glenney in the records, graduated in 1901, *The Medical Directory, 1905*, p. 1420.

[187] See https://civilrecords.irishgenealogy.ie/churchrecords/images/deaths_returns/deaths_1900/05762/4627926.pdf (accessed 6 February 2021).

[188] *Freeman's Journal*, 16 January 1901. Thomas Conroy was convicted of assault and ill treatment of his children on 22 June 1900, then resident at 70 Montgomery Street: Mountjoy Prison General Register Male 1899–1901, 1/43/1 number 4.

[189] *Dublin Daily Express*, 2 November 1904.

[190] See http://www.census.nationalarchives.ie/reels/nai003687108/ (accessed 31 January 2021).

Thomas Coughlan, who was described as 'an imbecile' in the inquest records and as being 'unable to give rational answers' in the DMP report. At 8 p.m. Kelly came out of Hayes's public house and spotted her daughter Mary with another child named Margaret Brodie. She instructed her daughter to go home and look after the infant. When they got there they found the child with its head submerged in a bucket of water, and a neighbouring woman came to their assistance.[191] The verdict and rider spared the mother further sanction: 'Died from being immersed in a bucket of water in the house 20 Charles St, and we have no evidence to show how she came there.'[192] Byrne had very little patience for negligent mothers and encouraged the jury to add a rider of gross neglect on the part of the mother, but it declined the opportunity.[193] Unlike the fate of the dispersed Conroy family, the Kelly family remained intact and Jane reported in 1911 that seven of her eight children were still living.[194]

Unmarried motherhood and concealment of pregnancy were typical attributes of alleged infanticide cases in Ireland, as they were elsewhere, especially for women who wanted to present a good moral reputation for future marriage and employment prospects. Verdicts in the coronial courts were highly sensitive to these social norms and were often left open or sufficiently vague so as not to implicate the mother. I have discussed elsewhere how this was what Elizabeth T. Hurren terms 'discretionary justice' in operation and how the contours of it differed from Irish urban to rural areas.[195] With respect to Dublin City, discretionary justice relied heavily on the ability to evoke the sympathy of the coroner's jury and whether or not the mother could prove good moral character or portray innocence of the ways of the world. Needless to add, social class and occupation played a very significant role in these discretionary cases. Beyond the immediate neonatal context, infant deaths were viewed in a different legal light as concealment of pregnancy was no longer an issue. Nonetheless, prevailing social conventions and personal opinions of jurors held sway.

Mothers found guilty of child neglect, dire poverty notwithstanding, could expect no sympathy from the DMP or the coroner's court. The Hegarty family of 6 Newcomen Court was berated for not feeding their 4-month-old son properly. Their neighbour Mary Coffey of 9 Newcomen Court stated how she had to step in several times as 'the mother was part of the time incapable of taking care of child'.[196] An anonymous letter signed by 'an eye witness' sent to the Summerhill Station stated that the parents were a 'drunken pair, that all they can get is too little for drink' and that they had three other children who died from neglect. The

[191] NAI/1901/128 Inquest on the body of Delia Kelly, 9 May 1901.
[192] NAI/1901/128, reports dated 9 May 1901.
[193] *Freeman's Journal*, 10 May 1901; *Newry Reporter*, 13 May 1901.
[194] See http://www.census.nationalarchives.ie/reels/nai000077448/ (accessed 31 January 2021).
[195] Breathnach and O'Halpin, 'Scripting blame'.
[196] NAI/1900/226 Inquest on the body of Joseph Hegarty, 29 August 1901.

DMP investigated the claims and found that the child had been under medical care for the previous month and Dr McGrath, 130 North Strand, prescribed for it three weeks prior—he signed a death certificate and defended the parents, stating that they had done as much as they could. The report also stated that the Hegartys had four living children—all were healthy but two had indeed died. What probably piqued the coroner's suspicion was that the parents had made arrangements with the Cemetery Office for a swift burial and the infant was insured with the Prudential Burial Society. The DMP put a delay on the burial in order to investigate the circumstances.[197]

'Baby Farming in the City'

Charges of neglect could be levied against parents at any stage but it was more likely to accrue in the post neonatal context and more pointedly in cases where children were placed 'out to nurse'. An accidental death of a nurse child brought other less savoury childcare practices to light. Unmarried mother, Kate Fay had her son George at the Westmoreland Lock Hospital on 22 August and his birth was registered by the 'occupier' on 10 September 1900.[198] Implied in the location of birth was that she was suffering from venereal disease.[199] It seems that she had not planned on keeping her child and she put him out to nurse with Ellen Timmins at 12 Gloucester Place to whom she made regular payments of the agreed sum of 5s. per week.[200] She stated in evidence that she got married and moved to Galway, but none of the timeframes match. Kate Fay said George was out to nurse for nine months when he died in early October, but on census night 31 March 1901 he was with her at Purdon Street, Dublin, and she was returned as unmarried.[201] Timmins, who was employed during the day as a cook in a brothel at 33 Lower Tyrone Street, sub-let the nursing of the child to Kate Higginbottom, to whom she paid 2s. a week. A newspaper account described the case as one of 'Baby Faming in the City' and stated that Fay 'knew perfectly well that witness (Timmins) was working during the day'.[202] Higginbottom who described herself as a married 30-year-old roomkeeper at 5.2 Ayres Court, had two sons, aged 17

[197] NAI/1901/226 Inquest on the body of Joseph Hegarty, 29 August 1901.
[198] NAI/1901/254 Inquest on the body of George Fay, 4 October 1901; for the birth record for George Fay, see https://civilrecords.irishgenealogy.ie/churchrecords/images/birth_returns/births_1900/01986/1764847.pdf.
[199] Laurence M. Geary, ' "The wages of sin is death": lock hospitals, venereal disease and gender in prefamine Ireland', in Margaret Preston and Margaret Ó hÓgartaigh (eds), Gender and Medicine in Ireland, 1700–1951 (New York, 2012), pp. 165–73.
[200] See http://www.census.nationalarchives.ie/reels/nai003684720/ (accessed 9 January 2021).
[201] See http://www.census.nationalarchives.ie/pages/1901/Dublin/North_Dock/Purdon_Street/1276882/ (accessed 9 January 2021). Living at 10 Purdon Street, she states she was unmarried.
[202] Irish Daily Independent, 5 October 1901.

and 1.[203] On the ill-fated day, she gave George Fay a piece of beef fat to suck and later noticed he was turning black. She ran to Dr Cohen with the child—on the way she suffered a weakness and Mary Jane Murphy of 54 Talbot Street, who happened to be nearby, took the child and ran to the doctor. Timmins had the child under treatment for sores, it was well nourished and there was no suspicion—it was an accidental case of asphyxia.[204] There was nothing to indicate cruelty towards the child,[205] and there was no allegation of mistreatment, but Dr Byrne took a particularly dim view of Ellen Timmins's profiteering.[206]

In stark contrast with 'baby farmers' operating outside official notice, 'nurses' who were registered with the local authority had the comfort of the law on their side when children died under their care. Francis Doran was 'out to nurse' with Catherine Smith, 4 Bethesda Place, Dorset Street when he died of 'inanition due to non-assimilation of food'—at about 4 weeks old he weighed a mere 4.5 lbs. The child was born at Holles Street Maternity Hospital and at about 13 days old his mother put him out to nurse under the alias Nicholas Murray. Catherine Smith proudly stated in evidence that she had been child-minding for twenty years and none had died under her care.[207] She acted responsibly when she noticed how poorly he was, and brought the child to the doctor. He was entered into the workhouse under the name Nicholas Murray, and Dr Caleb F. Powell (visiting surgeon NDU) noted that his body had a complete absence of fat, which raised alarms.[208] It seems to have been a genuine case of failure to thrive.[209]

Low-level operators were hidden in plain sight until things went badly wrong and the law could do little to root out or sanction those who were cold and calculated about their business. Unscrupulous 'baby-farmers' had no qualms about cutting their losses by starving the child when payments lapsed. Described in the *Freeman's Journal* as a case of a 'Shockingly Emaciated' child, Teresa Carr weighed a mere 8.5 lbs at 2 years of age when she died of 'Exhaustion caused by the hectic fever, the result of pleurisy.' Dr John Burgess clarified to the court that her weight was only slightly above a normal birth weight.[210] She was under the care of Elizabeth Dempsey and when her mother's payments stopped 'neglect – gross carelessness' ensued. It is unclear how long she was under Dempsey's care but a Celia Carr was recorded as living with the Dempsey family in the 1901 census,

---

[203] See http://www.census.nationalarchives.ie/pages/1901/Dublin/North_Dock/Gloucester_Place/1275041/ (accessed 9 January 2021).

[204] *Evening Herald*, 4 October 1901.

[205] NAI/1901/254 Inquest on the body of George Fay, 4 October 1901: http://www.census.nationalarchives.ie/pages/1901/Dublin/North_Dock/Gloucester_Place/1275041/ (accessed 9 January 2021).

[206] *Belfast Newsletter*, 5 October 1901, did not name any of the actors.

[207] *Irish Independent*, 8 October 1900.

[208] Workhouse admission and discharge records, B.G. 78 v. G book 80 (17 November 1899, no. 801)—v. G book 84 (27 August 1901, no. 3560), entered 1 October, died 4 October 1900.

[209] NAI/1900/131 Inquest on the body of Francis Doran, 6 October 1900.

[210] NAI/1901/117 Inquest on the body of Teresa Carr, 20 April 1901.

where Elizabeth is documented as Eliza.[211] Dr Burgess was of the firm belief that Teresa Carr could have rallied had she been properly attended to by a doctor, but the law was weak in this area. Those prosecuted under the Prevention of Cruelty Act for unnecessary suffering were simply guilty of a misdemeanour.[212] Technically, there were no legal obligations for guardians to seek medical attention until the 1908 act. Dr Byrne warned Elizabeth Dempsey that any statements she made could be used in formal proceedings against her, should it be brought before the courts.[213] Inspector Dixon and Sergeant Travers were present on behalf of the DMP and she declined to comment.[214] Optical character recognition software limitations notwithstanding, my searches in newspapers for any case or prison sentence against Dempsey have not proven fruitful. It seems that she got away with her appalling treatment of a helpless infant, which, judging by similar cases, would have amounted to little more than a fine had it progressed to the courts.

The case of Joseph Reilly was similar in that he weighed 11 lbs at 14 months, or approximately half what he should have weighed at that age. That case was taken further because the child had visible signs of appalling levels of utter neglect—he was blind from an ulcerated protruding iris. Dr Powell, who was a well-seasoned NDU doctor and had seen some of the worst cases of neglect in the course of his work, estimated that the child had been 'suffering frightfully' for 'a considerable time' from malnutrition and want of medical care. Mr McCloy of the NSPCC issued summons against the foster parents Richard and Kate Reilly of Larkhill Baldoyle. It was revealed that Kate Reilly had received the child in the most dubious of circumstances.[215] She stated that she answered an advert in the newspaper and was advised to go to a 'certain place' on 20 March 1901 to get the child.[216] Reilly said that she did not know who the parents were and surmised that the man she met was a student who gave her £5 for its keep. That amount of money was only going to last so long, so it was clearly a short-term money-making plan and the case that followed was described in the newspapers as one of 'Alleged Baby Farming'.[217] She had the child for about a year when it entered the NDU on 18 March—Dr Powell thought it the worst case of neglect he had ever seen.[218] At Coolock Petty Sessions, Mr Tobias prosecuted for the NSPCC—the Reillys were committed for trial and bail was set in the amount of £20 and two sureties of £10.[219] Richard Reilly was charged with the wilful neglect of a child and sentenced to three months at the City of Dublin Commission, 5 August 1902; Kate was

---

[211] See http://www.census.nationalarchives.ie/reels/nai003762820/ (accessed 8 January 2021).
[212] An Act for the Prevention of Cruelty to, and better Protection of, Children, 1889, c. 4.
[213] See https://civilrecords.irishgenealogy.ie/churchrecords/images/deaths_returns/deaths_1901/05729/4616636.pdf (accessed 8 January 2021); *Evening Herald*, 20 April 1901.
[214] *Evening Herald*, 20 April 1901; *Freeman's Journal*, 22 April 1901.
[215] *Freeman's Journal*, 15 April 1902.   [216] *Belfast Newsletter*, 8 April 1902.
[217] *Belfast Newsletter*, 15 April 1902.   [218] NAI/1902/61, inquest dated 7 April 1902.
[219] *Belfast Newsletter*, 15 April 1902.

sentenced to twelve months—she was released 3 August 1903.[220] The jury censured the newspaper for its part in facilitating the transaction.[221]

Conclusion

Deaths occurring in domestic contexts must be viewed from life cycle perspectives. The range of medical problems leading to cause of death were highly sensitive to age and those concerning children placed mothers under police and NSPCC suspicion. There were several cases where compassion was shown, especially towards poor mothers who were doing their best, but any mention of alcohol or excess brought with it severe judgements and admonishing riders. In cases involving alcohol abuse, there was no acknowledgement of addiction-driven despair and poverty; instead, child death was generally regarded as a personal moral failing on the part of mothers.

This chapter has provided ample evidence of the fact that deaths both in child and older cohorts are emblematic of considerable fear of official gazes by the poorest strata of Dublin society. Many adults suffered chronic illness in silence because they could not afford to be ill and there were general high levels of tolerance of poor health in the community. It is hard to imagine that Elizabeth Ormsby's death from pulmonary haemorrhage was not preceded by other telltale signs of serious pulmonary disease.[222] The same can be said of the child and youth tuberculosis cases. In the male breadwinner model, mothers were expected to look after everything in the domestic setting and they were the first to be blamed when things went badly wrong. The next chapter moves to a discussion of deaths outside the front door, where the burden of blame was distributed to community as opposed to maternal responsibility.

---

[220] NAI, PRIS/1/10/27 Register of remand prisoners, Kilmainham, no. 813; NAI, PRIS/1/44/3 General register of convicted female prisoners, Mountjoy, no. 3253.

[221] *Dublin Evening Telegraph*, 5 August 1902; *Freeman's Journal*, 6 August 1902.

[222] NAI/1902/19 Inquest on the body of Elizabeth Ormsby, 5 February 1902; *Freeman's Journal*, 6 February 1902.

3

Deaths Outside

Public and Workplace Settings

Streetscapes, the world beyond landings, hallways, and the front door, were really important spaces for children's play and were natural extensions of tenement life.[1] For adults it was the world of work, hawking, getting and spending, company, drinking, and entertainment. As a social space for all age cohorts the streetscape, whether by day or by night, offered equal measures of safety and danger. Figure 3.1 shows the breakdown of the 260 deaths of people who died outside of domestic or institutional spaces, the majority of which, 109, were at, or because of accidents in, workplace settings. Fourteen of the bodies 'found outside' were of unknown infants; three were considered stillborn with untied umbilical cords and six exhibited signs of unskilled attendance at birth. 'Mary Church' was found in Fairview church by a woman named Mary Ryan who testified that she 'got the baby christened by Father Caffrey'—it was deemed to have been born prematurely; the male infant body found at Trinity College Dublin was considered 'mummified', so no medical cause of death could be ascertained; and the remainder were as a result of exposure, starvation, and nephritis.[2] A further three children were identified: Joseph Wall (discussed in Chapter 2 in the context of family breakdown and child neglect, but enumerated here because he collapsed 'outside'; he is not included in the 307 domestic deaths) and two male infants found within a day of one another failed to thrive following alleged infanticide attempts—both cases will be discussed in Chapter 4.[3] As the causes of death range from violence to neglect, discussion of the remainder of those in the 'found' and institutional categories are dispersed throughout the book and do not constitute a discrete section.

Outside the front door, people were exposed to a different range of risks from road traffic accidents to drowning and workplace accidents.[4] This chapter groups together deaths according to these three overarching causes and begins by

---

[1] Drew Gray, *London's Shadows: The Dark Side of the Victorian City* (London, 2010), p. 126.

[2] NAI/1900/47 Inquest held on the body of 'Mary Church', 23 June 1900; NAI/1901/142 Inquest held on the body of an 'Unknown' male infant, 18 May 1901.

[3] NAI/1900/62 Inquest held on the body of Patrick Hanlon, 10 July 1900; NAI/1900/63 Inquest held on the body of John Jordon, 11 July 1900.

[4] Anna Davin, *Growing Up Poor: Home, School and Street in London, 1870–1914* (London, 1996), pp. 63–8.

Ordinary Lives, Death, and Social Class: Dublin City Coroner's Court, 1876–1902. Ciara Breathnach, Oxford University Press. © Ciara Breathnach 2022. DOI: 10.1093/oso/9780198865780.003.0004

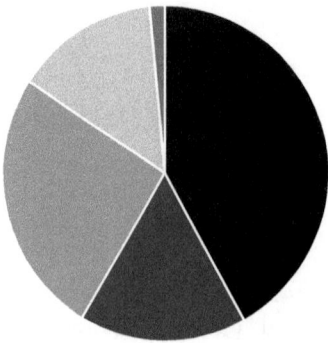

■ Work ■ Drowned ■ Found outside ■ Knocked down ■ Accident Outside

Figure 3.1 Deaths outside

discussing the deaths of people knocked down on the streets, and what patterns in city life can be discerned from them. It discusses some non-fatal cases and their outcome in the courts to exemplify the power dynamics that were at play on the streetscapes. Distinction in the first instance is made between cases of those who were knocked down by horses and trams. Trams posed risks to pedestrians but also to horses and drivers. As a result of modern transportation innovations, horse-drawn vehicular traffic was displaced to smaller streets, which had a particular impact on children. The second section focuses on the accidental deaths by drowning in the city's waterways. Implicitly understood in deaths by drowning was the potential for foul play; ten cases are of unknowns, or unidentified bodies, three of which were adults. Deaths by drowning associated with occupational hazards are enumerated separately and dealt with in the final section in this chapter on work-related accidents. Cases with evidence of self-harm of adults in waterways are discussed in greater detail in Chapter 4. Most of the 109 workplace deaths were of adult men working predominantly in the transportation and construction industries. Poor men and women tended to work in some of the most dangerous jobs, had little choice in the work they did, and were not fairly compensated. Many were caught in deadly poverty traps—there are a number of instances of those who went to work, or conducted 'out work' at home, despite the fact that they were literally dying on their feet. Living 'hand to mouth' made the world outside the front door every bit as constrained as their domestic spaces.

Road Traffic and Transport Accidents

Like most other European cities Dublin was a palimpsest of various built environment movements from the Wide Streets Commission and canal building of the late eighteenth century to the electrification of trams of the late nineteenth century.[5] According to O'Carroll-Burke, engineering was central to material state formation, and he contends that although innovations occurred experimentally, they were systematic. The experimental trajectory of the rail and tram system is borne out in the coroner and judicial court records, which show haphazardness and very uneasy shifts motivated by commercial interests that were enabled by parliament. There was no sense of a grand plan. Modernity, from the perspective of the coroner's court, mapped uncomfortably to the human geography of the city and the years I investigate here were ones when the full impact of the electric tramlines took effect.[6] Map 3.1 shows an outline of the tramlines, and demonstrates the way in which the network had monopolised space on the streetscape by 1900. Public right of way was not affected by the various tramways acts from the 1860s but tramway companies were given powers over the usage of their lines by other vehicular traffic.[7] This power came at some considerable costs and a duty

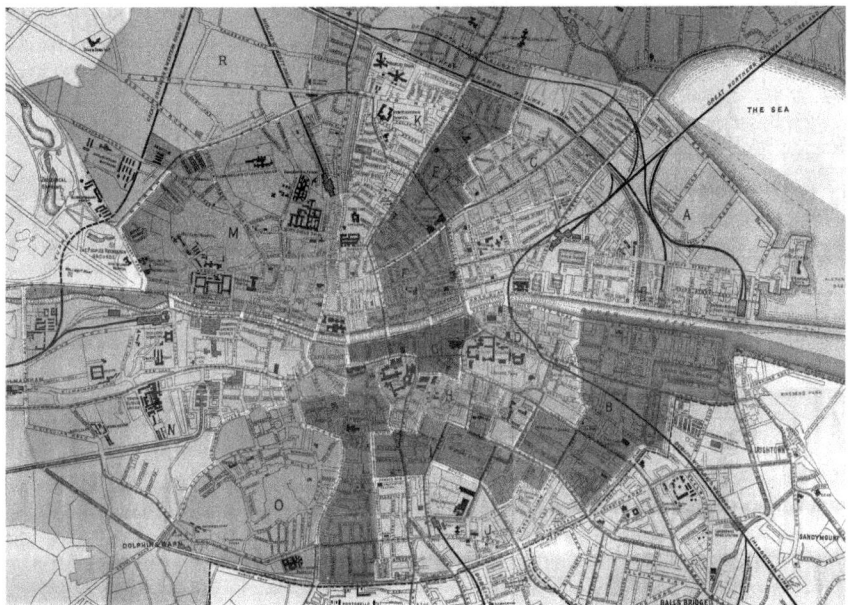

Map 3.1 Map of the City of Dublin and its environs

Note: I am grateful to Nicholas Field, University of Toronto Library.

Source: *Thom's Directory* 1900, for a colour version of this map see https://collections.library.utoronto. ca/view/mdl:G5784_D7_F7_10_190—191— (accessed 21 November 2021). Image courtesy of the Map & Data Library, University of Toronto.

---

[5] Christine Casey, *Dublin: The City Within the Grand and Royal Canals and the Circular Road with the Phoenix Park* (New Haven, 2005), pp. 119–20.

[6] Patrick Carroll-Burke, 'Material designs: engineering cultures and engineering states – Ireland 1650–1900', *Theory and Society*, 31:1 (2002), pp. 75–114 at 78, 89.

[7] Tramways (Ireland) Act 1860 (23 & 24 Vic.) c. clii; Tramways (Ireland) Act 1861 (23 & 24 Vic.) c.cii; The Dublin Tramways Act, 1871 (34 & 35 Vic.) c. c. lxxxviii, s. 36 (rights of public access

to maintain road surfaces, which was not always attended to properly. From 1860 to 1893, the following companies were permitted to establish tramlines and horse-powered omnibus trams: the Dublin Tramways Company, incorporated 1871; the North Dublin Street Tramways Company, incorporated 1875; the Dublin Central Tramways Company, incorporated 1878; the Dublin Southern Districts Tramways Company, incorporated 1878; the Dublin United Tramways Company Limited, incorporated 1881; and the Blackrock and Kingstown Tramway Company, incorporated 1883.[8]

Of the overall sample, there are thirty-seven cases of people who were killed in road traffic and transportation accidents (twenty-one adults and sixteen children), of whom the oldest was aged 8 and the youngest was 1 year and 5 months.[9] In terms of jury riders, the child deaths on the streetscape show a different range of attributes to those occurring in domestic spaces and, remarkably, they do not single out mothers as being to blame. Fourteen of the pedestrian incidents involved trams and trains, which are often used interchangeably in the records. The majority, twenty-one, involved hackney vehicles (also termed floats or vans), which were horse-drawn vehicles operated by a driver. Despite the fact that cycling was a well-established pursuit by 1900, only two cases concerned bicycle accidents.[10]

Although there were no witnesses to the accident, it was assumed that 8-year-old Samuel Henry Jenkins sustained injuries while cycling near his home down Kingsland Avenue on 25 May 1901. He was discovered in an unconscious condition with the bicycle strewn nearby.[11] The second cycling death concerned an open road collision near Lucan, when 30-year-old bootmaker James Nolan was on a Sunday cycling excursion. He sustained a serious head injury and his medical treatment was not comprehensive, but it was found to have been a purely accidental death.[12] One passenger death occurred on a steamer, which was investigated

preserved); Dublin Southern District Tramways Act 1893 (56 & 57 Vict.) c. ccxx; Dublin United Tramways Act 1896 (59 & 60 Vict.) c. ccxxiii.

[8] D. Stewart, 'Dublin city passenger transport services', *Journal of the Statistical and Social Inquiry Society of Ireland*, 1955, p. 136.

[9] The Verdict in the case of Edward O'Connor was very specific: 'Died from internal haemorrhage. From rupture of liver caused by the accidental passing of a cart over its body. We exonerate the driver from all blame. We consider the person in charge of the child should be censured. And we recommend the parents of the child to the kind consideration of the owner of the cart': NAI/1900/64 Inquest on the body of Edward O'Connor, 13 June 1900. (Not clear from the inquest who was in charge of the child.) The driver of the cart John Clarke was arrested at the scene.

[10] Brian Griffin, 'Cycling and gender in Victorian Ireland', *Éire-Ireland*, 41:1–2 (2006), pp. 213–41.

[11] NAI/1901/148 Inquest on the body of Samuel Henry Jenkins, 29 May 1901; *Freeman's Journal*, 30 May 1901.

[12] NAI/1901/266 Inquest on the body of James Nolan, 17 October 1901; *Freeman's Journal*, 18 October 1901; *Irish Daily Independent*, 18 October 1901. Nolan was on the correct side of the road, when he met an oncoming cyclist, Mr Moonan, who went the wrong direction as they extended road user courtesies to one another. Nolan was brought immediately to the Richmond Hospital where his head wound was dressed by a medical student, but he was not detained. When his condition deteriorated the following day he was seen by a dispensary doctor, Dr Maughan who advised that the case

as a homicide and is discussed in Chapter 4.[13] According to the annual reports, in 1900, 245 tram cars and a total of 2,236 so-called hackney vehicles (183 job carriages, 1,116 outside cars, 617 cabriolets,[14] seventy phaetons, and five stage carriages) were licensed by the DMP.[15] Commensurate with the expansion of tram lines there was an increase in the number of carriages to 255 in 1901, and there was a net decrease of 76 hackney vehicles in the same timeframe.[16] Licensing of hackney carriages was an important revenue stream for the DMP, which involved the inspection of road worthiness. The carriage district extended to a ten-mile radius from the General Post Office on Sackville Street, now O'Connell Street.[17] David Toms argues that with the exception of a select few multiple licence holders, the majority of Cork 'jinglemen' were precariously employed and subject to intense scrutiny under city by-laws.[18] Most Dublin H-car drivers shared the same profile and were lower-paid workers with inconsistent work. Their livelihoods depended on fast transportation times, minute knowledge of the city, and all aspects of social life. In many cases they were the first responders to emergency situations and with generosity and without hesitation they transported the injured and dying to hospital.

Being directly associated with the DMP, H-car drivers were subject to intense scrutiny. They could be charged with numerous offences like geographically specific permissions relating to licensing, and more common forms like drunkenness, furious driving (endangering animal health), public disorder, careless driving, cruelty to animals, and furious driving to public danger. If convicted they faced fines, suspensions, and revocations of licences, and if the offence was criminal in nature they could be imprisoned. Both vehicles and drivers were supposed to hold a licence and a badge—very often, H-cars were not driven by the licencee but by an employee of theirs whose horsemanship skills may have been lacking. Proceedings were taken against 1,772 persons under stage and hackney regulations in Dublin in 1901, and 610 were dismissed offhand.[19] Nationally, the

---

was hopeless and a clergyman be called. One of the jurors laboured the point of potential medical mismanagement but, it was argued by Dr Byrne, that the gravity of the situation was unlikely to have emerged until later. A further point to note is that head injuries from cycling accidents were relatively new to the emergency medical environment and the procedures for best practice were not well described. E.B. Turner, 'A report on cycling in health and disease. VIII. Training and racing', *The British Medical Journal*, 2:1854 (11 July 1896), pp. 98–9; E.B. Turner, 'A report on cycling in health and disease. IX. Cycling accidents', *The British Medical Journal*, 2:1856 (25 July 1896), p. 203.

   [13] The professional water faring deaths are accounted for in the workplace accidents section.

   [14] These were 'four-wheelers'— job carriages had two horses, phaetons were four-wheeled and doorless. *Dublin Metropolitan Police: Evidence taken before the Committee of Inquiry, 1901* [Cd. 1095], p. 10.

   [15] Dublin Carriage Act 1853 (16 & 17, Vic.) c. 112.

   [16] *Statistical tables of the Dublin Metropolitan Police for the year 1901* [Cd. 1166], p. xiii.

   [17] BPP, Report of Chief Com. of Police for Dublin Metropolis on Dublin Tramways Bill, May 1873 [189].

   [18] David Thomas, 'The Hackney carriage in Cork: vehicle of a Victorian Irish city 1854–1902', *Irish Economic and Social History*, 45:1 (2018), pp. 136–54.

   [19] *Statistical tables of the Dublin Metropolitan Police for the year 1901* [Cd. 1166], p. 12.

five-year average from 1896 to 1900 of offences against the stage and hackney carriage regulations brought before the Courts of Summary Jurisdiction was 3,628 per annum.[20] Needless to add, horses were unpredictable in their behaviour, especially if they were being driven by strangers. If we cast our minds back to Dr Byrne's first case, it was a sudden stop that caused the breaching to break and thus John Healy was thrown from his perch on to a cobbled stone street, which led to his death. H-car horses were large work animals akin to drafts, shires, or Clydesdales, and were a formidable presence on the city streets.[21] Writing about animal cruelty in the mid-nineteenth century, Juliana Adelman observes that their treatment was indicative of 'the city's progress'.[22] While animal cruelty was not as much an issue by 1900, bar a few cases of horses being driven 'furiously' and the odd prosecution under the Contagious Diseases acts, technological progress presented a new set of challenges as the city transitioned to electric and motor power.[23] A once-thriving sector was on the verge of obsolescence and collapse. It took its toll on mental health too, as the next chapter dealing with suicide shows.

In accordance with the Dublin Traffic Act 1875 all vehicles were to proceed on the left side of the road 'within four feet of the kerbstone where possible'.[24] Speed limits were set at twelve miles per hour for all traffic, from pushbikes to horses and trams. Although some operators were reticent to move from horse-drawn omnibuses to electric trams, technological advance was forced when the Dublin Southern Districts Tramway made the shift under the imprimatur of a local act in 1893.[25] Derided in works by W.B. Yeats and James Joyce as a ruthless business tycoon, William Martin Murphy was the managing director of the Dublin United Tram Company (DUTC), which by 1900 owned most of the lines radiating from the Nelson's Pillar Terminus on Sackville Street.[26] Murphy was an MP from 1885 to 1892 and used his power to wield considerable concessions for the rail and tram transportation network from which he personally profited.

In 1897, an act was passed to permit the electrification of the DUTC lines from Nelson's Pillar to Clontarf, and it quickly swallowed up its competition through

---

[20] *Judicial Statistics, Ireland, 1900* [Cd. 725, 682], p. 50.

[21] *Commission on horse breeding, Ireland. Reports by the commissioners appointed to inquire into the house breeding industry in Ireland* [C.8651 C.8652], pp. 6–7.

[22] Juliana Adelman, *Civilised by beasts: animals and urban change in nineteenth-century Dublin* (Manchester, 2020), p. 41.

[23] *Freeman's Journal*, 4 August 1900: case of a Catherine Speckman charged with having eight horses affected with parasitic mange.

[24] Dublin Traffic Act 1875 (38 & 39 Vict.) c. cxcv.

[25] Dublin Southern District Tramways, 1893 (56 & 57 Vic.) c. ccxx.

[26] Scott Kaufman, '"That Bantry jobber": William Martin Murphy and the critique of progress and productivity in "Ulysses"', *European Joyce Studies*, 21:21 (2011), pp. 210–23; Andy Bielenberg, 'Entrepreneurship, power and public opinion in Ireland: the career of William Martin Murphy', *Irish Economic and Social History*, xxvii (2000), pp. 25–43.

acquisition.[27] The Board of Trade was responsible for ensuring that dangers to the public were kept to a minimum and it regulated the speed at which traffic could travel.[28] Maximum tram speed was retained at twelve miles per hour and that rate was lower in villages and towns.[29] On Thursday, 26 July 1900 the northbound tram service linking Dublin City to the East Pier at Howth opened as a fully electrically powered service. Journey time was shortened to thirty minutes and the full ticket cost 5d.—this meant that it ran consistently, with regularity, and at pace.[30] The last of the horse-drawn trams was retired on 13 January 1901 when a section of the Southbound, Sandymount line, from Northumberland Road to the Star of the Sea, was electrified.[31] The trams were powered by stations located in Ringsend and Clontarf.[32]

Not only did the tramlines occupy their own immediate space, they pushed other road users out and created congestion problems elsewhere. When trams broke down they requisitioned even more space. For example, on Thursday, 14 June 1900 when the tram wire on the Rathmines route snapped near Saint Stephen's Green, it caused disruption to traffic and a diversion was put in place using the Hatch Street line. In that instance, the prompt actions of tram works ensured that no additional injuries occurred.[33] On another Sunday evening, at about 8 p.m. in July 1900, an electric cable snapped near College Green (Figure 3.2) and a live wire emitted sparks on a very busy route—the newspaper report also revealed that a similar episode occurred on Camden Street earlier that afternoon.[34] Later in the month, at 5 p.m. on a Sunday evening, the same thing happened on Upper Sackville Street just a few hours after another live wire incident on Talbot Street. Emergency crews were despatched to repair the faults and the ripple effect of such events consumed other resources like the DMP, which was tasked with keeping the public at bay.[35] Trams regularly derailed and often collided with one another. On 23 May 1900, the Clonskea and Terenure trams crashed at the top of Dawson Street in the city centre, hours after another accident involving a horse-drawn float and a tram occurred on South Great George's Street.[36] Signal failures and the sharing of single lines, for example at Dollymount, were another source of accidents.[37] Tram drivers were error prone too—some missed the stops or overshot them; to compensate they stopped too abruptly, and passengers standing to alight were thrown forward or to the ground. These cases

[27] Dublin United Tramways (Electrical Power) Act 1897 (60 & 61, Vic.) c. ccxxxvi.
[28] Tramways and Public Companies (Ireland) Act 1883 (46 & 47 Vict.) c. 43. s. 23.
[29] *Royal Commission on Irish Public Works. Second report of the Royal Commission on Irish Public Works* [C.5264 C.5264-I], p. 33.
[30] *Irish Daily Independent*, 27 July 1900; Tramways (Ireland) Act, 1900 (63 & 64 Vic.) c. 60.
[31] *Evening Herald*, 14 January 1901.
[32] *Evening Herald*, 16 January 1901; *Irish Daily Independent*, 13 February 1901.
[33] *Freeman's Journal*, 15 June 1900.   [34] *Freeman's Journal*, 9 July 1900.
[35] *Freeman's Journal*, 23 July 1900.   [36] *Freeman's Journal*, 24 May 1900.
[37] *Freeman's Journal*, 23 August 1900.

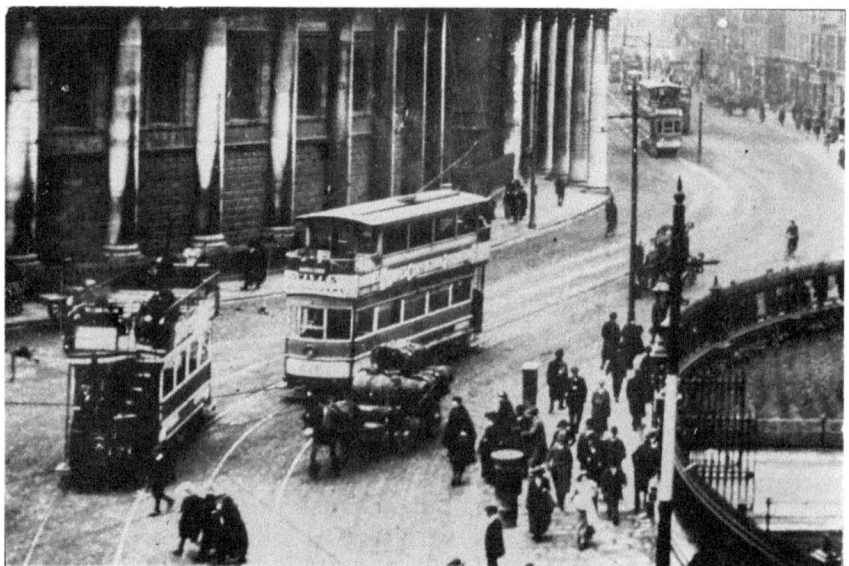

Figure 3.2 View of College Green, with Trinity College Dublin to the right, facing towards Sackville Street

Note: I am very grateful to Berni Metcalfe and Glenn Dunne, NLI, for providing me with this 'pandemic' copy.

Source: NLI/TRAM36. Image Courtesy of the National Library of Ireland.

ended up in the courts and in cases where the DUTC admitted liability they usually challenged the extent of injuries caused.[38] The DUTC was no stranger to the coroner, the police, and the city courts and it always had very strong legal representation.[39]

H-car, van, and float drivers came into regular conflict with the trams and these cases usually ended up before the Recorder of Dublin, Frederick Richard Falkiner (1891–1908), who was not always sympathetic to their plight.[40] In November 1900, the Recorder pointed out how it was unfair of H-car drivers to place all responsibility for stopping or yielding right of way on the 'motormen', when the horse-drawn cars were dimly lit or had no lighting at all—in such cases the bare minimum of damages were awarded against the tram company.[41] 'Restive horses' proved to be difficult for both H-car drivers to control around trams and for tram drivers to predict. A case coming before the City Sessions in October 1900 placed the onus on tram drivers to slow down in order to avoid collision. The case concerned a collision that occurred in Fairview on 6 September 1900 on

---

[38] *Evening Herald*, 18 June 1900.   [39] *Evening Herald*, 1 February 1901.
[40] *Dictionary of Irish Biography* entry by Patrick M. Geoghegan, https://doi.org/10.3318/dib.002998. v2 (accessed 20 November 2021).
[41] *Evening Herald*, 19 November 1900.

the Howth-bound line—the H-car driver did his utmost to make the dray move but failed in his endeavour. He claimed that the horse was frightened by the electric tram and, in anticipation of the horse moving, the tram driver did not try to stop. An award of £20 was made against the tram company.[42] There were two other personal injury claims brought before the Recorder that day—one was dismissed and another was adjourned. These were regular incidents. Another case of a non-fatal accident that occurred on the Terenure line revealed something more of road-user expectations. A 'motorman' witness to a crash between a tram and a horse-driven float testified that 'The plaintiff seemed to expect that the tram would stop and let him ahead.' The Recorder added that there was an onus on the people to take personal responsibility around trams especially during the summer when they 'were running like blackbeetles', and that in cases of collisions he would 'give fair play to both sides'.[43]

While most claims against the DUTC were in the order of £50 or less, in February 1901 it was sued for £6,000 in damages for life-changing injuries suffered by Martin Fitzgerald, an influential spirit grocer in Middle Abbey Street. Fitzgerald sustained injuries to his spine and fractured his thigh when his horse fell on the Grafton Street tram line, and he was 'flung out violently' from his trap. He suffered from chronic pain and was described as a 'hopeless cripple' as a result of the injuries.[44] Several H-car drivers, whose own vested interests were undeniable, gave evidence *in nisi prius* before Justice Gibson and a special jury as to the negligence of the tram company and the slippery road surface.[45] The matter of responsibility for sanding the tracks to improve traction for horses was sent before the Queen's Bench for review in 1899 and it decreed that the DUTC was responsible under section 37 of the Dublin United Tramway and Electrical Power Act 1897. Indeed, earlier legislation, the 1870 Tramways Act, already placed liabilities on the company for all accidents and damages. Fitzgerald was eventually awarded £1,000 in damages. The DUTC appealed the case, the verdict, and the amount awarded, but it was later unanimously upheld by the King's Bench Division on 12 June 1901.[46] I cite this case because it gives an impression of the power of the DUTC and the resources it took to mount a case against such a powerful entity.

A raft of cases came before the City Sessions suing for personal and animal injuries and damages to property.[47] While there were undoubtedly some bogus claims, in the main, the DUTC was deemed to be at fault. Newspaper headlines about tram accidents ranged from 'serious' to 'dreadful', and 'terrible'. They often

---

[42] *Evening Herald*, 27 October 1900.   [43] *Freeman's Journal*, 29 October 1900.
[44] *Freeman's Journal*, 1 February 1901.
[45] *Evening Herald*, 5 February 1901; *Irish Daily Independent*, 5 February 1901; *Freeman's Journal*, 6 February 1901.
[46] *Freeman's Journal*, 13 June 1901.   [47] *Freeman's Journal*, 30 October 1900.

concerned serious injuries or loss of limbs.[48] In its half yearly report in February 1901, the Clontarf and Hill of Howth Tramroad Company accounted for an expenditure of £386 paid in compensation and legal costs, as against £667 in profits. New procedures were put in place with respect to insurance and indemnification but it recognised the inexperience of the staff as a major factor in accidents during the first few months of operation from 26 July 1900.[49] In July 1901, the DUTC, a much larger operation, revealed that it had paid £6,338 in compensation in the previous year—the *Evening Herald* reported how some of these cases were maliciously motivated and that personal attacks had been made on the Company Chairman, William Martin Murphy, whose ruthless business practices made him deeply unpopular in several quarters.[50] Murphy thrived because his sphere of influence was vast and many others profited from his endeavours. Proximity to tram stops had a positive impact on property values and its potential was not lost in the newspaper advertisement for the sale of 'McDowell's of Rathfarnam', a medium-sized licensed premises.[51] The Carmelite College at Terenure, which specialised in the training of young men for the legal and medical professions, mentioned in its advertisements that it had an electric tram stop outside its gate.[52] Being located on a tram line was a key selling point for business, and a job that was advertised at the Lucan Spa Hotel, which also boasted sulphur baths and a mild climate.[53] Progressive attributes aside, the primary function of the tramway system was for the mundane purposes of the everyday. Tramcar drivers had much to contend with. The populace was unversed in how to behave around such innovations and there were numerous cases of pedestrians being knocked down every year—some were fatal. When such cases occurred drivers were arrested at the scene.

Tramcar-related deaths could occur in a few ways—through being knocked down, or by falling from or getting caught up in the mechanism itself. Each tram had a 'motorman' or driver and a conductor on board whose job it was to direct the driver and to collect the fares. Similar to what Stephanie Rains has observed about the social composition of train usage in the 1850s, electric trams provided two main functions: first, the vital movement of workers in and out of the city and second, as a facilitator to the rise in leisure time.[54] With a trend towards excursions on holidays and weekends, the newspapers commented on the importance of the rail and tram service to bringing people to key attractions like Dublin Zoo, which was 'thronged' on Easter Monday 1900, and to the equally crowded seaside

---

[48] *Freeman's Journal*, 8 January 1901: 'Serious Tram accident. Child's Leg Cut Off. Charge Against a Motorman'; *Freeman's Journal*, 14 January 1901: 'Terrible Tram Accident. Man's Legs Broken'.
[49] *Irish Daily Independent*, 27 February 1901.   [50] *Evening Herald*, 31 July 1901.
[51] *Freeman's Journal*, 11 June 1900.   [52] *Leinster Leader*, 15 September 1900.
[53] *Freeman's Journal*, 22 November 1900.
[54] Stephanie Rains, *Commodity Culture and Social Class in Dublin 1850–1916* (Dublin, 2010), pp. 9–10.

resorts like Malahide and Kingstown.[55] In what it described as the 'excursion of the season', for 3s. 6d. the Irish Temperance League advertised an alcohol-free trip from Belfast to Dublin Zoo using a combined train and tram journey, which offered a Temperance Fête in the equation.[56] These seasonal excursions were not as important as another thriving economy that the tram facilitated, that of carousing, and the entitlement of bona fide traveller to a drink once they travelled three miles from where they were normally resident, and permitted purveyors of alcohol at 'destination' resorts like Howth to get around the licensing laws.

Within weeks of its opening, the Howth tram saw its first serious accident and subsequent fatality of 23-year-old William Duffy. It seems an altercation occurred with James Kelly, the tram conductor of the Dublin-bound tram when Duffy, who had taken drink, attempted to smoke a pipe inside the carriage. Although Duffy was clearly out of order, what followed was an extraordinary act of senseless violence: James Kelly pushed Duffy out of the moving train. Some fellow passengers claimed that he fell under the carriage they were travelling in but later forensic examination showed that it was the Howth-bound train (travelling in the opposite direction) that inflicted the injuries and neither driver noticed—the excuse given was that it was dark. Duffy initially survived his terrible injuries and was deposed while in hospital. He gave the following account:

> I was in Howth on yesterday 29th inst and I travelled home by the tram. I left Howth to the best of my opinion about 9 or 9½ pm. I cannot say for certain if Christopher Doyle is the man who drove the tram. I am not able to say if James Kelly was the conductor of the tram. I had a little sup of drink taken no doubt. I am not certain that James Kelly is the man but he is like him. As far as I remember I was pushed off the tram at Kilbarrack but I cannot tell by whom. The tram was in motion at the time. I had no dispute with any person on the tram. I remember paying 3d. for my ticket between Kilbarrack and Baldoyle...I do not know how much drink I had taken but I was not too drunk. I do not remember being taken into the tram after the accident nor anything more until I awoke here in hospital last night.

There were several witnesses who could identify James Kelly. Mary Hanlon deposed that she knew Duffy well, and saw the whole affair unfurl before her. Prior to his attempts to smoke, witnesses stated that he had annoyed the conductor by getting up repeatedly and asking where his stop was. When he tried to light the pipe Kelly was heard shouting 'get down and bedamned to you', and he pushed Duffy. After he was thrown off, Hanlon's brother James Mulroy had words with the conductor about his behaviour. Kelly threatened to 'do the bloody same' to him, and tried to stop him from pulling the emergency bell. In their tussle the bell was pulled. The driver stopped the tram, came back to investigate but resumed the journey within minutes. Arthur Hanlon, Mary's husband, got out at that point; he stated in evidence that he 'had a call of nature' and, after the tram had left without him, he heard Duffy moan. Hanlon discovered him between the tram lines at Kilbarrack—his left foot was all but severed from his leg and the entire length of his right leg had several deep gashes. He was removed from the tracks with the assistance of the DFB and rushed first by tram car to the city, and then by Corporation Ambulance to Jervis Street Hospital on 29 July 1900.[57] Under cross-examination at the City Commission, Mary Hanlon contended that she felt that the tram had run over something and she was asked why she did not mention it prior to then. It appears that she felt intimidated; she said that she had her child to mind, her brother had intervened, and that they had done enough. Both Kelly and Christopher Doyle the motorman were arrested that night and brought before Clontarf Petty Sessions on 2 August 1900.[58] Duffy died on 3 August from 'shock and haemorrhage' and his case came before the coroner's court on 4 August, where Gerard Byrne appeared for the tram company. The jury recommended that it 'take into consideration the relatives of the deceased'.[59] After Duffy died, both the driver and conductor were charged with homicide.[60] James Kelly was committed for trial on 8 August 1900 at a sitting of a Special Court of Petty Sessions held at the Town Hall in Clontarf—his case was adjourned from the County Sessions to the City of Dublin Commission on 16 October 1900.[61] Kelly was defended by Timothy Harrington MP and instructed by Gerard Byrne. Despite several witness statements, they convincingly argued that Duffy was not pushed and that it was the outbound tram that caused his death. Kelly was acquitted of all charges and continued, it seems, to work for the tramway company for at least another year.[62]

Gerald Byrne, counsel for the DUTC, regularly appeared at the coroner's court to discredit witnesses and to get matters on the record, especially in cases that involved the excesses of alcohol. William Redmond died after being hit by the Howth tram near Sutton and his four limbs were broken with the impact. Like Duffy, he too was conveyed to Jervis Street Hospital. In his DMP witness statement, he admitted to having a few pints in Howth and took responsibility for being on the track. Gerard Byrne made every effort to challenge the veracity of

---

[57] NAI/1900/87 Inquest on the body of William Duffy, 4 August 1900; *Freeman's Journal*, 30 July 1900; *Irish Daily Independent*, 30 July 1900; *Evening Herald*, 30 July 1900.

[58] *Irish Daily Independent*, 3 August 1900.

[59] NAI/1900/87 Inquest on the body of William Duffy, 4 August 1900.

[60] *Freeman's Journal*, 6 August 1900.

[61] NAI, County Dublin Commission on 16 October 1900; *Irish Daily Independent*, 9 August 1900.

[62] *Irish Daily Independent*, 17 October 1900. It seems he was still a conductor living in Tramway Cottages, Clontarf East, in 1901: http://www.census.nationalarchives.ie/reels/nai003674836/ (accessed 21 November 2021).

the evidence given by Duffy's comrade, a precariously employed retired fisherman, William Langle, who had been out of work for five weeks. Implied in this line of questioning 'What has a hulking fellow like you been living on for the past five weeks?', was that Langle lacked respectability or was involved in forms of criminality and that, by association perhaps, Redmond kept low company. Langle replied how he could 'live on a pint of porter and a penny bun every day' and survived 'on a shilling or sixpence that I get'. A juror stepped in to Langle's defence and Dr Louis Byrne corrected him stating that he had no right to interject like that.[63] Gerard Byrne tried to convince the jury to return a verdict of accidental death and wryly added, 'the Tram Company never turned a poor helpless widow away from their doors...But evidence showed that there was no responsibility, as admitted by the deceased, who stated before his death no one was to blame but himself.' The jury found the DUTC guilty of not properly lighting the line, recommended the widow to the kind consideration of the company, and exonerated the motorman.[64]

Poor understanding of tram speeds coupled with miscalculated risk caused 85-year-old Catherine Lindey to suffer fatal injuries as she crossed the road outside Trinity College Dublin between 5 p.m. and 6 p.m. on Christmas Eve 1900.[65] As both Map 3.1 and Figure 3.2 show, it was a very busy thoroughfare. Dr Keogh, resident surgeon, Dr Steevens' Hospital, happened upon the accident. He ran to her aid and, assisted by some passers-by, had the woman lifted into cab no. 910 driven by the owner, Michael Evans, badge 1147. Keogh accompanied her to the nearby Mercer's Hospital. She had general bruising all about her body, a wound on the right side of her head and suffered such serious injuries to her hand that one of her fingers had to be amputated. Her general health was poor, she had bronchitis, and she died a week after the accident from cardiac failure. In the interim, DMP Constable James Cooke brought the tram driver to the hospital and 'confronted him with the deceased. She said he was the driver and that it was partly her own fault and declined to charge him.' The jury added a rider exonerating the driver and appealed for compensation for her family.[66] The absence of a conductor was deemed by the jury to be the primary factor in the accident that led to Henry Dennison's slow demise. When he was getting off the tram at Kimmage Road station his right foot turned under him and he fell to the ground. Not realising that Dennison was in difficulty on the track the tram driver backed up a little and caught his foot—his shoe was torn and it broke skin. He was assisted home to his brother's house and when his condition deteriorated he

---

[63] NAI/1901/242 Inquest on the body of William Redmond 14 September 1901; *Freeman's Journal*, 16 September 1901.
[64] *Irish Daily Independent*, 16 September 1901; NAI/1901/242 Inquest on the body of William Redmond, 14 September 1901.
[65] *Freeman's Journal*, 2 January 1901.
[66] NAI/1901/1 Inquest on the body of Catherine Lindey, 1 January 1901.

ended up at the Meath Hospital having his leg amputated. Like Catherine Lindey, he considered himself to blame when he was interviewed in hospital by the DMP.[67]

The tussle for space between trams and H-cars was a perennial problem, especially when new systems and lines were being embedded. Clear lines of distinction were made between the motormen and the tram companies in all fatal cases. James Hanlon, H-car driver, badge no. 203 was driving H-car licence number 825 when he collided with the Howth tram on Talbot Street. Bernard Murphy, tram driver, and conductor, James Heart, were in charge of electric tram 175. In somewhat of a rare occurrence, the step of Hanlon's H-car got caught up in the passing tram, which witnesses estimated was going at a rate of 15 mph. Hanlon was thrown and suffered fatal head injuries.[68] Murphy and Heart were charged with carelessness and negligence in the management of a tram.[69] The Howth line was clearly a very problematic one—James Burke died when his horse and car collided with a tram on the Howth Road.[70] He was rushed to Jervis Street Hospital but refused to permit his leg to be amputated and died three days later—Dr Carrol O'Sullivan was of the opinion that he could have lived had he agreed to the surgery. One witness, Michael Keohane of 45 Carlingford Road, Drumcondra, claimed the tram was poorly lit and driving too fast at 9 or 10 mph. Gerald Byrne appeared as counsel for the tram company and argued that were the tram going that fast it would have smashed through the horse car. Witnesses stated that they did not 'hear the gong' but the coroner's jury was of the opinion that the driver was not to blame.[71] The jury rider was typical in its opinion of such cases; it attached 'no blame to anyone' and his relatives were recommended to the DUTC.

Children were a serious risk factor for tram drivers, they were both oblivious to dangers and too small to be in the conductor or the driver's line of sight. The day after James Hanlon's death, 2-years-and-9-month-old Christopher Gaines was struck by the Inchicore-bound electric tram car no. 159. It was driven by John Smullen, who was subsequently arrested.[72] Gaines was in the charge of his two older sisters, aged 12 and 10, when he was crossing High Street near the 'Chapel' (St Audeon's). He was so severely injured that he died at Jervis Street Hospital shortly after admission at 5.45 p.m. No blame was attached, and his family was recommended to the kind consideration of the tramway company.[73]

---

[67] NAI/1900/113 Inquest on the body of Henry Dennison, 12 September 1900.

[68] NAI/1900/122 Inquest on the body of James Hanlon, 1 October 1900.

[69] James Heart was still a tram conductor a year later: http://www.census.nationalarchives.ie/reels/nai003777672/. The only Bernard Murphy listed in the Dublin census was returned as a lorry driver in 1901: http://www.census.nationalarchives.ie/pages/1901/Dublin/Fitzwilliam/Gannons_Cottages/1306367/ (both accessed 31 October 2021).

[70] NAI/1900/106 Inquest on the body of James Burke, 6 September 1900; *Evening Herald*, 6 September 1900.

[71] *Freeman's Journal*, 7 September 1900.

[72] *Warder and Dublin Weekly Mail*, 6 October 1900.

[73] NAI/1900/123 Inquest on the body of Christopher Gaines, 1 October 1900.

A second inner-city tram case was that of 3-year-old Patrick Harbourne who was in the charge of his 6-year-old bother when tragedy struck on Talbot Street. It was a late-summer Saturday afternoon and the two boys were on their way to buy a halfpenny worth of ice cream when he was knocked down by the tram coming from Howth. He was immediately brought to Jervis Street Hospital and the 24-year-old-driver, William Buggy, was subsequently arrested for 'carelessness and negligence'.[74] The coroner's jury exonerated him from all blame and in their rider recommended the parents of the child to the kind consideration of the Dublin Tram Company.

Suburban tram lines on narrow streets and roads caused accidents too: Joseph Manning aged 2 years and 3 months lost all his left toes when the Inchicore tram crossed over his foot near his home at Mount Brown in Kilmainham—his leg was later amputated but he survived his injuries.[75] That should have been a clarion call to parents and guardians in the area to take better precautions, but the following year Kathleen Waters, aged 5 years and 6 months ran out her own front door at 39 Old Kilmainham oblivious to the danger. The motorman James Fox was brought before the Southern Police Court for careless driving but it was proven that he was in no way to blame.[76] Witnesses stated that they were satisfied that the driver did everything to stop the tram but in the process the child's body was dragged for about twenty feet. She died from the 'shock' of her injuries. The coroner's jury was very sympathetic to the driver and added a rider that exonerated him from all blame and appealed to the tram company to compensate her relatives.[77] It is difficult to ascertain what monies were paid in individual cases as they rarely came before the courts—settlements were made privately and the records of the DUTC are not extant.[78] Although such experiences could be traumatising for drivers these were good jobs and most continued with that work. For example, William Buggy, James Heart, and James Fox were all listed as tram drivers in the 1911 census.[79] The evidence presented in the coroner's court and the riders had a bearing on whether or not cases proceeded from criminal charges to convictions. The burden of proof for manslaughter or murder charges was high and even the

---

[74] NAI/1901/203 Inquest on the body of Patrick Harbourne, 5 August 1901; *Evening Herald*, 3 August 1901.

[75] *Irish Daily Independent*, 24 July 1900.

[76] *Evening Herald*, 27 November 1901. Only one James Fox was returned as a tram driver in the 1901 census and he was from County Wicklow: http://www.census.nationalarchives.ie/reels/nai003698505/. In 1911 he was married with one child and was in the same occupation: http://www.census.nationalarchives.ie/reels/nai000113696/ (accessed 31 October 2021).

[77] NAI/1901/299 Inquest on Kathleen Waters 26 November 1901.

[78] Some Dublin Southern District Tramway Company business records are held at Bristol Archives, but do not contain evidence of compensation payments. I am grateful to Nicola Hole, Archives Assistant, Bristol Archives for her research on my behalf. I am also grateful to Reverend Dr Norman Gamble, Archivist of the Irish Railway Record Society, for his insights and advice on the matter of records survival and compensation matters.

[79] Census return for William Buggy: http://www.census.nationalarchives.ie/reels/nai000095399/ (accessed 9 October 2021).

case of James Kelly, who was seen to push a passenger from a moving train, did not meet the threshold of a true bill being found. The tram companies were powerful and wealthy, and their ability to pay compensation to relatives of the deceased meant that employees had greater protection.

'A murder of children playing about': H-Car Deaths

Communal parenting with everybody and nobody looking after each individual child, and an assumption that children at play would look after one another, often led to fatal consequences.[80] The following three cases occurred within three weeks of one another: on 26 July 1900, 17-month-old John James Allen was knocked down by a horse and cart near 63 Church Street. According to two eye-witnesses there was 'No one in charge of the child'; he suffered fracture of the skull and laceration of the brain.[81] In the following month, two 6-year-old girls, Elizabeth/ Ellen Green/Greene[82] and Bridget Fitzpatrick, were both knocked down, on 30 July at North King Street and on 16 August at Townsend Street, respectively. The same injuries were described.[83] In all three 'child' cases discussed here the jury exonerated the driver from all blame. It is interesting to note that Allen's mother was not castigated in a jury rider as in the cases of burns occurring in domestic settings but her whereabouts was investigated. Ironically, urban public space and its layers of biopower surveillance in the form of police, public health inspectors, clergy, and neighbours offered mothers small freedoms as the public at large shared responsibility for child safety. Streets were what Patrick Joyce terms a 'socially neutral space'.[84] He differentiates between streets as thoroughfares, and lanes and alleys, which he contends (citing Martin Daunton) had a degree of 'social privacy' associated with 'the experience of space prior to the intervention of the municipality'.[85]

With the expansion and electrification of the tramlines, other vehicular traffic was displaced, and even in cases where drivers made poor decisions, they were exonerated. For example, John Begg, the driver of a hay-laden cart was exonerated

---

[80] Hester Barron and Claudia Siebrecht (eds), *Parenting and the State in Britain and Europe, c.1870–1950 : Raising the Nation* (Basingstoke, 2017).

[81] NAI/1900/78 Inquest on the body of John James Allen, 26 July 1900; Denis Kelly and Mary Kelly, 64 Church Street; the cart was property of Irish Sterilised Milk, Ice and Cold storage Co Limited, Island Bridge and driven by Martin Keating 66 Church Street; *Freeman's Journal*, 27 July 1900, reported the story and in its telling the exonerated driver was unnamed.

[82] NAI/1900/80 Inquest on the body of Elizabeth Greene, 30 July 1900; *Irish Daily Independent*, 31 July 1900; witness statements dated 30 July 1900; the cart was property of Philip Mahon, Newtown, County Dublin, was driven by John Begg, Drishogue, Ballyboghil, and was carrying a load of hay.

[83] NAI/1900/98 Inquest on the body of Bridget Fitzpatrick, 16 August 1900; driver of 'brewers dray' was not named—it was noted that he saw the child and shouted at her to get back.

[84] Patrick Joyce, *The Rule of Freedom: Liberalism and the Modern City* (London, 2003), p. 151.

[85] Joyce, *The Rule of Freedom*, pp. 88–9.

by the jury even though he ventured down North King Street with a load of hay that was far too wide for the width of the street. John Smyth, an eye-witness from 141 North King Street, testified that the hay was overhanging the cart and occupying three quarters of the pathway. He was driving at pace towards Capel Street too close to the narrow footpath and in the process hit three people: a woman named Margaret Byrne was wheeling her child in a perambulator down the street—the cart knocked her down and threw her child out of its pram, and another child named Elizabeth Green was fatally injured.[86] The driver was charged with wilful negligence in the management of a horse and cart—he was brought before the City of Dublin Commission on 1 August 1900 but, despite his prior convictions, no bill was found against him.[87]

In marked contrast with these three north inner-city cases, when 6-year-old Patrick Byrne was knocked down on John Dillon Street in the south side, the jury returned the expert medical advice as the verdict, but recommended the mother to the 'kind consideration of the van owners'. There was little difference between the circumstances of this and the other three cases, which merits comment. Anne Lynch of 21 Meath Street witnessed the accident and claimed that she called out to the driver three times, but he was going too fast to stop. Although there were no public safety or first aid campaigns to raise awareness of what to do, her reaction was immediate and innate—she picked up the unconscious child and took a split second decision to run to the doctor at 20 High Street (a distance of 328 yards or 300 meters, it was to Dr Abraham Tarleton's residence as it happened). Unfortunately, the doctor was out and by then Constable John Quigley 166A (Chancery Lane police station) came on the scene. They went together in a cab to Meath Street Hospital.[88] Dr Patterson pronounced life extinct on arrival as the child had suffered a punctured lung. On leaving the hospital, Lynch and Quigley met the driver who asked about the child—it was at that point he was arrested, charged, 'and given the usual caution'.[89] The driver claimed that the boy was one of several playing football in the street and that he did all he could to 'pull up' but was unable to stop in time. He also alleged that the child ran under the horses' feet.[90] While there was no evidence of alcohol consumption, the driver was charged with manslaughter and the van owners (Messrs Cooney, 56–60 Back Lane, at John Dillon Street, a mustard, laundry blue and black lead manufacturing

---

[86] *Freeman's Journal*, 31 July 1900; *Irish Daily Independent*, 31 July 1900.

[87] NAI, Dublin Crown Files at Commission, August 1900, Queen v John Begg, manslaughter. Begg was no stranger to the courts, he was fined £1 for assaulting his son in January 1900, and £2 for assaulting his wife in May that year—he defaulted payment and was sent to Kilmainham gaol for a month. NAI, CSPS1/09020 Swords Petty Sessions Register, case 29, 9 Feb 1900 and case 101, 23 June 1900.

[88] NAI/1900/190 Inquest on the body of Patrick Byrne, 10 December 1900.

[89] NAI/1900/190 DMP report dated 10 December 1900.

[90] NAI/1900/190 DMP report dated 10 December 1900.

company), were asked to compensate his mother.[91] Local knowledge of the financial situations of families and indeed commercial entities played a large discretionary part in how jury riders were composed. Unlike the north inner-city case of John James Allen, the whereabouts of Barbara Byrne at the time of the incident was not brought into question. Although it was not mentioned in the court records, the census shows that Mrs Byrne was respectable because she had the gravitas of being a widow and was deserving because she had four other dependant children.[92] The driver Martin Keating was brought before the August Commission but no bill was found against him.[93] Cases like his were almost a time-wasting exercise as they were routinely dismissed.

When driver Edward Byrne was charged with 'negligently managing the vehicle' and causing the death of 17-month-old William O'Brien on 3 July at 10 a.m. he told Police Constable Hugh McDermott 31B Lad Lane: 'I could not help it. I did not see the child until I had passed over it. There were a murder of children playing about.' What is unusual in this case is that the child's mother, Bridget, had placed him in the care of an older child 'for a few minutes' when it walked out into the street. They lived at 24 South Cumberland Street and the child's presence at Harcourt Street some twenty minutes' walk away was described as 'by some unexplained means'. It is not clear where Bridget O'Brien was when she placed the child under another child's care but small children wandering abroad was not an unusual sight in Dublin. Witness to the accident, Mary Dooley of 1 Hamilton Row, testified that the 'driver pulled up immediately on my shouting. The float was going very slowly. I did not see any children near the deceased at the time of the accident.'[94] The jury rider exonerated the driver from all blame, but an appeal was made to his employers Messrs Wells and Holohan, Harcourt Place for kind consideration and compensation to his family.[95] The company was represented at the inquest by W.T. Sheridan, solicitor, who said he would convey the jury recommendation to them.[96] Edward Byrne was brought before the Southern Police Court and exonerated because of the coronial court verdict of accidental death.[97] Compensation was very much a discretionary matter. Following the death of his

[91] '56 to 60, Back Lane, Cooney's manufacturing, manufrs. of mustard, laundry blue, blacking and black lead manufacturing company': *Thom's Directory, 1901*, p. 1359.

[92] See http://www.census.nationalarchives.ie/pages/1901/Dublin/Merchants_Quay/John_Dillon_Street/1304462/ (accessed 20 December 2018).

[93] NAI/Dublin Crown Files at Commission, 1 August 1900: *King v Martin Keating*, manslaughter.

[94] NAI/1901/179 Inquest on the body of William O'Brien, 3 July 1901.

[95] *Freeman's Journal*, 4 July 1901.

[96] A similar set of circumstance caused the death of Mary McKenna: NAI/1901/225 Inquest on the body of Mary McKenna, 28 August 1901: 'Rupture of splenic vein and liver the immediate cause of death being internal haemorrhage and shock'. Vanman, George Wetterfield, 11 Gullestin Place Rathmines was charged with carelessness and negligence in the management of a horse yoked to a laden mineral water van. Child was from 6 Werburgh Street and crossed road in front of the van which was going at a slow pace but could not stop in time—she died shortly after reaching Adelaide Hospital. Driver was sober.

[97] *Evening Herald*, 3 July 1901.

son, Robert McKenna tried to take an action against Thomas McKinley H-car owner for damages in respect of his son's death. The child suffered a scalp wound on 22 December and died eight days later at the Meath Hospital. One of McKinley's employees knocked the child down.[98] Because the coroner's verdict exculpated the driver, the Recorder dismissed the case.[99]

An obvious question that emerges from this cohort of cases is why people did not hear impending danger. The answer seems to lie in a combination of factors, from the competing sounds of the cityscape to poor road-user awareness. In his discussion of the location of Quaker Meeting Houses in eighteenth-century Philadelphia, Richard Cullen Rath traces how one site was closed owing to the disturbances of street noise. He contended that despite the introduction of innovations like noise-reducing paving for wheels, the sound of horseshoes on cobble-stoned streets created greater levels of noise than modern motorcars.[100] The Dublin streetscape of the early twentieth century was very different to Philadelphia of the eighteenth, where several other ambient noises of bells, street traders, children at play, horses, barking dogs, trams, and trains probably drowned out the shouts of pull up, and the names of the children who were being called back by parents and others nearby. In a special edition of *Urban History* on the history of music in 2002, Peter Borsay drew distinction between music and sound and questioned the threshold at which both became noise.[101] Historians of aural culture are very naturally drawn to the place of music and the past, and how acoustic architecture emerged. The streetscape, by contrast, has not received the same level of attention. John Picker argued in 2012 that the 'auditory landscape of the past' had been largely ignored by scholars of social and literary history, and since then little has changed. With respect to Dublin, literary scholars of Joyce and O'Casey might contest that claim strongly, but perhaps social and urban historians are still guilty of this charge.[102] There is a marked difference between listening and hearing, and while I am not casting any aspersions on the auditory health of the victims discussed here, if the evidence of warning sounds is taken into account, then maybe varying degrees of deafness was a factor. What is more likely is that unsupervised children who had no sense of danger were inured to the sounds of it. For them the streetscape was as much their home as the tenements they came from and there was safety in numbers. In all the cases discussed here, the victims were in the company of other and usually older children with a

[98] NAI/1901/2 Inquest on the body of Patrick McKenna, 1 January 1901.
[99] *Evening Herald*, 19 February 1901.
[100] Richard Cullen Rath, 'No corner for the devil to hide', in John Streane (ed.), *The Sound Studies Reader* (Abingdon, 2012), pp. 130–40 at 137.
[101] He asked, 'Where is the boundary between music and sound? On which side of the divide lies the ritual use of "instruments" like drums and bells, or the cries of street traders?' See Peter Borsay, 'Sounding the town', *Urban History*, 29:1 (2002), pp. 92–102 at 97.
[102] John Picker, 'The soundproof study', in John Streane (ed.), *The Sound Studies Reader* (Abingdon, 2012), pp. 141–51 at 144.

responsible adult not too far away. What is most striking about these deaths is that parents were not prosecuted for neglect. All drivers were arrested at the scene or shortly thereafter, and any imputation of drink taken could elevate the charge from dangerous driving to manslaughter. Bill Luckin argues that the whole area of drink driving was governed by ambiguous legislation and much was left to the discretion of coroners, lower courts, and juries to decide the more complex issue of when inebriation posed personal and public risk.[103] Luckin concludes that, irrespective of social class, anyone convicted under manslaughter charges for drink driving offences between 1890 and 1920 were simply unlucky.[104] Motor cars had yet to make their mark on the Dublin streetscape—when introduced they posed several new risks to other road users, especially pedestrians.

Accidental Deaths in Waterways

Dublin City's physical geography was defined by its waterways: the bisection of the river Liffey gave rise to its north/south divide and the man-made Royal and Grand Canals marked two of its four outer perimeters, the others being the North and South Circular Roads. As such, the streetscape also encompassed waterways, and deaths associated with drowning and suspected suicides are very significant in these data. Of the total number of fifty-seven cases of death by drowning only three involved adult females—one was an unknown case of a woman aged about 30 and the other two were of named individuals—all three reports included evidence of intent to self-harm.[105] Excluding suspected suicides and work-related deaths by drowning, thirty people drowned either accidentally or while swimming. Seven were cases of unknown adult men found floating, so it was not possible for investigating DMP constables or the jury to ascertain how they ended up in the water. A dearth in swimming skills combined with poor awareness of the risks associated with deep water, strong currents, and tides, gave rise to most of the male deaths in the canals, the river, and near Clontarf, which was the most accessible seafront to residents of the north inner city. Coronial court juries regularly pointed to the fact that the city's waterways lacked comprehensive public safety signage and life-saving devices.

Associational culture surrounding water sports invariably did not extend to the working classes.[106] Ronan Foley contends that even in fishing communities in the

---

[103] Bill Luckin, 'Drunk driving, drink driving: Britain, c.1800–1920', in Tom Crook and Mike Esbester (eds), *Governing Risks in Modern Britain: Danger, Safety and Accidents, c.1800–2000* (Basingstoke, 2016), pp. 171–94.

[104] Luckin, 'Drunk driving'.

[105] NAI/1900/7 Inquest on the body of an unknown woman, 26 April 1900.

[106] *Freeman's Journal*, 22 July 1901. Newspaper reports of the Pembroke Annual Gala, held in late July 1901, indicate that the teams competing were drawn from Dublin University, Pembroke Swimming Club, and the Dublin Swimming Club, all-male elite clubs that had membership subscriptions associated with them.

West of Ireland the sea was a fearful entity and swimming was not part of the 'vernacular coastal cultures' and he traces the rise of mass participation to the 1940s.[107] Further to this, the bathing houses along the Dublin coastline and membership of swimming clubs were the preserve of the middle and upper classes.[108] Lifesaving skills were more common to the elite in Ireland. Although the Royal Humane Society (established 1776, London) had a presence from the early nineteenth century, very few awards for bravery were presented by the Lord Mayor of Dublin on its behalf.[109]

Working-class women and girls were unlikely to engage in pursuits that involved undressing in public, particularly in built-up areas surrounding the Grand and Royal Canals. The positioning of the canal system as a primary transport artery was usurped by the railways in the latter half of the nineteenth century, and it was not properly maintained from dredging and foliage perspectives. That state of neglect was a possible factor in the death of Isaac Grey, who had gone for a night swim in the Grand Canal with two other men. He had taken no drink and unlike the other casualties in this cohort of deaths, he was a good swimmer. It was reported in Grey's inquest that the DMP had been trying to stamp out the practice as the canal was full of mud and weeds. To deter what it regarded as unsafe practices, the DMP had prosecuted four swimmers in the previous month, presumably under nuisance or parks, common, and open spaces legislation.[110] The unprotected canal banks posed year-round dangers—Dominick Nolan, aged 7 from 63 St Joseph's Place, Lower Dorset Street was out playing by the Royal Canal near Binn's Bridge, Drumcondra, with another little boy, named Thomas Glennon in November 1900, when he went missing. Nolan was a good walking distance from his house and was missing for three days before his body was recovered.[111] Thomas Gartland's body was also found at Binn's Bridge: he was last seen on 7 December 1901—it was a dark and stormy night and his wife testified that he had been drinking heavily of late.[112] Irrespective of his drinking habits, that two deaths occurred in precisely the same place a year or so apart indicates that greater efforts should have been made to protect the public from

[107] Ronan Foley, *Healing Waters: Therapeutic Landscapes in Historic and Contemporary Ireland* (Farnham, 2010), pp. 116, 120.

[108] Fergus Barron, *Swimming for a Century* (Dublin, 1993); *The Irish Times*, 27 November 1893. The Irish Amateur Swimming Association was established in Belfast on 25 November 1893, when the Leinster and Ulster Swimming Association agreed to adopt the organised races and maintain the rules of the parent body in Britain.

[109] For example, James A. Abbott of 23 Merchant's Quay who tried to save a man from drowning in the Liffey on 15 June 1901: *Evening Herald*, 9 August 1901. Thomas Longmire received a certificate for his attempt to save Ellen Moriarty. Christopher Love, *A Social History of Swimming in England, 1800–1918: Splashing in the Serpentine* (Abingdon, 2015), p. 104; Ciarán McCabe, 'Humane society movement and the transnational exchange of medical knowledge', *Journal of the Royal College of Physicians of Edinburgh*, 49:2 (2019), pp. 158–64.

[110] *Irish Daily Independent*, 31 July 1900; *Irish Daily Independent*, 31 July 1900; *Dublin Daily Nation*, 31 July 1900.

[111] NAI/1900/165 Inquest on the body of Dominick Nolan, 13 November 1900.

[112] NAI/1901/304 Inquest on the body of Thomas Gartland, 9 December 1901.

exposed and dangerous waterways. Further to these drowning deaths caused by slipping into the canals, 14-year-old John Kenny drowned when he slipped off a makeshift boat made from planks while he was out was rowing on a pond off Ossory Road with two other boys.[113]

With sad predictability, every July and August warm weather combined with a rise in the Irish Sea temperatures created an increase in the number of young men and boys dying in drowning accidents. A heatwave hit Dublin in the first week of July 1901 and the weather remained 'fine' for the rest of month.[114] In mid-July 1901, Kevin Quinn went with his friend James Spence to Curley's Hole on the North Bull to swim. Bull Island was not a natural formation—it appeared following the construction of sea walls in the late eighteenth and early nineteenth centuries. Part of the rationale for the sea walls was to channel the force of the river to assist with dredging, and the net result was that the stretch of water at the mouth of the River Liffey leading to the Irish Sea was treacherous—it was not a suitable bathing area for inexperienced swimmers, especially at ebb tide.[115] When Quinn got into difficulty, Spence tried to save him but his efforts failed. Quinn, in his panic, grabbed him by the neck, which left Spence with no option but to extricate himself and call for help. Samuel Wright, a passer-by, swam out to assist in the rescue but to no avail—Quinn did not resurface. It was described in evidence by District Inspector Stewart as a 'treacherous place, in fact a regular quicksand', where several young men had drowned over the years; he asked the jury to make a recommendation that it be marked out so that 'boys coming out from the city should keep clear of it'.[116] With the redrawing of the metropolitan boundary, enacted January 1900, commencement date 15 January 1901, Clontarf Township became part of the city, and the jurors questioned why the DMP did not patrol the area.[117] In the week that followed, a few letters were published in newspapers in an effort to force the authorities to do something about the problem: 'Year after year we hear of drowning accidents in this ill-fated hole, and still nothing is done to protect that stranger visiting Clontarf.'[118] The jury recommended the gallant conduct of James Spence of 49 Summerhill and Samuel H. Wright of 33 Drury Street to the Royal Humane Society. Quinn was one of ten children and a plumber's son, and unusually for his social class, his funeral notice was published in the *Freeman's Journal*. His funeral moved from his family home at 11 North William Street to Glasnevin Cemetery, where he was buried.[119]

---

[113] NAI/1901/275 Inquest on the body of John Kenny, 29 October 1901.
[114] *Evening Herald*, 9 July 1901.
[115] P.G. Kennedy, 'Violation of sanctuary', *Studies: An Irish Quarterly Review*, 38:149 (March 1949), pp. 37–45.
[116] *Irish Daily Independent*, 16 July 1901; NAI/1901/186 Inquest on Kevin Quinn dated 15 July 1901.
[117] Dublin Corporation Act 1900 (63 & 64 Vict.) c. 264 s. 4.
[118] *Evening Herald*, 20 July 1901.   [119] *Freeman's Journal*, 16 July 1901.

On the eve of the well-advertised Clontarf Regatta, which was described as an aquatic event, Dublin national school children received their summer holidays.[120] To mark the occasion a few boys headed from the north inner city towards Dollymount Strand, to go for a swim. It was ebb tide when Thomas Curley, aged 12, got into difficulty—he was only able to swim a little. He called out to his friend James O'Connor who was by then on the shore, but a passing woman warned him not to re-enter the water as it was too dangerous. Two men, Joseph Ledwidge and Edward Thair, went to Curley's rescue and they recovered his body within an hour. He was subject to coronial inquiry after he drowned in the same place as Quinn.[121] It occasioned further letters to the newspapers about whether the Port and Docks or the Board of Trade was responsible for erecting a sign and some safety equipment.[122] Both Curley and Quinn were working-class boys whose schools were unlikely to have been participants in the physical education programmes offered in the elite boys' schools like Belvedere College—neither could swim properly.[123]

The city's more immediate waterways also claimed a few lives that summer: Denis McGuirk, aged 69, jumped in the River Liffey while drunk and threatened to kick anyone who would stop him. He got into difficulty and drowned.[124] Nine-year-old Thomas Rogers from 6 Newfoundland Street was playing around the docklands area with a neighbour, William Kirwan, on 2 August. He was reported missing on 5 August and his body was recovered from the River Liffey on 7 August 1901. In a tale that combines child's play with the normality of a 9-year-old contributing to his family survival through begging, Kirwan revealed how he left the deceased as he was trying to get some grain from a vessel and he did not see him again.[125] On the same day Kirwan's body was recovered, Nicholas O'Kelly, aged 10, drowned in the Royal Canal while swimming with Thomas Leonard, aged 11. O'Kelly got into difficulty and Leonard tried to save him—they both got into difficulty. Edward Moore was passing by and he saved Leonard, but by the time he realised there was a second boy in the water it was too late. Police used grappling irons to drag the canal and discovered the body later that day.[126] A few weeks later, 8-year-old Patrick Quelch died in the Grand Canal while swimming with

[120] *Evening Herald*, 22 July 1901.

[121] *Irish Daily Independent*, 22 July 1901; NAI/1901/193 Inquest on Thomas Curley dated 20 July 1901.

[122] *Evening Herald*, 23 July 1901.

[123] Charlotte Bennett, '"Help to win the war" or "Ireland above all"?: Remobilisation, politics, and elite boys' education in Ireland, 1917–18', *Irish Historical Studies*, 44:166 (2020), pp. 326–48. Curley's father was a labourer in a corn store: http://www.census.nationalarchives.ie/reels/nai003813905/ (accessed 26 July 2021).

[124] NAI/1901/166 Inquest on the body of Denis McGuirk, 20 July 1901.

[125] NAI/1901/207 Inquest on the body of Thomas Rogers, 8 August 1901; *Evening Herald*, 8 August 1901.

[126] NAI/1901/206 Inquest on the body of Nicholas O'Kelly, 7 August 1901; *Evening Herald*, 7 August 1901.

friends.[127] Nine accidental drownings occurred between June and August 1901. Shared features in all cases were the dearth in swimming skills, the absence of life-saving skills and equipment, and the lack of policing of dangerous water-fronts. The authorities shirked responsibilities towards the public with respect to water safety. After these deaths the matter of training the DMP in first aid and in resuscitation methods set out by the Royal Humane Society was raised in questions with the Chief Secretary, George Wyndham, but he did not address the matter properly in his response.[128] With public pressure brought to bear, in August 1901 the Dublin Port and Docks Board eventually agreed to place lifebuoys along the North Bull.[129]

Workplace Deaths

Workplaces were the scenes of horrendous accidents. Falling from heights in boats and on building sites were very common causes of serious injury; workers were also at risk of goods, concrete, bricks, and building debris falling on top of them. In this sample of coronial court cases, a total of 109 deaths were caused by, or occurred at, work. Of these deaths, forty were as a result of falls, twenty-two people were sick and died while at work, nineteen were crushed, hit, or caught by mechanical devices, fourteen drowned (another was crushed in a lock gate and drowned as a result), nine were knocked down, two died because of goods falling on top of them, and there was one death each from choking, fire, and suicide (the latter is also counted here because of its workplace location and links to cause of death, but will be discussed in the penultimate chapter).[130] Greer and Nicholson contend that in occupational accident terms, males aged between 13 and 18 were the most at-risk group, but the average age of ninety-nine male deaths in this sample is 39 (in four cases ages were not given).[131] Only six cases involved women, and of these, four cases were as a result of chronic illness. Simon Purdue posits that men were at the greatest risk of injury in Belfast because they conducted the most dangerous jobs;, for instance the maintenance of heavy machinery.[132] Although the male Dublin workforce did not face the same intensity of occupational hazards as their Belfast compatriots in the shipyards of Harland and Wolff

---

[127] NAI/1901/215 Inquest on the body of Patrick Quelch; *Irish Daily Independent*, 20 August 1901.
[128] *Irish Daily Independent*, 12 August 1901.   [129] *Weekly Irish Times*, 10 August 1901.
[130] NAI/1901/279 Inquest on the body of Jane Boylan, 2 November 1901: 'Jane Boylan, 64, servant at brothel. Asphyxia the result of food accidentally entering the trachea Worked at 4 Lr Tyrone St a brothel for previous 5 yrs. Harry Looney who resides in charge of brothel reported that she was found by Louisa Williams a prostitute, Mrs Lawless was the owner.'
[131] Desmond Greer and James W. Nicholson, *The Factory Acts in Ireland, 1802–1914* (Dublin, 2002), p. 137.
[132] Simon Purdue, 'Giving life and limb for empire: gender and occupational health in industrial Belfast, 1870–1914', *Irish Historical Studies*, 43:164 (2019), pp. 220–36 at 234.

they still encountered the risks of being crushed by heavy machinery and of items falling on them. According to this dataset, shipping and construction were the most dangerous sectors. Dock workers were at risk of falling into the water and into a ship's hold but were equally at risk of goods falling from a height on top of them from overloaded cranes and faulty hoists.[133] Falls from ladders and badly structured scaffolding were the biggest risk factors for construction workers.

Despite the series of factory acts passed throughout the nineteenth century, health and safety precautions were seriously deficient. Preoccupied with regulating the hours women and children could work in the textile industry, initially the acts only applied to larger sites, until the Factory Acts (Extension) Act 1867 broadened the remit to workshops and sites with over fifty employees. A factory inspectorate was established in 1833 but it was limited in its operation. Under the 1844 act, dangerous machinery was to be fenced off—this workplace safety measure raised awareness of the dangers and this undoubtedly saved many lives.[134] The acts also concerned sanitary conditions, ventilation, and overcrowding on larger sites. The 1901 Factory Act had several further provisions to 'protect life and limb', including certificates of fitness to work for children and women four weeks post-partum.[135] Settlement of disputes with respect to wages and damages under the amount of £10 could be dealt with in courts of summary jurisdiction under the Employers and Workmen Act, 1875.[136] Employees could take claims against employers under the 1880 Liability Act.[137] Injuries had to be serious and occasion a minimum of a fortnight off work, but if the employee was found to be negligent then the employer did not have to provide any compensation. Major advances were made in labour rights when the Workmen's Compensation Act (WCA), 1897, stipulated that, if in the course of workplace duties employees suffered injuries, they were entitled to payments.[138]

For the purposes of the Factory Acts' inspection and reporting, Ireland was coupled with Scotland. Reflecting industrial patterns, the country was divided into 'North' and 'South Ireland' and the reports lack specificity. According to Greer and Nicholson, 1,588 of a total number of 240,003 workers reported accidents in 1900—645 were of Class A or serious nature caused by 'mechanical power', while the 922 Class B accidents were ones that caused workers to miss more than three days of work.[139] Cause of death 'by accident or negligence' statistics were published nationally, and by gender and age in the annual reports of the

---

[133] *Annual Report of the Chief Inspector of Factories and Workshops, for 1900 (Factories—Shops—Workshops: Annual Report)* [Cd. 668], p. 111.

[134] Factories Act 1844 (7 & 8 Vic.) c. 15.

[135] NA, The Factory and Workshop Act, 1901; *British Medical Journal*, 2 (1901), p. 1871; Greer and Nicholson, *The Factory Acts in Ireland*, p. 69; Factory and Workshop Act, 1901 (Edw. VII) c. 22.

[136] Employers and Workmen Act 1875 (56 & 57 Vic.) c. 54.

[137] Employers' Liability Act, 1880 (43 & 44 Vic.) c. 42.

[138] Workmen's Compensation Act, 1897 (60 & 61 Vic.) c. 37.

[139] Greer and Nicholson, *The Factory Acts in Ireland*, p. 137.

Registrar General (ARRGs).[140] The Registrar General extracted figures for Dublin for the purposes of the 1900 report and provided average statistics for the eleven years from 1888 to 1899, but that was a one-off occurrence.

Differentiation must be made between employees of established companies and those who were self-employed, low-paid workers, and casual labourers, particularly where ill-health is concerned. The Committee on Dangerous Trades concluded in 1899 that there must have been several deaths that were listed as being from natural causes when the root of the medical issue was industrial in nature. It cited cases of lead poisoning as an example.[141] Cardiac disease caused fifteen people in this sample to die at work—whether they were oblivious to their chronic health condition or ignored symptoms was not always recorded. What is certain is that they were drawn from the class of people who could not afford to lose a day's wage. Four of the cardiac deaths were coupled with a pulmonary complication. There were five deaths associated with ruptures of blood vessels, one case of peritonitis and three cases concerned tuberculosis (one kidney and two pulmonary, the latter being coupled with cardiac causes). Occupations included general labourer, shop girl, grocer's assistant, night watchman, H-car driver, servant, and corporation messenger, all of which were low-paid workers, with an average age of 46 for twenty-two of the twenty-three cases for which age was given. Medical cause of death has received attention in Chapters 1 and 2, but it is important to reiterate how vulnerable to poverty these precarious workers were. Joseph Bruce is included here as he died on his return home following a day of exertion at work: he is among a cohort of people who ignored their personal health concerns so he could continue to earn a wage. Dr George Taylor noted a long list of potential causes of poor health—Bruce's lungs were described as emphysematous, and his heart and kidneys both had evidence of extensive disease. A labourer in the employment of Mr Malcolm, contractor, of 24 Eden Quay, Bruce was on his way home to 23 Northumberland Road when he started to spit up blood at Grattan Street. Even with his long list of medical problems, he had not been attended to by a doctor.[142] That he was not at work when he died, and that he was more than likely a casual worker meant that his relatives' claim to compensation was weak. Sarah Hamilton's death from 'cardiac failure due to thrombosis of coronary artery' occurred while working in a field in Cabra. Aged 65 and of no fixed abode, she was engaged in a casual labour arrangement—her co-worker Bridget Murray who was also 'weeding in a field in Cabra', spotted her suffering a weakness. She was literally dying on her feet while conducting backbreaking work.[143] Her case is indicative of the vulnerability of older women to

---

[140] *Thirty-seventh detailed annual report of the Registrar-General (Ireland), 1900* [Cd. 697], p. 155.
[141] *Dangerous Trades Committee. Final report of the Departmental Committee appointed to inquire into and report upon certain miscellaneous dangerous trades (1899)* [C.9509], p. 6.
[142] NAI/1900/16 Inquest on the body of Joseph Bruce held on 3 May 1900.
[143] *Evening Herald*, 25 May 1900; NAI/1900/28 inquest on the body of Sarah Hamilton dated 24 May.

abject poverty in a city where stability was difficult for a single wage earner to achieve. She was identified by Esther Travers of 9 Ward's Hill, who shared a similar socio-economic profile of being unemployed and aged 60. Travers had a lodger, 59-year-old Catherine Davis, who provided her with much-needed cash income.[144] When accidents happened to self-employed or casually employed workers they had few recourses, such as the 'elderly' William Slye (aged 64) a carman who died at the Meath Hospital on 28 January 1901 from sepsis eleven days after he suffered a compound dislocation of the left foot.[145] The rest of this section discusses cases of workers who had more, albeit hard-won, job security in the breweries, docks, the building site, and the factory.

Guinness's Brewery was one of the city's biggest employers and eight men died on company properties over the two-year period discussed here. The first death was that of Patrick Gargan who suffered major internal bleeding as a result of lacerations to his liver when he was accidentally caught between a wagon and a wall at Guinness's Brewery on 5 November 1900. Technically this was a railway accident, the nature of which I will discuss further below.[146] He was single and had only been employed there for two months prior to his accident. Guinness provided his father with a donation of £10 which included a £3 burial allowance and a contribution of £10 was given towards a memorial for him.[147] The brewery was undergoing expansion at the turn of the century and the seven other deaths were associated with construction and renovation. William Kerr, a slater in the employment of Samuel Bolton, builders of Rathmines, was on a scaffold seventy-three feet from the ground when he fell a distance of about twenty-three feet into an iron tank on 22 February 1901.[148] A few weeks later, William McKay, who was in the employment of Messrs McCullagh and Nearne, Painters, Saint Stephen's Green, was engaged in painting the interior of a new building at Rainsfort Street when he fell from a plank about fifty feet from ground.[149] A tarpaulin was spread ten feet from ground to protect Guinness employees working beneath and it gave way as he fell.[150] In an effort to reposition liability, Hugh McLaughlin, a foreman at McCullagh and Nearne, made the point that it was Guinness workers who erected the tarpaulin. McKay fell through the safety net and on top of a heap of 'hoop iron' and all of his vital organs suffered major trauma. He was sent straight to Dr Steevens' Hospital at 4.15 p.m. but such was the extent of his injuries that there was little Dr Dobbin could do for him: he died at 5.30 p.m.[151] The jury rider

---

[144] See http://www.census.nationalarchives.ie/reels/nai003802950/ (accessed 19 October 2021).

[145] NAI/1901/27 inquest on the body of William Slye, 30 January 1901.

[146] NAI/1900/160 Inquest on the body of Patrick Gargan, 9 November 1900; *Freeman's Journal*, 9 November 1900; *The Irish Times*, 9 November 1900.

[147] GDB/PE01/008872. I am very grateful to Eibhlin Colgan, Archive Manager, Guinness Archive, Dublin, for this information.

[148] *Irish Daily Independent*, 22 February 1901; NAI/1901/51 Inquest on the body of William Kerr, 22 February 1901.

[149] *Freeman's Journal*, 29 March 1901.   [150] *Freeman's Journal*, 29 March 1901.

[151] NAI/1901/90 Inquest on the body of William McKay, 28 March 1901.

was deliberately oblique: 'we consider that proper precaution was not taken to protect the lives of the men'—it did not allocate responsibility for compensation to either company. Another painter, Henry Farrell, died in a similar manner at a different Guinness site, falling from a flimsy scaffold and ladder rig, but without a safety net. The jury in that instance placed the responsibility on the sub-contractor and Farrell's employers: 'we consider the ladder did not project sufficiently far above the scaffold to be safe, therefore it was not put up in a workmanlike manner. And we recommend the relatives of the deceased to the consideration of the employers Messr Sibthorpe.'[152]

The most devastating workplace incident in this sample occurred on Guinness Brewery property on Easter Monday 1902.[153] Three men, named Henry Tobin, Joseph Birmingham, and William Owens, were crushed when they were removing a concrete floor—there could have been an even greater toll had two others not escaped. The men had been working on the adjustment of a floor height and the supporting girder was removed two days before. Irrespective of where responsibility lay, an illogical and flawed construction method was permitted to prevail on a Guinness site. Under the charge of Owens, who was described as an experienced scaffolder, the men made a plan to remove the floor from below, not above as recommended by Thomas Kelly, who was the foreman of the Guinness work team. Kelly was absent when the incident occurred. Perhaps there was some false comfort in knowing that the floor remained standing in the absence of a girder for two days. That fateful day, two of the men, Birmingham and Tobin, commenced work under the concrete floor and Owens took a sledge to the remaining supports. Inevitably, the floor gave way—Birmingham and Tobin were 'shockingly crushed' and died instantly. Owens was also crushed—he was alive but was unable to speak and died on arrival at Dr Steevens' Hospital.

The verdict was that all three died from 'Shock & haemorrhage from the accidental falling of a concrete floor in Portland St'; in the rider there was an expression of concern for worker's safety but no allocation of blame: 'And we consider the girder forming part of the support of the floor in question having been removed on Saturday and the deceased being allowed to resume work on Monday morning without any supervision whatever we must express the opinion that proper care was not used.' It was a makeshift construction team, comprising men from different companies and a high likelihood that they had no prior experience of working together. Birmingham, who was identified by his brother Myles, worked for Messrs W. Becket of Percy Place works and Owens and Tobin for Messrs Bolton Rathmines. All three inquests took place on 2 April 1902. Tobin's son Henry was the subject of a coroner's inquiry on 15 May 1900—his death from

[152] *Evening Herald*, 9 August 1901; NAI/1901/210 Inquest on the body of Henry Farrell, 9 August 1901; *Irish Daily Independent*, 10 August 1901.
[153] *Freeman's Journal*, 1 April 1902.

convulsions raised few eyebrows. The related DMP report showed that this was a solid working-class household that settled in tenements around James' Street. They were decent and respectable and there was no suspicion of foul play.[154] His wife Mary, a room keeper according to the census, was left to fend for four children under the age of 12. Dr Robert E. Halahan described the extent of Tobin's injuries as 'mutilated to a frightful extent'.[155]

Inspired by the concepts of paternalistic human resource management, Guinness had begun to develop a comprehensive cradle to grave medical system in the 1870s. Preoccupation with social mobility evidenced by strategic purchases and careful measures of benevolence characterised early Guinness family philanthropy efforts. For example, the purchase and gifting by Edward Guinness of Saint Stephen's Green to the people of Dublin in 1876 undoubtedly assisted in achieving his later honours.[156] In keeping with the example set by other members of the so-called 'Beerage', successive generations of the Guinness family married and bought their way into the nobility from the early nineteenth century. But by 1900 obscene wealth coupled with a then deeply entrenched family tradition of philanthropy meant that the family had unparalleled influence both in Ireland and at Westminster.[157] Guinness became part of a growing number of industrialists who had taken on the philanthropic ethos of employee well-being and a private system of social welfare.[158] Whatever moral imperatives might have existed, apart from Gargan, who had been employed for a mere two months, the rest of the fatalities were legally not the responsibility of the brewery.[159] Aside from a brief entry in the Brewery Annual Report citing the coroner's court verdict of insufficient supervision there is no mention in the Guinness records about the three Portland Street deaths.[160] In all six construction/renovation-related deaths located at Guinness properties the men were not recommended to the kind consideration of the brewery. Third-party contractors ('undertakers') were subcontracted to do the work and therefore were responsible for the men they

---

[154] See http://www.census.nationalarchives.ie/pages/1901/Dublin/Ushers_Quay/James_s_Street/ 1302129/ (accessed 24 June 2021).

[155] NAI/1902/54 Inquest on the body of Henry Tobin; NAI/1902/55 Inquest on the body of Joseph Bermingham; NAI/1902/56 Inquest on the body of William Owens, 2 April 1902.

[156] Saint Stephen's Green (Dublin) Act 1877, 1877 (40 & 41 Vic.) c. 134.

[157] Following his death in 1868, Sir Benjamin Lee Guinness's estate was worth £1.1 million: see Patrick Lynch and John Vaisey, *Guinness's Brewery in the Irish Economy 1759–1876* (Cambridge, 2011), p. 182.

[158] Andy Bielenberg, 'Late Victorian elite formation and philanthropy: the making of Edward Guinness', *Studia Hibernica*, 32 (2002/3), pp. 133–54.

[159] NAI/1900/160 Inquest on the body of Patrick Gargan, 9 November 1900; letter from the Inspectors of Factories and Workshops responding to the Coroner's request to attend the inquest at Dr Steevens' Hospital, 8 November 1900.

[160] GDB/CO04.11/0001.05, 'Annual Reports 1902 A. Guinness Son & Co. Ltd', Guinness Archive, Diageo Ireland. I am very grateful to Eibhlin Colgan for this reference.

employed.[161] It is unclear what settlements, if any, were made. The eighth, and final, death at Guinness's Brewery was that of Michael Conroy, who worked for contractors Messrs Wilson and Company Brewers Engineer, Somerset, and his was the only case where equal liability was levied by a coroner's jury rider. Between 7 a.m. and 8 a.m., 16 January 1902, he fell from a height of just over ten feet through a hole in the floor at Rainsford Street. He suffered a skull fracture and died later that day at Dr Steevens' Hospital. As both parties shared liability, the jury recommended his widow, mother, and relatives to the kind consideration of both Guinness and the contractors.[162]

Brewing and distilling were significant economic growth areas and there were two further deaths at other locations. In what appears to have been a direct employment contract, the jury requested 'kind consideration' of the widow and children in the case of Christopher Kelly, who died from serious head injuries when he fell from a scaffold at Jameson's Distillery in Bow Street on 26 September 1900.[163] The final case was one of clear employer responsibility. Patrick Fagan was oiling cogs at the Phoenix Brewery, James Street, when he got caught in the machinery. His right arm and a portion of his jaw were torn away. He somehow managed to walk outside and was taken by H-car to Dr Steevens' Hospital where he died at 5.45 a.m. the following day.[164]

There were a number of single casualty construction incidents. For example, John Bradley died when he fell from a scaffold at the gasworks. William Causea, the site foreman, testified that he had twenty years' experience and instructed that no expense be spared in the construction of the scaffold. He declared that he had tested it for 13 cwt as well as the weight of four men a fortnight prior. Four men were on it when one of the wires holding the scaffolding in place snapped. Legal representation for the Gas Company emphatically stated that the contractors, Messrs Piggot and Company of London, were fully responsible.[165] John Doyle was engaged in concreting the top of a third storey wall of the Tercentenary Building under construction at Trinity College Dublin when his accident occurred. He went to investigate the delay on the delivery of building materials and fell through the open space through which they were hoisted. He was employed by contractors Emery and Sharp, Great Brunswick Street.[166] The jury verdict of accidental death was returned in both instances, which was an import-

---

[161] *Brennan v The Dublin United Tramways Company* [1901], 2 IR 241. Brennan lost an eye while working for the DUTC—the Recorder of Dublin found in favour of applicant. DUTC appealed and it was argued that as Brennan was working for a contractor on ancillary (non-essential) work, the decision should be reversed.

[162] NAI/1902/9 Inquest on the body of Michael Conroy, 18 January 1902.

[163] NAI/1900/121 Inquest on the body of Christopher Kelly, 28 September 1900.

[164] NAI/1901/237 Inquest on Patrick Fagan, 9 September 1901.

[165] *Irish Daily Independent*, 29 May 1900; NAI/1900/31 Inquest on the body of John Bradley, 28 May.

[166] NAI/1900/115 Inquest on the body of John Doyle, 19 September 1900; *Freeman's Journal*, 20 September 1900.

ant factor for future negotiation and litigation purposes. If it was found that workers were negligent, then the law was firmly on the side of employers. For example, Patrick Quinn's widow received no compensation after his fall. He was conducting brickwork on a third-floor wall and it gave way while he was 'in the act of putting a piece of timber out the window'. He fell to the second floor and debris fell on top of him. Henry A Lundy, architect of 38 Dame Street claimed when he was inspecting the premises that he noticed the 'deceased was working in a very dangerous manner'. Quinn was taken by Corporation Ambulance to Dr Steevens' Hospital and attended to by Dr Dobbin.[167] The case for compensation came before the Recorder of Dublin on 25 January 1901 and findings were against the widow on account of the deceased's 'serious and wilful misconduct'.[168]

Crushing incidents in factories were usually deemed accidental, but employers leaned heavily on the factory inspectorate to show that their machinery was properly maintained, and that they were not at fault. Patrick Connolly died shortly after his left leg was completely severed off from four inches above the knee. The DMP report speculated that while he was trying to take water from underneath a flywheel his trousers got caught. Dr Crinion and Fr Breen were sent for. He had been tending to the same machine for seven years; his father was normally the operator but he was on sick leave. Patrick Connolly had been the sole operator for about three days when the accident occurred.[169] It was stipulated that the machine had recently passed full inspection but the jury recommended his relatives for compensation.[170] Similarly, Mr Nolan, representing the Inspector of Factories, deemed the electric goods lift that caused a death at Switzers to be in perfect working order.[171] The newly installed lift had been 'handed over' by the contractor but construction workers of Messrs Booth Brothers were instructed to continue to bring goods via the stairs. Some of the men defied the direct orders and a man named Doyle used his penknife to pick the lock to the lift. Mechanic's assistant James Nolan was seriously injured when he looked over the guard rails and his head got caught by the lift, which was being operated by Thomas Brophy. No blame was attached to anyone.[172] Mr Bellhouse, Inspector of Factories, gave evidence in the case of baker Joseph Tierney who suffered from lacerated wounds on three fingers of the right hand and compound fractures of both forearms when he was taking dough out of a drum. Bellhouse stated that the machine should have been stopped and Mr O'Rourke, the bakery owner, said that he regularly gave

---

[167] NAI/1900/186 Inquest on the body of Patrick Quinn, 6 December 1900.

[168] 'M'Cabe v. The Corporation of Dublin', New Irish Jurist and Local Government Review, 1 (1900–1), p. 88.

[169] NAI/1901/112 Inquest on the body of Patrick Connolly, 17 April 1901.

[170] NAI, Workmen's Compensation Act (WCA), Dublin, Book Awards & Applications 1898–1904, p. 115. According to the WCA register his parents spent seven months dealing with the matter of arbitration—it was resolved to their satisfaction plus costs measured by the court.

[171] NAI/1901/18 Inquest on the body of James Nolan, 21 January 1901.

[172] Evening Herald, 21 January 1901.

advice to that effect. Complacency often set in with experience and while Tierney should have been more attentive to safety matters, others testified to the fact that in practice the machine 'was practically never stopped'.[173]

A few industrial accidents occurred because general noise levels drowned out shouts of warning. James Curran's death occurred after he was struck by a crane at the main drainage works at Pigeon House Fort on 21 September 1900 while trying to repair a 'hopper'. As it involved a potential manslaughter charge, the case was carefully observed by the DMP. The crane operator, James Finnegan, volunteered evidence at the inquest and DMP Inspector Grant interjected to say that he was going to arrest him for careless driving. Grant was taken to task by Mr Clay, solicitor on behalf of Messrs Pearson and Company, contractors to Dublin Corporation, for trying to make a state trial out of an inquest. Finnegan was cautioned by Dr Byrne about implicating himself, but he proceeded to state that he did not hear his co-worker Michael Reardon calling out to him. Reardon testified that he instructed Finnegan to 'to keep the grab in the boat, I don't know if he heard me'. He reiterated the matter by stating: 'Owing to the crane operating it was impossible for the crane man to hear me on account of the noise.'[174] Finnegan was treated the same as H-car drivers in cases where people were knocked down, and he was charged on remand the following day at the Southern Police Court for carelessness in the management of a steam engine.[175] The case was held over until 6 October so the Resident Surgeon, Dr Taylor, who had attended to the case at Sir Patrick Dun's Hospital could give evidence. Diagrams of the crane and the hopper showed that even if Finnegan had seen the men on the hopper, he could not have stopped in time, and the manslaughter charge was dismissed.[176] Noise levels caused George Murray to mishear the lift operator saying to steer clear while loading and unloading goods at Jacob's Biscuit Factory. Instead of staying back as instructed, he put his head into the shaft, and it got caught. He suffered spinal cord injuries which caused immediate paralysis but he was conscious and he asked his co-worker John Duff of 142 Townsend Street to call a priest, which he did not do—instead, they carried him to the Adelaide Hospital where he was detained.[177] The DMP report claimed 'there is no culpable negligence attached to any person'. Three days after his accident, on 21 September, a priest was called and last rites were administered.[178] The jury found the death was accidental but recommended the widow, Julia, who lived with their family at Athy, Co Kildare, to the kind consideration of Messrs Jacob, which undertook in the coroner's court

---

[173] NAI/1901/46 Inquest on the body of Joseph Tierney, 18 February 1901; *Irish Daily Independent*, 19 February 1901.

[174] NAI/1900/125 inquest on the body of James Curran, 3 October 1900; *Evening Herald*, 3 October 1900.

[175] *Evening Herald*, 4 October 1900.   [176] *Evening Herald*, 6 October 1900.

[177] *Irish Daily Independent*, 25 September 1900; NAI/1900/118 Inquest on the body of George Murray, 24 September 1900.

[178] *Evening Herald*, 24 September 1900.

that 'the matter would receive the attention of the firm'.[179] The amounts of these out of court settlements were, and continue to be, commercially sensitive and undisclosed.

The workplace also encompassed waterways, and deaths associated with shipping and boating are significant in these data. A total of twenty-six deaths occurred on boats or on docksides, fourteen of which were from drowning; five from falls; two deaths each were caused by crushing, being knocked down, and illness; and one was owing to goods falling on top of a worker. Thomas Tully died in the hull of a steamer after he was struck by a bag of grain that slipped out of its rope when it was being lowered into a canal boat.[180] The only person of colour in these data was Donald McDonald, a cook on board the *Royalist* who drowned after he fell into the water. He was described as a New York native. People heard cries for help at about 9.30 p.m. on 31 January 1902 and his body was recovered ten days later.[181] Schooner Captain Robert Johnston died on 24 January 1901 from immersion in the water after he got caught in the lock gate of the Spencer Dock, North Wall. He had multiple injuries and his death was from drowning, but he is counted here under crushing.[182]

Some of the drowning cases relate to occupational hazards of working on the waterways, but some were characterised by calamitous drinking sessions. I include them here as opposed to under the earlier accidental drowning section because they are intrinsically work related. In the first instance, the public house was a key part of the culture of getting dock work and drinking together was an important part of crew camaraderie. The following cases raise serious questions about the proof of the alcohol consumed as well as contemporary perceptions of drunkenness. Typical of accidents while 'drinking on the job' was the case of Daniel Dent, a 24-year-old sailor of 17 Cambridge Street, who was employed on the *Avoset*, a vessel that was moored in the Canal Basin. His wife Catherine reported the case and documented that he was working with the skipper Martin Whelan of 14 Cambridge Road, and Daniel Clarke of 34 Irishtown Road that day, 'overhauling the yacht'.[183] They spent some part of the day drinking. The witness statements recount a pub crawl of 'drink in Nolans [sic] public house 25 Upper Grand Canal St, they left about 1.30 p.m. and went home to dinner, and on their way they called at Byrne's public house, 16 Thorncastle St., Ringsend, where they

---

[179] *Irish Daily Independent*, 25 September 1900. It is likely that this Julia Murray at Belan, Kildare was his widow, and they had seven children. See http://www.census.nationalarchives.ie/reels/nai000898152/.

[180] NAI/1900/70 Inquest on the body of Thomas Tully, 17 July 1900; *Freeman's Journal*, 18 July 1900.

[181] NAI/1902/23 Inquest on the body of Donald McDonald, 12 February 1902.

[182] NAI/1901/21 Inquest on the body of Robert Johnston, 24 January 1901.

[183] NAI/1901/129 Inquest on the body of Daniel Dent, 11 May 1901; DMP Report dated 10 May 1901, Peter Byrne, SS, Irishtown E Division (DMP number not recorded). Both 17 Cambridge Street and 34 Ringsend Road are listed as tenements: *Thom's Directory, 1901*, p. 1694.

had another drink.'[184] They proceeded at 3 p.m. to go to Cassidy's, 8 Thorncastle Street, and after that drink they went back to the yacht to lock it up. This necessitated a journey out and a return to shore in a punt. On the return journey, Patrick Clarke got in first and Dent 'overbalanced himself' while getting in—in the process he capsized the punt and both were thrown into the water. Thomas Cullen, the captain of a nearby yacht the *Prima Dona* rescued Clarke and rowed towards Dent who was struggling to hold on to the bottom of the punt. Unfortunately, Dent lost his grip and sank. Clarke admitted that they had consumed both ale and porter, 'they had five or six drinks during the day', but pleaded that they were not drunk and that the 'deceased was sober & competent to mind himself'.[185] This was a persistent trope in all of the cases involving alcohol, and it was a major category of interest in the deaths of young and able-bodied men. The verdict was of 'accidental drowning in Grand Canal Basin'.[186]

Londoner John Ivors was a fireman on board the SS *Portaferry*—it left John Rogerson Quay on 1 December and was due to return on 9 December. He had been out for a drink on 30 November with his shipmates and failed to report for work on 1 December. The crew waited for him for a few hours but eventually they had to commit to the schedule. In short, he was not missed by relatives who thought he was at work and his body was found on 7 December with no identification on him.[187] Peter Brady, a 22-year-old single sailor returned from the city under the influence of drink on the evening of 8 February 1902 but was not drunk according to his comrade Edward Nolan.[188] As he boarded the *Ethel of Preston* at Sir John Rogerson Quay he slipped and fell off the ladder which extended from the ship to the quay wall. Nolan tried to catch him, but he sank immediately.[189]

Three cases occurred at Tedcastle McCormick & Company Coal merchants: John McInerney fell sixteen feet into the hold of the SS *Cumbria* while unloading goods on 14 January. He died a fortnight later of meningitis following a fracture of the skull.[190] John Herbert died of blood poisoning after he was run over by a steam crane—he suffered a terrible injury to his right thigh. The driver of the train was exonerated and Herbert's relatives were recommended to the company for 'kind consideration'.[191] Another Tedcastle employee, John Brophy, fell into the River Liffey and drowned after he had left work one evening. He was seen by two

---

[184] 8 Thorncastle Street is listed as business address of James Cassidy, grocer and spirit merchant, 12l: *Thom's Directory, 1901*, p. 1695; 16–18 Thorncastle Street is listed as the business address of Joseph Byrne, family grocer and spirit merchant, 21l: *Thom's Directory, 1901*, p. 1695.

[185] NAI/1901/129 Evidence of Patrick Clarke dated 11 May 1901.

[186] NAI/1901/129 Verdict dated 11 May 1901.

[187] NAI/1900/187 Inquest on the body of John Ivors, 10 December 1900.

[188] *Irish Daily Independent*, 11 February 1902.

[189] NAI/1902/21 Inquest held on the body of Peter Brady, 10 February 1902.

[190] NAI/1901/26 Inquest on the body of John McInerney, 29 January 1901; *Evening Herald*, 29 January 1901.

[191] NAI/1901/151 Inquest on the body of John Herbert, 4 June 1901.

men falling into the river while 'apparently asleep'—the witnesses mounted an immediate rescue campaign but to no avail.[192] The jury recommended that the place be better protected.

When crushing accidents happened at sea there were few medical recourses—Simon Rooney's left leg got caught in a crank of the SS *City of Hamburg* and was amputated from the knee down. The ship was en route from Rotterdam to Dublin via Belfast on 15 January 1901 with a cargo and a crew of seventeen men. He was brought to Jervis Street Hospital, where he died and was identified by his mother Amelia.[193] Glasgow man John Henderson was aboard the *Denia* when it encountered heavy seas while passing Copeland Island outside Belfast Lough. He suffered a rupture of the bladder and fracture of the pelvis from accidentally falling on the crank shaft of the engine during the swell but did not complain immediately. Once his shipmates realised how grave his condition was, they made for Dublin—he died at Sir Patrick Dun's Hospital on 20 December 1901.[194]

Railways

All accidents occurring in the operation of railways or on railway premises had to be reported to the Board of Trade—this included passenger incidents and deaths. Railway worker accidents were limited to those that prevented them from working for more than five hours in the days following the incident.[195] Eleven deaths of railway and one tram worker death occurred in this two-year period. In addition to the usual reporting mechanisms, the coroner had to make a return within seven days after the inquest to the 'principal Secretaries of State'.[196] In what was described as an 'extraordinary accident in Westland Row', Patrick Collins died while trying to repair overhead tram wires. He and his brother Edward were on a raised horse-drawn platform conducting the repairs when the unattended horses 'took fright and bolted'.[197] Both men were thrown to the ground and, while Edward suffered no injuries, Patrick suffered a skull fracture and subsequently died.[198] The jury considered that DUTC did not have sufficient men on the job, which was a regular complaint in workplace accidents—in Collins's case someone

---

[192] NAI/1901/315 Inquest on the body of John Brophy, 20 December 1901; *Evening Herald*, 20 December 1901.
[193] NAI/1901/17 Inquest on the body of Simon Rooney, 16 January 1901.
[194] NAI/1901/317 Inquest on the body of John Henderson, 23 December 1901; *Evening Herald*, 23 December 1901.
[195] *Railway accidents. Returns of accidents and casualties as reported to the Board of Trade by the several railway companies in the United Kingdom During the three months ending 31st March 1901, in pursuance of the Regulation of Railways Act (1871), 34 & 35 Vict. cap. 78; together with reports of the inspecting officers, assistant inspecting officers, and sub-inspectors of the Railway Department to the Board of Trade, upon certain accidents which were inquired into* [Cd. 774], p. 8.
[196] Huband, *A Practical Treatise*, pp. 282–3.   [197] *The Irish Times*, 4 July 1900.
[198] *Irish Daily Independent*, 3 July 1900.

should have been holding the horses steady.[199] Jurors in the case of railway shunter Patrick McCormick also cited the insufficient number of staff as the leading cause of his death. Nobody witnessed the accident that occurred while he was at work at Kingsbridge Station. Shortly after his removal to Dr Steevens' Hospital he died from internal bleeding following an accident while in the discharge of his duty. It was assumed that he got caught between two carriages. The jury recommended the widow and children to the kind consideration of the Railway Company and exonerated the drivers from all blame.[200] The following day, another case came before the coroner: Michael O'Brien, an 18-year-old machinist suffered major head trauma at the Inchicore Rail Works when he was struck by a twelve-stone pulley. Like all other railway worker cases, his came under the remit of the Board of Trade, but the inspector had to attend another urgent matter and was not present for the coronial inquiry—the jury considered the rope used to hoist the pulley unfit for purpose.[201]

In the first three months of 1901, three passengers were killed entering or alighting trains. In the same period, four so-called 'servants' were fatally wounded, two in falls from engines and one each in shunting and overhead bridge incidents.[202] Although the reports only present statistics and high-level locational data at a UK level, the shunting death corresponds with the death of James Walker at Amiens Street Station on 7 January 1901.[203] Citing the strong anti-union bias of rail companies, Geraghty and Rigney argue that organisation among rail workers did not make proper progress until the 1880s.[204] Leckey estimates that 53 per cent of men eligible had joined the Irish Amalgamated Society by 1897.[205] Walker was a member of the Amalgamated Society of Railway Servants and Mr Walter Hudson, a trade union secretary, was present at the inquest on behalf of the railwaymen.[206] Hudson stated that the matter of shunting was a 'most vexed one'.[207] There were no witnesses to the accident, his body was almost severed in two, and Dr Dunne of Jervis Street Hospital maintained that his death was instantaneous. It was apparently a well-lit area; his wife was recommended to the kind

[199] NAI/1900/55 Inquest on the body of Patrick Collins, 4 July 1900.
[200] NAI/1901/80 Inquest into the death of Patrick McCormick, 19 March 1901; *Irish Daily Independent*, 20 March 1901.
[201] NAI/1901/82 Inquest into the death of Micheal O'Brien, 20 March 1901; *Evening Herald*, 20 March 1901.
[202] *Railway accidents* [Cd. 774], p. 12.
[203] NAI/1901/8 Inquest into the death of James Walker, 9 January 1901.
[204] Hugh Geraghty and Peter Rigney, 'The engineers' strike in Inchicore Railway Works, 1902', *Saothar*, 9 (1983), pp. 20–31.
[205] Joseph J. Leckey, 'The railway servants strike in Co. Cork, 1898', *Saothar*, 76:2 (1976), pp. 39–45 at 40.
[206] *Evening Herald*, 9 January 1901; *Irish Times*, 8 January 1901.
[207] *Evening Herald*, 9 January 1901.

consideration of the Great Northern Company.[208] Railway porter Thomas Dempsey had to go into a badly located coal vault as part of his daily duties at the busy Kingsbridge (now Heuston) Station. On 15 February 1901, he was descending the stairs to enter the vault when he got caught by a carriage being pushed by four men. His upper body was pinned to the platform. Typical of shunting accident injuries, he suffered internal bleeding from a rupture of his liver. Dr Louis Byrne went to view the location of the vault and considered it extraordinary that what was described as a 'regular death trap' had an egress onto a main train line and was perplexed as to how the railway company could permit it to be there and how the Board of Trade could have passed it. The jury rider exonerated the men who were pushing the carriage from all blame and considered the railway company guilty of gross negligence.[209] Engine drivers were also at risk of being run over or injured, like Thomas Cummins who suffered devastating injuries when he was accidentally run over by a train at the Howth terminus on 9 November 1900. The jury strongly recommended his wife and children to the kind consideration of the Great Northern Railway Company.[210] Engine driver Laurence Lawlor died from a fracture of the skull caused by accidentally striking against O'Neill's Bridge near Carrickmines station on the Dublin and Wexford Railway train on 17 December 1900. Lawlor was attempting to fix a break in the engine box when the accident happened. He died three days later at the Meath Hospital—his relatives were not explicitly recommended to the kind consideration but we can assume that some compensation was paid.[211]

A Royal Commission was appointed in 1900 to consider the high numbers of deaths and injuries on the railways in the UK. Given the enormous concessions granted to private rail companies over several decades, with respect to right of way and compulsory purchase of land, it recommended that the state should intervene to encourage them to comply with safety measures. It recommended that the law be changed to ensure that all accidents occurring to rail servants in the course of their duties be reported to the Board of Trade. As the regulations stood, only accidents occurring on railway lines were subject to reporting instruments.[212] The amounts paid to dependants of railway servants in individual cases are unclear.[213]

---

[208] *Amalgamated Society of Railway Servants, register dated 1898–1899*, MSS.127/AS/2/3/8 accessed via findmypast.co.uk; *Evening Herald*, 8 January 1901.

[209] *Evening Herald*, 18 February 1901; NAI/1901/45 Inquest on the body Thomas Dempsey, 18 February 1901.

[210] NAI/1900/162 Inquest on the body of Thomas Cummins, 12 November 1900.

[211] NAI/1900/199 Inquest on the body of Laurence Lawlor, 22 December 1900; *Irish Daily Independent*, 24 December 1900.

[212] *Royal Com. to inquire into Causes of Accidents, Fatal and Non-fatal, to Servants of Railway Companies and Truck-Owners. Report, Minutes of Evidence, Appendices* [Cd.41 Cd.42], pp. 11–12.

[213] I am grateful to Reverend Dr Norman Gamble, Archivist of the Irish Railway Record Society, for his insights and advice.

Compensation: 'Compo' Culture

Workmen's compensation was big business and there was no shortage of insurance and assurance societies in the Irish market. The Absolute Assurance company took out a regular advert in the *Freeman's Journal* offering employer's liability as part of its array of policies; the Patriotic Assurance company, established in 1824, advertised its range of products less frequently.[214] The superintending Factory Act inspector for the Scotland and Ireland division observed in his report of March 1901 that 'The Irish are an impressionable and emotional people, they are quick to see...'which way the wind blows". They are also a highly litigious one, which is but another form of national pugnacity.'[215] His biases are not borne out in the coronial court or the county court records. Very few cases were as a result of employee negligence, the nature of injuries were frightful, and compensation was not a given. Relatively few cases came before the county courts under the Workmen Compensation Act 1897 and the Employer Liability Act 1880—there were thirty of the former and one of the latter in Dublin City for 1900.[216] The report stated that the number should be viewed with caution: 'they leave untouched the great body of cases of compensation to workmen. In the majority of cases, compensation is settled by agreement or by informal arbitration, no memorandum is registered, and no official information therefore is available.'[217] According to the 1897 act, contributions towards funerals could not exceed £10 and it set a baseline payment of a minimum payment of £150 to dependants for workplace deaths. The process could be arduous and claims had to be made within six months of the accident. First, the aggrieved parties had to serve notice in writing on the company with the particulars of the accident and the amount in salary normally received. These matters could be and were contested by employers, especially if inflated salary estimates were included. A committee comprising employer and workmen initially decided settlements but if cases were still in dispute then the case could go to an arbitrator. If that did not work, the final recourse was the county court, where a judge could appoint an arbitrator.

It is unclear if families received any compensation from the aforementioned builders as the business records are not extant. An important judgement was handed down in 1900 following the appeal of an award to a widow whose husband died while conducting what was termed 'third term alterations'. A county court had awarded her £245 under the act but that decision was reversed in the court of appeal on the grounds that the work he was doing was neither construction nor repair. The House of Lords reversed the judgement and argued that if the

[214] (Absolute Security) *Freeman's Journal*, 2 August 1900; (Patriotic Assurance) *Freeman's Journal*, 15 August 1900.
[215] *Annual Report of the Chief Inspector of Factories and Workshops, for 1900 (Factories—Shops—Workshops: Annual Report)* [Cd. 668], p. 341.
[216] *Workmen's compensation* [Cd. 816], p. 37.   [217] *Workmen's compensation* [Cd. 816], p. 3.

work added materially to the structure of a building then it came within the meaning of the Workmen's Compensation Act 1897.[218] Some indicators of amounts awarded in compensation can be gleaned from newspapers and court of appeal records. For example, in October 1902 the case of Mrs Ellen Delaney was heard by the Recorder of Dublin, Sir Faulkner, at Kilmainham courthouse. Her husband was employed by contractors Mrs McLoughlin & Harvey of Dartmouth Road in works at Guinness's Brewery and he died following a fall from a lift in July 1902. Mrs Delaney claimed £280 in compensation from his employer and was awarded £260 11s. following negotiations.[219]

Coroner's jury riders recommending compensation to relatives often fell on deaf ears. Those who were wholly or partly dependent on lost earnings were eligible to apply. Following Christopher Kelly's death in September 1900, his wife Ellen filed a notice for £150 in compensation under the act. She and their two children were wholly dependent on his wage. While the case was ongoing, she sent her son Joseph to live with her sister-in-law in Dublin, and her daughter Mary Kelly, aged 8, was sent to Limerick Junction. The notice to claim is extant, but the outcome of her case is unclear, and it may have included an out of court settlement. Ellen was returned as a hawker in the 1901 census and was at least reunited with her daughter Mary Jane and lodging at 6.6 Swifts Alley, but Joseph was still with his aunt indicating that her finances were possibly still precarious.[220] Patrick Fagan's relatives also had to take a case under the WCA, against the Phoenix Brewery, which contested the particulars of the notice and the case went to arbitration at the county court.[221] Documented as William in the WCA records, his three dependants were awarded £40 between them in equal amounts and £5 in costs.[222] Joseph Tierney's mother applied for £195 in compensation from O'Rourke's Bakery, under the WCA on behalf of herself and her two daughters, to whose support he contributed. The amount was calculated with respect to his potential earnings of £296 8s. over the following three years.[223] James Nolan's parents took a case under the WCA based on his weekly earnings of 17s. per week in the amount of £132 12s.[224] As his dependant, Sarah Berry made an application

---

[218] *Irish Daily Independent*, 11 December 1900.

[219] *Irish News and Belfast Morning News*, 3 October 1902.

[220] NAI, WCA, Applications for Arbitration & Notices, 1900–1901. Case of Ellen Kelly v Messrs John Jameson & Son Ltd. It came before the recorder 15 November 1900. This case does not have a number as subsequent cases like Fagan's in 1901. Ellen and Mary Jane Kelly: http://www.census.nationalarchives.ie/pages/1901/Dublin/Arran_Quay/Church_Street/1336968/; Joseph Kelly was still living with his Aunt Mary Jane Keogh at 56.2 Church Street.

[221] NAI, WCA Applications for Arbitration & Notices, 1900–1, 1901 no 139. CBB 26 *Fagan v. Phoenix Brewery*.

[222] NAI, WCA Book Awards & Applications 1898–1904, p. 132. Money was divided between Kathleen, Margaret, and Mary Anne Fagan. This is likely to be his family living at 28.4 Usher's Quay: http://www.census.nationalarchives.ie/reels/nai003793344/ (accessed 20 November 2021).

[223] NAI, WCA March 1901. Case of *Tierney v Rourke* request for arbitration.

[224] NAI, WCA, No 134 15 October 1901. Case of *Nolan v Booth Brothers* request for arbitration.

under the WCA against Tedcastles for the loss of Michael McEneney's wages.[225] She was partially supported by him, and received weekly sums in respect of his £1 earnings from 8 February 1901.[226]

Dock workers operated in gangs, were paid in hourly rates, and were often highly exploited by their 'ganger' (foreman). It was their high death rates that led to their eventual inclusion in the Factory Acts.[227] It is unclear what compensation relatives received but the following case provides an indication of the amounts paid. When Henry Williams drowned off the Wicklow coast while serving on a Board of Trade steamer on 31 May 1900, T.M. Healy made inquiries as to how his parents might be compensated. Following inquiries to the Irish Lights Department, Gerard Balfour sanctioned a payment of £50 to his parents.[228] In a case that concerned a labourer who died from falling off a plank on ship in dry dock, in June 1901 the House of Lords overruled a lower court by deeming the docks constituted a factory.[229] Drowning victim Edward Hanlon's accident occurred in Spencer's Dock on 9 January 1901 and it was not until July that year that his wife Mary successfully sued the North City Milling Company for damages at the City Sessions in the amount of £150 on behalf of herself and her eight minor children. She was awarded £50, and £100 was to be invested for the children as wards of court.[230] The case opened debate as to whether a dock constituted a factory, and noted how the employers of seamen were not liable to pay compensation.[231] The ruling in the Hanlon case aided future claimants—Thomas Hogan's widow had to take her case to the county court. He was engaged in unloading a coal boat, SS *Ellor*, with another man, when they both fell off a plank. His employer denied costs, and said his wages were 7s. not 30s. a week and the act did not apply to his contract. She was awarded £150 when the case was finally settled on 6 February 1902 after two adjournments and a case to the court of appeal.[232]

In 1900, eighty-three workmen's compensation cases came before the county courts and seventy-four were decided by the judge. Awards in favour of the

---

[225] NAI, WCA, Book/Requests for Arbitration, 1899–1909, March 1901, p. 103. It is unclear what their relationship was—she may have been his sister, but her maiden name on her marriage certificate was recorded as McNeily; he was recorded as McInerney in the coroner's records NAI/1901/26: https://civilrecords.irishgenealogy.ie/churchrecords/images/marriage_returns/marriages_1887/10820/ 5946120.pdf. When she made the claim, Sarah Berry was still married with four children and living with a lodger: http://www.census.nationalarchives.ie/pages/1901/Dublin/Trinity/Petersons_Lane/ 1311260/.

[226] Case of Michael McEneaney, March 1901, NAI, WCA Book Awards & Applications 1898–1904, p. 103.

[227] Greer and Nicholson, *The Factory Acts in Ireland*, p. 237.

[228] *Irish Daily Independent*, 13 July 1901.   [229] *The Irish Times*, 25 June 1901.

[230] *Evening Herald*, 26 July 1901; *Irish Daily Independent*, 27 July 1901; NAI, WCA, Applications for Arbitration & Notices, 1900–1, WCA no, 121 CBB 74 *Hanlon v Dublin North City Milling Co.*

[231] 'Docks as factories and the Workmen's Compensation Act – *Hanlon v. North City Milling Company*', *New Irish Jurist and Local Government Review*, 2 (1902), pp. 74–5.

[232] NAI, WCA, Book Awards & Applications 1898–1904, p. 130.

plaintiffs could be paid in lump sums or weekly sums.[233] The matter of workmen's compensation was complicated and much depended on the benevolence of employers and whether worksites met the technical definition of a factory. Most cases were settled by agreement but some went to county court. Railway and tram deaths were dealt with separately, and in the absence of company records it is not possible to ascertain individual payments. Four railway deaths in 1900 resulted in lump sums totalling £666 being paid to dependants following a hearing before a judge at county court, nine factory deaths resulted in £290 being paid (eight had dependants), and three building-related deaths resulted in payments of £145 to dependants. A further two railway cases were settled by agreement between parties and resulted in a single £300 lump sum payment.[234] In 1901, six railway deaths resulted in a total award of £778 8s. for the dependants, approximately 10 per cent of which was paid in legal costs.[235]

Conclusion

Outside the front door an array of dangers posed threats to life. For children, spaces for play were limited and each of the concentric circles radiating out from their households of origin embodied increasing levels of risk. In the absence of safety devices, landings, hallways, and front and back steps were all potentially treacherous to small children, and streets and waterways were fraught with problems. In this chapter, I took a multi-method approach, using life cycles and gender to examine how accidents occurred and how blame was apportioned. What is quite apparent is that when municipal authorities or powerful industrialists were clearly culpable for the lack of public safety measures or unsafe work environments, jurors were circumspect and slow to allocate blame. Juries all too readily singled out and censured mothers for accidents in the home, even when it was clear that they were victims of systemic disadvantage and cyclical poverty. Dublin City was small and few jurors would risk their own personal reputation by speaking out against the elite—reprisals could be meted out both directly and indirectly. Riders that pleaded for compensation did so obsequiously and, with the exception of a handful of WCA records, in the majority of cases it is unclear what lasting impact they had. A manifestly unfair process, it rendered some families penniless until such a time as compensation was paid. In the interim, some families disintegrated. Moreover, employers not only had the law on their side; they could also afford to pay for legal representation.

---

[233] *Bulletin of the Bureau of Labor*, Issues 50–55 (U.S. Government Printing Office, 1904), p. 164.

[234] *Workmen's compensation. Statistics of proceedings under the Workmen's Compensation Act, 1897, and the Employers' Liability Act, 1880, during the year 1900* [Cd. 816], pp. 34–5.

[235] *Workmen's compensation. Statistics of proceedings under the Workmen's Compensation Acts, 1897 and 1900, and the Employers' Liability Act, 1880, during the year 1901* [Cd. 1210], p. 33.

4

Unnatural, Suspicious, and Violent Death

Crime classification has caused perennial problems for the historiography of criminality and convict lives and, with respect to suspicious and violent deaths, elements of these problems both replicate in and emanate from the coronial courts. Accidental and sudden deaths from natural causes are not difficult to determine from the verdicts and indeed the evidence in the cases discussed here, as there is a distinct absence of foul play. By contrast, medical opinions on suspicious and violent deaths, while factual, can also be highly subjective and open to jury interpretation. Some violent deaths are unambiguously described in the verdicts and usually involve grievous bodily harm resulting in death at the hands of persons known or unknown to the police but others occupy a medico-legal grey area. Irish coronial court records have a broad range of cases that are definitely suspicious, and potentially the result of violence, but lack of evidence or eye-witness testimony makes them difficult to categorise definitively, especially in cases where the jury returned open verdicts. In assessments of suspicious circumstances, much depended on whether or not the medical witnesses explicitly stated foul play and if the jury unequivocally accepted their professional assessment. Even when impossible-to-self-inflict wounds were described in post-mortem reports, juries could, and did, as this chapter will show, cite lack of evidence of foul play.

As a court of record, suspected cases of suicide and, to a lesser extent, infanticide invariably reached conclusion in the coroners' courts. The quality of witness statements had a bearing on outcomes, and the ultimate deciding factor in terms of criminality was the fervour of policemen to investigate further and prosecute in the criminal courts. Pursuit of perpetrators in criminal courts cannot be used as an unquestionable barometer of criminal intent either; H-car drivers, for instance, were always arrested at the scene of a collision and prosecuted for endangerment or manslaughter but none of the cases discussed in Chapter 3 resulted in their conviction in the criminal courts as the cause was invariably determined as accidental. The cases of potential infanticide in the sample exemplify the problems associated with classification. Take, for example, the events leading to the discovery of the body of a male infant found drowned in the Ringsend Basin on 3 November 1900.[1] It surely involved an act of physical violence, whereas another case of an infant who died from 'shock due to exposure

---

[1] NAI/1900/152 Inquest on unknown male infant, 3 November 1900; *Evening Herald*, 3 November 1900.

Ordinary Lives, Death, and Social Class: Dublin City Coroner's Court, 1876–1902. Ciara Breathnach, Oxford University Press. © Ciara Breathnach 2022. DOI: 10.1093/oso/9780198865780.003.0005

and haemorrhage from the umbilical cord the result of neglect' involved deliberate inaction, of not tying the cord and leaving the child exposed to the elements to
bring about death.[2]

With the caveat of blurred lines, I have identified sixty-three cases across a
spectrum of physical violence and criminality, ranging from evidence of negligence in the case of vulnerable children to more explicit criminal intent with
aforethought and malice. Perhaps the neatest way of discussing these cases is by
gender and life cycle, and both criteria can be correlated with varying degrees of
violence. By adopting these frameworks, discussion can be divided into three
primary focus areas: thirteen deaths of infants under the age of 1 (one gender
unknown), twenty-one potential suicides, and twenty-nine cases associated with
interpersonal violence (see Figure 4.1). Twenty-eight of the sixty-three (nine suicide, three infanticide, and fourteen cases of interpersonal violence) cases were
female. Following the thematic and spatial formula used in the preceding chapters, coupled with quantitative evidence, this chapter is also threaded with a more
in-depth discussion of the centrality of alcohol consumption to coronial court
inquiries.

Infanticide in Ireland has received considerable attention since 2012, notably in
works by Elaine Farrell on the late nineteenth century, and Clíona Rattigan on the
early twentieth century.[3] As thirteen of the cases in this sample of suspicious
deaths concern infanticide, with causes of death that range in order of degrees of
criminality from neglect to mutilation, it merits some further discussion here

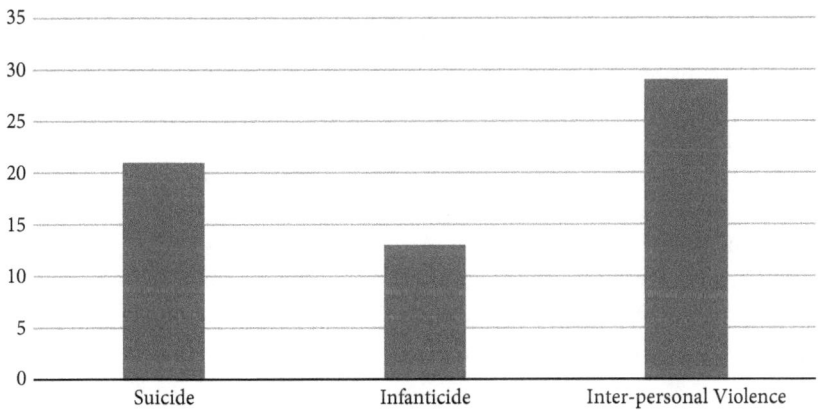

Figure 4.1 Violent deaths, infanticide, suicide, and inter-personal violence
Source: NAI/Dataset 1900–2.

---

[2] NAI/1901/216 Inquest on unknown male infant, 21 August 1901.
[3] Elaine Farrell, *Infanticide in the Irish Crown Files at Assizes, 1883–1900* (Dublin, 2012); Elaine
Farrell, *'A Most "Diabolical Deed"': Infanticide and Irish Society, 1850–1900* (Manchester, 2013); Clíona
Rattigan, *What Else Could I Do: Single Mothers and Infanticide, Ireland 1900–1950* (Dublin, 2012).

because of the critical role the coroner's court played in the legal process. Procedurally, the discovery of an infant body initiated a different course of action to that of an adult case. According to statute, the first duty of the coroner's court was to determine whether or not the child was born alive and the verdict, in most cases, determined the judicial outcome.[4] The second section of this chapter examines cases where suicide was the most likely cause of death. Instances of apparent suicide or *felo de se* (directly translated as felon of self), legally fall under the category of foul play and there are twenty-one cases that either yielded verdicts of 'temporary insanity' or simply ignored the evidence of suicidal tendencies. Some of these cases involved alcohol, which had a strong bearing on the verdict. Irrespective of how suicide was viewed in moral and religious terms, under Irish law it was considered a criminal act until 1993; attempted cases were prosecuted in the courts and there are ten verdicts of people whom the coroner's jury considered to have been 'of unsound mind' or 'temporarily insane' when they committed the act: one was considered a 'dangerous lunatic', a further six glossed over evidence of suicidal tendencies, three were unclear verdicts, and the final case included here was one that the DMP considered to be suicidal. In these cases of ambiguous verdicts the evidence of self-harm was ignored possibly to spare relatives the stigma associated with mental health problems, the implications for burial, or for financial reasons like the forfeiture of insurance policies.[5]

If viewed on a continuum of varying degrees of violence then at the more extreme end of this sample are, without question, some of the most gruesome and tragic cases in these data. The final section of this chapter examines twenty-nine cases of inter-personal violence, fourteen of which involved female victims. Eleven or the majority of the male cases arose from what I am terming a brawl of which nine involved alcohol consumption. These cases differ greatly from premeditated assaults and were often random one-punch episodes that resulted in a fatality. Coroners' courts were the first stage in the legal process in suspicious cases and my research has led to a depressing set of revelations about some of the most vulnerable women and, by association, children in Dublin City. Despite the advance of the 'civilising process', Irish law had little to no victim focus unless acts were premeditated, particularly heinous, or committed by people of prior bad character.[6] Under the Offences Against the Person Act 1861, murder was a capital offence,[7] but the state rarely brought murder charges; most of those convicted and

---

[4] Mark Jackson, *New-Born Child Murder: Women, Illegitimacy and the Courts in Eighteenth-Century England* (Manchester, 1996), p. 143.

[5] Scottish Widows' Fund and Life Assurance Society's Act 1882, 1882 c. lxxv; Norwich Union Life Insurance Society Act 1868, 1868 c. cxlviii; Georgina Laragy, '"A Peculiar Species of Felony": suicide, medicine, and the law in Victorian Britain and Ireland', *Journal of Social History*, 46:3 (2013), pp. 732–43.

[6] Richard McMahon, Joachim Eibach and Randolph Roth Source, 'Making sense of violence? Reflections on the history of interpersonal violence in Europe', *Crime, Histoire & Sociétés/Crime, History & Societies*, 17:2 (2013), pp. 5–26.

[7] Offences Against the Person Act 1861 (24 & 25 Vict.) c. 100.

sentenced to execution had their sentences commuted.[8] Only two Dublin cases, that of Hannah Kavanagh in 1900 and John Toole in 1901 had 'death recorded' in the period under review here; the former was commuted to penal servitude and the latter was executed in Mountjoy prison for the brutal murder of Lizzie Brennan.[9]

With great frequency, light sentences were handed down in cases of gender-based violence giving a distinct impression that the victims' lives did not matter as much as the perpetrator's reputation or the potential pecuniary impact on dependant family were they punished fully. More often than not the state charged perpetrators with manslaughter which carried sentences of penal servitude for life and convicts were usually released on licence after serving about two thirds of their sentence.[10] Caroline Conley's contention that 65 per cent of those convicted for homicide served less than two years is difficult to substantiate and is not borne out in the General Prison Board files.[11] A typical sentence for manslaughter was seven years' penal servitude—Owen Corbally represents a case in point. Aged 33 and a labourer, in 1900 he was sentenced to seven years but was released on licence in 1905.[12] Only one of the cases discussed here resulted in a successful manslaughter charge, which speaks to the high threshold of evidence the state had to meet. There was no public outcry following most of these deaths; neither was there a call to arms to ensure justice.

Although the coroner's court is often dismissed in the English context 'as a quiet and curious backwater'[13] and the jury as 'low, base, ignorant, besotted, venal', it was a critical basis to the Irish criminal courts' process. This chapter offers a systematic way of examining how the coroners' courts operated as a crucial first step in establishing evidence of criminality vis-à-vis cause of death. As the vox populi, or voice of the people, jury riders in the coronial setting could be very powerful—they were indicative of the public appetite and support for conviction and sentencing in the criminal courts, especially in the context of capital offences. I have traced where possible how these cases move from the coroner's to the police, summary, and criminal courts in an attempt to establish patterns of inquiry and sentencing. Moreover, I show how verdicts in coronial courts were

---

[8] Carolyn Conley, *Melancholy Accidents: The Meaning of Violence in Post-Famine Ireland* (New York, 1999), p. 145.

[9] NAI, General Prison Board (GPB)/CN/G5 1900–2, 'Death Book', deaths in the 'Home Circuit and Dublin Commission'.

[10] Ciara Breathnach, 'Medical officers, bodies, gender and weight fluctuation in Irish convict prisons, 1877–95', *Medical History*, 58:1 (2014), pp. 67–86 at 77–8.

[11] Carolyn Conley, *Certain Other Countries: Homicide, Gender, and National Identity in Late Nineteenth-century England, Ireland, Scotland, and Wales* (Columbus, 2007), p. 17.

[12] NAI/GPB/PEN/1905/32 case of Owen Corbally.

[13] Joe Sim and Tony Ward, 'The magistrate of the poor? Coroners and deaths in custody in nineteenth-century England', in Michael Clark and Catherine Crawford (eds), *Legal Medicine in History* (Cambridge, 1994), pp. 245–67 at 245; Burney, *Bodies of Evidence*, p. 6.

subject to political, moral, and gender bias even when clear evidence of criminality was apparent.

Suspicious Infant Deaths

Overarching concerns with female morality, illegitimacy, fertility, and succession led to a few acts to ensure the protection of new-born infants, giving rise to what Arlie Loughnan terms an 'infanticide doctrine', which she posits was 'both inculpatory and (partially) exculpatory' and describes as 'an unusual legal construct'.[14] In order to understand the centrality of the coroner's court to the way in which infanticide was prosecuted in Ireland at the turn of the twentieth century it is worth outlining the emergence of the doctrine in the Irish context, which can be traced to 1623 and was the first act that made it a capital offence.[15] In an appeal to change the law as it stood in 1895, John Glaister reflected on how these seventeenth-century dictates placed 'the burden of proof' on putative mothers to show that the 'that the child was born dead'.[16] Although repealed in 1803 with Lord Ellenborough's Act, the emphasis on proof of a live birth was retained. It also stipulated that child murder was punishable under normal legislation as the 'major charge' but it permitted the jury to convict mothers on the lesser charge of concealment of pregnancy (as a precursor to intent), which carried a maximum sentence of two years.[17] Effectively, it made infanticide a non-capital offence and entrenched the importance of evidence of a live birth. Popular interpretations of the law, combined with other practical considerations, made the moment of childbirth a critical window of opportunity to evade detection for those intent on harm.

Immediate action or inaction at birth could bring about death; ten of the thirteen cases of potential infanticide discussed here were neonatal (Table 4.1, age 0). Infanticide was categorised as a misdemeanour under section 27 of the Offences Against the Person Act 1861 and, together with abandonment and concealment of pregnancy, crimes against infants constituted a very small percentage of cases in the criminal courts.[18] What perturbed some legal experts like John Glaister in

---

[14] Arlie Loughnan, ' "Strange" case of the infanticide doctrine', *Oxford Journal of Legal Studies*, 32:4 (2012), pp. 685–711 at 686–7.

[15] An Act to Prevent the Destroying and Murthering of Bastard Children (1623), c. 27.

[16] John Glaister, 'The law of infanticide: a plea for its revision', *The Edinburgh Medical Journal* [July 1895], pp. 1–18 at 2.

[17] Malicious shooting or Stabbing Act, 1803 (43 Geo. 3) c. 58 'Lord Ellenborough's Act'; Glaister, 'The law of infanticide', p. 5.

[18] Offences Against the Person Act 1861 (24 & 25 Vict.) c. 100 s. 27: 'Whosoever shall unlawfully abandon or expose any child, being under the age of two years, whereby the life of such child shall be endangered, or the health of such child shall have been or shall be likely to be permanently injured, shall be guilty of a misdemeanor, and being convicted thereof shall be liable...to be kept in penal servitude."

Table 4.1 Cases of alleged infanticide, suspicious infant deaths April 1900–April 1902

Surname	G	Age	Date of inquest	Cause of death	Place found	Suspicion	Trial
Unknown	M	0	01-May-00	Neglect at birth	Street	Yes	No
Carroll	F	0	28-May-00	Asphyxia	Home	Yes	No
Hanlon	M	3m	10-Jul-00	Non assimilation of food	Home	Yes	Yes
Jordan	M	4w	11-Jul-00	Non assimilation of food	Phoenix Park	Yes	No
Unknown	M	0	22-Sep-00	Drowned	Alexander/W	Yes	No
Unknown	M	0	03-Nov-00	Drowned	Ringsend/W	Yes	No
Barry	F		19-Nov-00	Asphyxia	Foley's Hotel	Yes	Yes
Stephens	M	0	20-Dec-00	Asphyxia	Home	Yes	Yes
Unknown	F		24-Jan-01	Drowned	Liffey/W	Yes	No
Gorey	U	0	05-Apr-01	Mutilation	Home	Yes	No
Unknown	M	0	03-Jun-01	Haemorrhage	Street	Yes	No
Finnerty	F	4m	15-Jul-00	Starvation and neglect	Home	Yes	
Unknown	M	0	21–Aug-01	Shock exposure and haemorrhage	Gully/W	Yes	Yes

the late nineteenth century was that 'to secure a conviction on the major charge is of the very rarest possible occurrence' to such an extent that minor charges of concealment of pregnancy predominated in the Irish courts.[19] Key to prosecutions under the 1861 act was proof that the child had been born alive and it is for such reasons that crimes associated with infant life are ambiguously returned under DMP reports and the Judicial Statistics, which in turn are difficult to correlate with the court records.[20] As the reported discovery of an infant body always occasioned a coroner's inquest, it makes methodological sense to work from the coronial court records through to the criminal courts to examine processes, procedures, and outcomes.

Leanne McCormick's work on reproductive knowledge and abortion in Belfast has shown that 'sectarian divisions in the city appear to have had a direct impact on networks of knowledge on how to terminate pregnancy'.[21] She argues that Roman Catholics there were less likely to have access to information about how to procure an abortion than Protestants. Very few charges of the procurement of abortion services were brought before the Irish courts where it seems, and I have argued elsewhere with Eunan O'Halpin, that neonaticide was a common way of dealing with unplanned pregnancy.[22] All but one of the thirteen cases in Table 4.1

---

[19] Glaister, 'The law of infanticide', p. 6.   [20] See Farrell, 'A Most "Diabolical Deed"'.
[21] Leanne McCormick, '"No sense of wrongdoing": abortion in Belfast 1917–1967', *Journal of Social History*, 49:1 (2015), pp. 125–48 at 125.
[22] Ciara Breathnach and Eunan O'Halpin, 'Scripting blame: Irish coroners' courts and unnamed infant dead, 1916–32', *Social History*, 39: 2 (2014), pp. 210–28.

resulted in some form of censure, accusation of neglect, or a criminal trial. Eight were of male infants, four were female, and one was gender unknown. Decomposition rendered infant bodies 'gender unknown' especially when they were left in water or, as in one case here, where the body had been mutilated and the genitalia were missing. With respect to name, unknown signifies infants whose bodies were discovered but no mothers or putative adults were identified—they account for six cases here, one of which was female.

Waterways were used to great effect in the act of killing and disposing of infant bodies. Kelly explains in his study of the early nineteenth century that waterways served a dual purpose of instrument for killing and method of disposal.[23] The coroner's court was where formal investigations into most unknown infant dead cases concluded. No arrests followed the discovery of three drowned infants shown in Table 4.1; these involved the cases of the male infants found in the Alexander and Ringsend Basins in September and November 1900, respectively, and a new-born female infant, who had been in the water about four or five weeks, found in the River Liffey at the North Wall on 24 January 1901.[24] Waterways were also used as sites of disposal, as happened with the male infant whose inquest took place on 21 August 1901. He was found in a gully opposite Saint Lawrence O'Toole's Roman Catholic church and was placed there sometime after 16 August—the date it had last been cleaned. The verdict was that the child had died from 'shock due to exposure and haemorrhage from the umbilical cord'.[25] Another unknown case was that of a male child who 'Died from haemorrhage result of the severing of the blood vessels of the neck said wound was caused by some person or persons unknown.' Post-mortem found 'a piece of calico was stuffed into its mouth to a considerable length and a portion of it protruded from the wound in the throat.'[26] Apart from the severance of the jugular vein and the windpipe there was evidence of non-skilled attendance at birth. Despite its discovery on a busy city centre street, the risks associated with concealment of pregnancy and of getting caught disposing of the body notwithstanding, nobody was apprehended for this gruesome case of what the newspapers termed 'a shocking discovery'.[27] As Table 4.1 shows in eight cases, mothers were identified and therefore could be held legally accountable. They will form the basis of the rest of my discussion on infanticide.

While most of the suspicious infant deaths here concern single women, married women also exhibited tendencies towards infanticidal behaviour. The second

---

[23] James Kelly, '"An Unnatural Crime": infanticide in early nineteenth-century Ireland', *Irish Economic & Social History*, 46:1 (2019), pp. 66–110 at 68.

[24] NAI/1900/116 Inquest on an unknown male infant, 22 September 1900; NAI/1900/152 Inquest on an unknown male infant, 3 November 1900; NAI/1901/23 Inquest reports on an unknown female infant, 24 January 1901.

[25] NAI/1901/216 Inquest an unknown male infant, 21 August 1901.

[26] NAI/1901/150 Inquest an unknown male infant, 3 June 1901.

[27] *Freeman's Journal*, 4 June 1901.

case in Table 4.1 concerned Mary Carroll, whose female infant died of asphyxia in May 1900. She was deemed innocent of any wrongdoing in accordance with the coroner's verdict. It was a highly peculiar case—her husband came home from work and purportedly knew or noticed nothing about her unassisted home birth, which occurred during the night at 22 Island Street while he slept. In the aftermath, she placed the infant's body in a box and mentioned nothing to her husband who went to work the following morning as normal—it was her landlord who alerted the authorities. The DMP report stated it was stillborn but Dr Thomas Neill, Assistant Master at the Coombe Hospital, found evidence of air in the lungs along with some mucous. The umbilical cord was cut but not tied. That she was married and her husband was in employment afforded her a veneer of respectability and the case was simply allowed to dissolve away as one of asphyxia to which the jury 'do not attach any blame to any one concerned': the affect being that it was not pursued into the police court. So common were coronial inquiries like this that it raised no newspaper attention and the death was not subsequently registered. By right, with asphyxia as cause of death, it should have reported by the coroner's office to the registrar, and it may have been, but some extra-legal discretion may have been exercised on the part of the registrar who was not obliged by statute to register a stillbirth. The 4-week-old male infant who was left to perish in Phoenix Park, was later identified by the maternity nurse at NDU as the child of Anne Jordan, born on 11 June. Jordan was absolved of wrongdoing by virtue of the verdict which was that the child died through non-assimilation of food and the shock of exposure.[28]

Such was the stigma associated with unmarried motherhood that young women like Kate Keller often relocated some distance away from their households of origin to maintain façades of chastity. Keller was a lodger at King's Inn in the latter stages of her pregnancy, and her landlady, a Mrs Sheahan, recommended that she employ the services of Mrs Bridget Curley of 6 Granby Place, Dublin City, to look after the child, Mary Margaret Finnerty.[29] Following the recommendation they agreed a rate of 2s. 6d. per week.[30] Shortly after the arrangement was made and Keller had returned to Oughterard, Curley wrote to her seeking to renegotiate the terms and asking for more money. A few days later she wrote again to state that the child's health had deteriorated and that she proposed placing the child in the 'Union'. Strong social resonances aside, the Dublin Union hospitals did not have a great reputation and were usually the last resort for the sick and dying poor. Keller immediately went to Dublin where she said she found her child filthy and lying, partially clothed with an old shawl, on brown paper. She

[28] NAI/1900/63 Inquest on the body of John Jordan, 11 July 1900.
[29] NAI/1901/188 Inquest on the body of Mary Margaret Finnerty, evidence taken at NDU on 15 July 1901.
[30] *Freeman's Journal*, 16 July 1901.

had little choice but to immediately bring the child to the NDU where she was assessed and weighed by Nurse Agnes Tyrell. When Keller had her child at the Rotunda it weighed 5.5 lbs.[31] At four months old Mary Margaret weighed 5 lbs. Dr Powell claimed that the child was starved to death and the assistant master reported the matter to the DMP. Dr Louis Bryne argued that the verdict of neglect was tantamount to manslaughter.[32] Curley was later brought before the Dublin City Commission on 6 August 1901, initially on a manslaughter charge (and why I include her here and not in Chapter two) but it ended up being a child cruelty case. Although it was a rarely employed term in Irish newspapers, the *Weekly Irish Times* described the case unequivocally as a case of 'Baby Farming in Dublin'.[33] Mary Bruton, ward mistress at NDU, described the child as verminous with 'hardly any flesh on it – nothing but skin and bone. It had every appearance of dying.'[34] Dr Caleb Powell used words like malnutrition and starvation to describe cause of death and stated she should have weighed between 10 lbs and 15 lbs.[35] Curley was found guilty of gross neglect of an infant under her care, and was sentenced to a mere nineteen days imprisonment.[36]

Concealment and Evidence of Foul Play by Mothers

Sarah Stephens, originally from Virginia in County Cavan, had been working for Lord Tweeddale in Scotland when she fell pregnant.[37] She returned to Ireland and her mother brought her from County Cavan to Dublin at the beginning of October 1900 and placed her under the care of Jane Couch of Mission Hall, 40 Lower Gloucester Street.[38] She instructed that her daughter should be taken to the Rotunda Hospital 'when the time would come'. If my crude genealogical investigations are correct then the Stephens' family professed as Church of Ireland, which enabled access to a Dublin network.[39] Mr Couch 'took lodgings for her at 36 Rutland St' for eight weeks prior to confinement—her landlady was

---

[31] *Freeman's Journal*, 16 July 1901.
[32] *Belfast Newsletter*, 16 July 1901.   [33] *Weekly Irish Times*, 20 July 1901.
[34] NAI, Dublin Crown Files at Commission, August 1901: *King v Bridget Curley*, evidence Mary Bruton dated 12 July; *Freeman's Journal*, 5 August 1901.
[35] NAI, Dublin Crown Files at Commission, August 1901. *King v Bridget Curley*, evidence Dr Caleb Powell dated 19 July.
[36] *Irish Daily Independent*, 8 August 1901; *Freeman's Journal*, 16 July 1901.
[37] NAI/1900/198 Inquest on the body of Male Infant, 20 December 1900—body is not identified as child of Sarah Stephens.
[38] *Thom's Directory, 1901*, p. 1439, notes George Arthur Couch, Missionary and T. Wyatt, Missionary, the latter lived at 40 Lower Gloucester Street with his family in 1901: http://www.census.nationalarchives. ie/reels/nai003760993/ (accessed 13 March 2021).
[39] See http://www.census.nationalarchives.ie/reels/nai000438551/; her father Richard was a Boatman: http://www.census.nationalarchives.ie/reels/nai003810567/ (both sites accessed 1 February 2020). It is highly likely that this return in the 1901 census is Sarah Stephens as the age 26 is roughly right, she was originally from County Cavan, and was working as a domestic servant in Dublin.

a woman named Eliza Merry. On the ill-fated night, Sarah Stephens claimed to be suffering from a sore throat and Eliza Merry made her some tea—she returned to check on her about ten minutes later and was refused entry to the room. Merry called for Couch about 7 p.m. and they entered the room together— Stephens was in bed and they both saw a bucket covered in a cloth 'and in the bucket an infant covered in water'. Couch went to the Rotunda Hospital, and the authorities there sent her to the Summerhill dispensary. There she met relieving officer Laurence Keogh who accompanied her to Summerhill police station. Dr Oulton eventually arrived at about 11 p.m., and he testified that after seeing the child's face submerged in water, he compassionately turned his attention to the mother. His testimony was as follows:

> I sat down beside the defendant and asked her was she willing I should examine her to see her condition. She said she was. On examination, I found that the afterbirth was not expelled. I removed it. She told me then that she was sitting on the bucket & that the child was born into it.

On his initial examination of the infant's body he found the umbilical cord was torn 4.5 inches from the navel. His post-mortem revealed that it was in fact a healthy child weighing 7.5 lbs. Dr Oulton stated that there was meconium passing from the bowel and urine in the bladder, both evidence he believed of a live birth. In medical jurisprudence the hydrostatic or lung flotation test was contested as an unreliable indicator of proof of life from the eighteenth century onwards but it still retained currency in Ireland and was used in this case.[40] He found water in the stomach and blood 'in the right carditis of the heart', evidence he claimed was consistent with asphyxia.[41] Contrary to the very strong evidence pointing to the fact that Sarah Stephens had killed her child, the coronial court jury proclaimed that the it 'Died from asphyxia caused by being immersed in a bucket of water in the house 36 Lower Rutland Street and have no evidence to show how the child was placed there.' Irrespective of the open verdict, she was brought before the Southern Police Court and charged with 'having unlawfully and with malice and aforethought killed and murdered her illegitimate male infant shortly after its birth'.[42] She was returned for trial at the City Commission in February 1901 but her appearance was postponed as she was listed in the 'Medical Officer's report of prisoners' as being 'seriously ill' and 'unfit for trial'.[43] Instead she was brought

[40] Mary Wessling, 'Infanticide trials and forensic medicine Wurttemberg', in Clark and Crawford (eds), *Legal Medicine in History*, pp. 117–45 at 134.
[41] NAI, Dublin Crown Files at Commission, *King v Sarah Stephens*. Evidence of Dr Oulton, 9 April 1901.
[42] *Evening Herald*, 8 January 1901; *Irish Daily Independent*, 9 January 1901.
[43] Report of the Mountjoy Female Prison MO, Dr Raymond Granville Dowdall: NAI, Dublin Crown Files at Commission, 5 February 1901.

before the next session on 9 April 1901 on the lesser charge of concealing the birth.[44] Her counsel, Gerard Byrne entered a guilty plea and requested that she be released to the care of a number of women who 'were kind enough to undertake to see after her'. She was bailed on 9 March 1901[45] and released 'on her own recognisances in £10 to come up for sentence when called on'.[46] Stephens's religious persuasion not only gave her access to a network of women willing to assist in concealing her pregnancy for social reasons—it also gave her access to the elite of Dublin society willing to act as guarantors. Anna McDowell Cosgrave, a Poor Law Guardian living at 5 Gardiner's Row,[47] and Mary Weldrick of 87 Great Britain Street,[48] also a guardian, both put up £10 each to secure her release. A number of factors worked in Stephens's favour—it was her first child, relatively speaking she was of rural origin, the sympathetic evidence of Dr Oulton (who had seen many similar cases), and the willingness of women of note to vouch for her spared her the full weight of the law.

Kate Barry, aged 22 according to the coroner's inquest, concealed her pregnancy too and it was her confession to her co-workers that led to her being found guilty of murdering her new-born female infant in Foley's Hotel, Wicklow Street on 17 November 1900.[49] Barry was a live-in cook who shared a room with two other hotel workers, Mary Buckley (with whom she shared a bed) and Ellen Boland.[50] All three retired at 10.30 p.m. on 16 November 1900 and shortly after that Barry got up and left the room. As she was 'a long time absent' Buckley and Boland got worried and went looking for her. They found her in the lavatory, which was locked; she assured them that she was fine, that there was no need to inform the mistress and she asked them to leave. Unsettled by the scenario, Buckley came back to check on her again five minutes later and claimed that on her return visit that she heard a baby cry. Buckley also claimed that although they shared a bed and had known one another for four months that she did not notice the pregnancy.[51] Barry confessed to Boland the following day that she had placed 'it in a box'. The matter was brought to the attention of the authorities. When the box was opened by Dr Charles Casey, he found the child wrapped in a towel, which Barry had used to block the airways.[52] Dr Thomas Stephens conducted the post-mortem and said it was a healthy child. The cord was torn near the umbil-

---

[44] *Evening Herald*, 6 April 1901; *Freeman's Journal*, 8 April 1901.
[45] NAI, Dublin Crown Files at Commission, *King v Sarah Stephens*, 9 April 1901.
[46] *Freeman's Journal*, 10 April 1901.
[47] See http://www.census.nationalarchives.ie/reels/nai003767706/ (accessed 18 January 2020).
[48] See http://www.census.nationalarchives.ie/reels/nai003759933/ (accessed 18 January 2020).
[49] NAI/1900/173 Inquest on the body of a female infant. Inquest is cited in Farrell but not traced to criminal courts: Farrell, 'A Most "Diabolical Deed"', pp. 54–5.
[50] NAI, Dublin Crown Files at Commission, 3 December 1900, *Queen v* Kate Barry. Evidence of Mary Buckley taken 24 November at the police court.
[51] NAI, Dublin Crown Files at Commission, 3 December 1900, *Queen v* Kate Barry. Evidence of Mary Buckley taken 24 November at the police court.
[52] *Freeman's Journal*, 20 November 1900.

icus 'and was ragged'; he conducted the hydrostatic test and believed it was born alive.[53] The coroner's jury found that the 'said newly-born infant was murdered by its mother, Kate Barry'.[54] She was indicted on 17 November, brought before the police court on 24 November and before Justice Madden on the second day of the December sitting of the City of Dublin Commission charged with manslaughter.[55] On 3 December she was described as an orphan and just 20 years of age. According to the newspaper accounts her defence argued that she was 'bereft of reason' after giving birth. The jury was convinced that Barry was 'not responsible for her act at the time'. She was found not guilty and discharged.[56] It is very difficult to correlate her case with the statistical tables returned by the DMP, which give broad figures and very little by way of a breakdown. In 1900, under Class I offences, two cases of murder of infants under 1 year were recorded and both were sent to prison; the two cases of abandonment of children under 2 were acquitted.[57] Figures are presented in aggregate and while the date of crime committed is given (and it is likely the apprehension on 3 December 1900 was Kate Barry) we cannot identify the perpetrators definitively as the jurisdiction of the DMP was greater than that of the city coroner's.[58] The duality of major and minor charges makes it difficult to understand how these crimes were categorised in the returns as the law permitted the lesser charge. Barry was charged with manslaughter and not the murder she was indicted for originally. In 1901 there were no cases of murder of persons under 1 year accounted for. The DMP statistical returns included sixteen cases of abandonment of which three were apprehended (one discharged), nine cases of concealment with two apprehensions (one was discharged, the other was sent to prison) and one female was apprehended and tried for manslaughter.[59]

Offering a sharp contrast to the cases of hapless, young, and single country girls was the case of Bridget Hanlon and Agnes Browne, who were both brought before the police court on 27 July 'on habeas corpus charged with infanticide'[60] and before the City of Dublin Commission on 1 August 1900 for the manslaughter of 3-month-old Patrick Hanlon at 59 Marlboro Street. While the coroner's jury found that the child died of inanition (or inability to absorb his food), the course of the subsequent investigation revealed malice aforethought and attempted murder.[61]

---

[53] NAI, Dublin Crown Files at Commission, 3 December 1900, *Queen v Kate Barry*. Evidence of Dr Thomas Foye Stephens, taken 24 November at the police court.
[54] *Freeman's Journal*, 20 November 1900.
[55] *Freeman's Journal*, 5 December 1900; *Irish Daily Independent*, 5 December 1900.
[56] *Irish Daily Independent*, 5 December 1900.
[57] *Statistical tables of the Dublin Metropolitan Police for the year 1900* [Cd. 615], pp. 4–5.
[58] *Statistical tables of the Dublin Metropolitan Police for the year 1900* [Cd. 615], pp. 6–7. According to the *Statistical tables of the Dublin Metropolitan Police for the year 1901*, p. x., the population of the DMP jurisdiction was 390,187.
[59] *Statistical tables of the Dublin Metropolitan Police for the year 1901* [Cd. 1166], pp. 2–4.
[60] *Freeman's Journal*, 28 July 1900.
[61] NAI/1900/62 Inquest report of Patrick Hanlon, 10 July 1900.

Witnesses Rosanna Rourke, Christopher Woods, and Anne Cassidy were all in the front drawing room of 59 Marlboro Street when they overheard the women make their dastardly plan in the back hallway. Rourke claimed that she heard a child cry and went out into the hallway where Hanlon and Brown were. She overheard Browne say 'whisht there is someone coming we'll wring the bloody child's neck' to which Hanlon responded 'I love my child I am the mother of the child'; this, the witness later speculated, was in an attempt to 'prevent violence to it'. Rourke intervened and advised giving the child some milk and Browne told her to 'mind your own business'. At that point she could see a pink flannelette cloth wrapped around its neck. Hanlon revealed to Rourke that she had just left the 'St James's Street Union' and she claimed to not know the two other women, whom she described as 'unfortunates who lived in 66 Montgomery St', but cursory research shows that she had entered the NDU and SDU with Brown on a few occasions earlier in 1900.[62] The party in the front room sensed something was very much awry—Anne Cassidy took the child from Browne's arms and brought it to Dr Dunne in Jervis Street, and later to the NDU hospital. There he was placed under the care of Visiting Surgeon Caleb James Powell on 6 July. A constable was called and Hanlon and Brown were arrested, the third unnamed woman escaped. The child subsequently died on 9 June from the 'shock' and bruises, the result of violence according to Powell.[63] Hanlon had her baby in SDU under Nurse Margaret Bayliffe and spent a month there post-partum with her child. She was unmarried and her mother Catherine also lived at the SDU so she had no support network outside of it and she fell in with 'unfortunate' company. Post-mortem found a complete absence of fat from all parts of the body, so it seems the child had been suffering the rigours of neglect and under-nourishment in the two months since they left the SDU. Both Hanlon and Brown were described in the newspapers as being from 'the unfortunate class', which often served as a euphemism for prostitute. Their actions accelerated the death of the child—they were brought before the City of Dublin Commission on 1 August 1900 charged with attempted murder but were convicted of manslaughter and sentenced to five years' penal servitude.[64] Compared to other cases discussed in this section and in the section on neglect in Chapter 2, it seems that their low social status had an impact on their treatment in the courts and beyond.

Prior character had a strong bearing on treatment during incarceration—normally, offenders proceeded through a series of phases, good behaviour coupled

[62] NAI, Dublin Crown Files at Commission, August 1900: deposition of Rosanna Rourke dated 7 June, indictment numbers 8 and 17. NAI. BG 79/G89, nos. 936–7; NAI, BG 78/ G80, nos. 2776–7, 13 January 1900; NAI, BG 79/G89 1648–9 28 February 1900; 6 April 1900 Bridget entered on her own to have her child NAI, BG 79/G89, no. 2863, child no. 3457 was born 24 April, and they left together on 6 June 1900.

[63] NAI, Dublin Crown Files at Commission, August, 1900: deposition of Rosanna Rourke dated 27 July 1900.

[64] *Freeman's Journal*, 4 August 1900.

with marks earned with the passage of time punctuated progress. Agnes Browne had four convictions for illegal possession of silver, drunkenness, and two counts of profane language. When some confusion about her previous convictions arose in her convict record, a letter dated 30 April 1901 stated that she rightly belonged in the 'old offender division' and not the 'select division'. Because of her prior convictions and despite having earned enough marks for release, her application to the 'refuge class' was denied in March 1903 and she was released on licence to the Model Lodging House on Benburb Street in November 1903. That licence was revoked when she was found drunk on a highway on 7 April 1904.[65] She was eventually released in July 1905 after serving over four years. Like Browne, Bridget Hanlon was denied entry to refuge class on 3 March 1903 'having regard to the Police report at the time of her conviction' which alluded to the fact that she was living in a brothel at the time. An inquiry into her character on 16 August 1901 stated that she 'was not a public or well-known prostitute and did not live in brothels or associate much with fallen women. She has lived from time to time for past few years in some of the "homes" for fallen women in the city and suburbs. She was not much known to the police.' For such reasons, she was released earlier than Browne on licence in December 1903 to her sister Mrs Rogers of Little Britain Street.[66]

The various cases accounted for here occupy part of a spectrum of child cruelty and murder (Table 4.2). To bring these cases where leniency prevailed into another light, it is worth dwelling on a contrasting case, whereby the law and the public appetite for punishment were at odds, and where evidence of prior good character was brought to bear. Hannah Kavanagh's case came before the county coroner as the body was found near Pigeon House Road but it stands in contrast with the city cases for two reasons: first, her child was 3 months old when she killed it and second, the fact that she was charged with, and convicted for, murder.

Table 4.2 Actions arising from infanticide, suspicious infant deaths April 1900–April 1902

Surname	First	Age	Cause of death	Married	Trial	Outcome
Hanlon/ Browne	Bridget/ Agnes	3m	Non assimilation of food	Unclear	Yes	5 yrs
Barry	Kate	0	Asphyxia	No	Yes	Acquitted
Stephens	Sarah	0	Asphyxia	No	Yes	Released 'on her own recognisance'
Curley	Bridget	4m	Starvation and neglect	No	Yes	19 days

[65] NAI/GPB/PEN/1905/51 penal file of Agnes Browne, B285.
[66] NAI/GPB/PEN/1905/77 penal file of Bridget Hanlon, B286.

She was described in newspapers as 'A poor creature, young, half simple…born into a family over which hung the dread shadow of insanity harassed by her parents for money, money, money: betrayed by the man who promised her marriage.… Has she no friend or brother to hunt this man out?'.[67] The case came before Christopher Friery, as coroner of the County Council of County Dublin, at the morgue on Londonbridge Road, who had 'called attention to the frequency with which infant children were being deposited in rivers and about lands in the neighbourhood of Sandymount'.[68] It seems that she arrived in Dublin pregnant and took up a position on 23 March 1900 in the household of Samuel Johnson Dodder Bank. She did not conceal her pregnancy when questioned about it, and she left her employment for a short while in June to have her baby at Holles Street Hospital. Predicated on the promise of marriage, on 19 June Kavanagh decided to keep the child; she placed it out to nurse with Bridget Whelan, Cambridge Place, on 30 June. When the promise of marriage was breached and financial pressure from home was brought to bear, Kavanagh decided to dispose of her child, which at 3 months carried with it a much higher prospect of being caught and apprehended. Whelan later testified that on 22 September Kavanagh called for the child and claimed that she had made arrangements for another woman to 'nurse the child'.[69] On 23 September an inquest was held on the body of a 3-month-old unknown infant found drowned in the River Liffey near the Coastguard Station at Pigeon House Road. Kavanagh was apprehended and tried for murder, and the jury returned a verdict of guilty with a recommendation to mercy. Mr Justice Gibson had little choice but to hand down the death sentence on 17 October 1900. He fixed her date of execution, by hanging, for 16 November 1900.[70] An appeal to mercy was made and her sentence was commuted on 19 October to penal servitude for life. She was discharged on licence in December 1901 to the care of the 'Discharged Prisoner's Aid Society'.[71] Kavanagh was convicted on 17 October and, unlike Hanlon and Browne, she was released after a year.[72]

Not all suspicious deaths in domestic contexts and with evidence of clear criminal actions resulted in apprehensions by the police, which brings us back to the perennial problem of classifications. The final case in this infanticide cohort concerned a double tragedy of Mary Gorey and her child. After her body was found, that of a mutilated infant was discovered too, in a room at 31 Findlater Street. When Joseph Malone 29D, Green Street, examined the scene of Mary Gorey's death he made a macabre discovery of 'a tin can containing a quantity of flesh and

---

[67] *Evening Herald*, 18 October 1900.   [68] *Evening Herald*, 27 September 1900.
[69] Sworn evidence of Bridget Whelan, 27 September 1900—she confirmed this sworn evidence on 2 October; *Irish Daily Independent*, 18 October 1900.
[70] NAI/GPB/CN/5 the Death Book recorded all execution cases—most death sentences were commuted.
[71] NAI, GPB/CRF/K-32–1900 (Criminal Reference File) document dated 22 December 1900.
[72] NAI, GPB/PEN/1901/115 Penal File of Hannah Kavanagh B287.

bones cut up into small pieces – also a soiled petticoat'.[73] Dr John Burgess had to face the grim task of itemising over two hundred body parts and he deposed on 5 April 1901 that the sex was not determinable.[74] Gorey, who had been 'in service' at a house on Stephen's Green up until seven weeks' prior, was living with her brother Christopher and his wife. A detailed post-mortem was conducted by Dr Burgess, who testified that she had been recently delivered of a child. The coroner advised that the jury return an open verdict as it hinged to such a large degree on the outcome of the adjourned inquest of Mary Gorey herself. The verdict in Gorey's case was 'Canonisation of the uterine veins after her confinement' but in the course of that inquiry it was revealed that she told her brother Christopher how she had taken poison on 31 March, which necessitated the examination of the contents of her stomach by the state laboratory. The poison was contained in a bottle that had been prescribed by Dr Dobbin for external use only. It was purchased at P. Carthy's chemist shop at 83 Queen's Street. Christopher Gorey claimed that he tried to get his sister to go to the hospital but she refused, stating that she felt fine. Sir Charles Cameron testified that although the contents of the bottles he was furnished with, if taken in sufficient quantities, were indeed poisonous, her stomach was empty save for some mucus. Only nine members of the jury agreed on the proposed rider, 'That Christopher Gorey acted inhumanly [sic] in not rendering medical aid to his sister'; seven were opposed to the motion. As the supporting number was under twelve, the coroner could not accept it. Instead, a verdict of death 'from want of proper attention after confinement' was returned.[75] Dr Byrne rarely commented on such matters but he added, 'Speaking personally, I certainly would not ask if she wanted a doctor, but I would get a doctor or bring her to hospital.'[76] Both Christopher and his wife claimed to know nothing of the pregnancy or the mutilated child's body. Although the child's genitalia and some of its face were missing, whether or not Mary Gorey had help in killing the child, chopping up the body or disposing of the missing parts was deliberated in the coroner's court but did not give rise to further legal action on the part of the DMP.

Infanticidal women were undoubtedly treated differently by the criminal courts. With the increasing pathologisation of the mental state of post-partum women as the nineteenth century progressed, they were invariably presented, as in the case of Kate Barry, as 'mad not bad' in the criminal courts.[77] The temporary insanity ruling or the 'McNaugten rules' devised in 1843 were not directly applied

[73] NAI, 1901/97 Inquest on the body of Unknown Infant, Child of Mary Gorey, 5 April 1901; *Irish Examiner*, 4 April 1901.
[74] NAI, 1901/97 Inquest on the body of Unknown Infant, Child of Mary Gorey, 5 April 1901.
[75] *Evening Herald*, 12 April 1901; *Freeman's Journal*, 13 April 1901; NAI/1901/96 Inquest on the body of Mary Gorey, 1 April 1901.
[76] *Evening Herald*, 12 April 1901.
[77] Loughnan, ' "Strange" case of the infanticide doctrine', p. 688.

in any of the cases discussed here but are implicit in the way some cases were allowed to fade away without repercussion. Loughnan argues that in tandem with changes to the law the pathologisation of the parturient woman emerged and thus puerperal fever/mania/insanity entered the medico-legal lexicon and what she terms 'manifest madness' gained traction.[78] So embedded was the mindset of leniency in neonaticide and infanticide cases that, with the exception of alleged prostitutes Hanlon and Browne, most of the cases discussed here barely resulted in prosecutions and, if they did, sentences were light.

Suicide: Law, Religion, and Traditions

In his response to the Dublin public health inquiry in 1900, Alderman Joseph Meade claimed that the suicide numbers were 'exceedingly low' but it is likely that his figures were based on officially recorded cause of death which underrepresented the full extent of the problem.[79] Suicide was routinely underreported in Ireland, which owed much to whether deaths came to the attention of a coroner and how the coronial courts categorised cause of death.[80] The advice given to coroners in 1864 on recording alleged suicide was that they were to include three classes of facts in the verdict: the first established the identity of the person involved, the second referred to the things employed to carry out the act, and the third was the medical perspective or a description of the physical injuries.[81] Part of the problem with suicide classification was that coroners' courts tended to use euphemistic language in verdicts that was both sympathetic to the deceased and their surviving relatives. Both Olive Anderson and Victor Bailey have argued in their respective work on English statistics that they are not a useful way to study the hermeneutics of suicide. Anderson's comprehensive work argued that age, gender, and place all impacted suicide rates.[82] Bailey based his work on a large body of coronial court records primarily from Hull in England, and advocated an ethnomethodological approach to court records.[83] McCarthy and Walsh adopted such an approach in an earlier article discussing suicide in Dublin from 1954 to 1963. They argued that the verdict of suicide was returned in less than half or 47.8 per cent of the likely number of 136 cases. Of the remaining 52.3 per cent, 'the verdict was couched in broad general terms, phenomenologically descriptive of the

[78] Loughnan, ' "Strange" case of the infanticide doctrine', p. 698.   [79] *Dublin Report*, p. 181.

[80] Dermot Walsh, 'Suicide in Ireland in the 19th century', *Irish Journal of Psychological Medicine*, 34:3 (2017), pp. 177–81.

[81] *A Statistical Nosology, Comprising the Causes of Death, Classified and Alphabetically Arranged, with Notes and Observations* (Dublin, 1864), pp. 55–60: https://babel.hathitrust.org/cgi/pt?id=uiug.30112059511607&view=1up&seq=67.

[82] Olive Anderson, *Suicide in Victorian and Edwardian England* (Oxford, 1987).

[83] Victor Bailey, *This Rash Act: Suicide Across the Life Cycle in the Victorian City* (Redwood City, 1998), pp. 3–4.

circumstances leading to death and excluding any consideration of motivation'.[84] The turn of the nineteenth century was no different and because the historiography of suicide is underdeveloped, this section begins by explaining why.[85]

Suicide in the nineteenth century occupied a legal grey area—the existing legislation had ramifications for both the burial rites and the property of the deceased. Unlike infanticide, which was specifically nominated in a series of acts and, in particular for our purposes, as a misdemeanour in the Offences Against the Persons Act 1861, the statutes pertaining to suicide and attempted suicide did so indirectly. Attempting suicide was considered an indictable felony under section 15 of the 1861 act and many cases came before the courts.[86] With the exception of the Summary Jurisdiction (Ireland) Amendment Act 1871 and its mention of attempted suicide, it was not explicitly stated in Irish homicide law and it was very much open to interpretation.[87] Although they were primarily courts of record, coronial courts were where suicides were assessed and categorised from a criminal perspective. Despite the fact that suicide was what Georgina Laragy terms 'a crime without punishment', it could bring a range of indignities, primarily to the posthumous handling of the corpse and pecuniary sanctions with regard to the estate of the deceased. Thus the role of the coroner's court with respect to suicide shifted from that of a court of record to being a locus of official categorisation for legal purposes. Only if the coroner's verdict found it was a deliberate act of self-murder while of sound mind could ignominious burial or financial penalties be levied. To fully understand the legal complexities of suicide it is necessary to look at a few factors: first, how it nestled into burial law, which was informed by canon law; second, the origins of its criminalisation; and third, why it is necessary to extricate Irish from English law as they were not in unison, mainly for confessional but also for cultural reasons. A further consideration is the interplay

---

[84] P. Desmond McCarthy and Dermot Walsh, 'Suicide in Dublin', *The British Medical Journal*, 1:5500 (4 June 1966), pp. 1393–6 at 1394.

[85] Georgina Laragy's monograph *Suicide in Ireland; 1823–1918; a social and Cultural history* will make important contributions to knowledge (forthcoming with Liverpool University Press).

[86] Offences Against the Persons Act 1861 (23 &24 Vic.) c. 100, s. 15 'Whosoever shall, by any means other than those specified in any of the preceding sections of this Act, attempt to commit murder, shall be guilty of felony, and being convicted thereof shall be liable...to be kept in penal servitude for life...'. Brendan Kelly, *Hearing Voices: The History of Psychiatry in Ireland* (Dublin, 2016); Criminal Law (Suicide) Act, 1993, no. 11: Suicide was decriminalised in Ireland in 1993.

[87] Summary Jurisdiction (Ireland) Amendment Act 1871, 1871 c. 76, summary procedure in certain cases of attempted suicide within police district of Dublin Metropolis, 1871 c. 76 s. 9: 'Where any person is charged before any of the divisional justices of the police district of Dublin Metropolis presiding in one of the public courts of the said district with having in any manner attempted to commit suicide, if the person charged shall confess the same, it shall be lawful for the justice to convict the person charged, and commit him to the common gaol or house of correction, there to be imprisoned, with or without hard labour, for any period not exceeding three months: Provided always, that if the person charged do not consent to have the case heard and determined by such justices, or if such justice be of opinion that the charge is fit to be made the subject of prosecution by indictment, rather than to be disposed of summarily, he shall, instead of summarily adjudicating thereon, deal with the case in all respects as if this Act had not been passed.'

between custom and law, the emergence of traditions surrounding self-murder, and how that filtered into supernatural beliefs.

Both canon and common law informed the ways in which the legal code of suicide evolved. Embodied primarily in the writings of St Augustine (354–430) in the *City of God* and later Thomas Aquinas (1225–1274) in his *Summa Theologiae*, canon law emerged firmly on the side of suicide as a form of murder and contrary to the sixth commandment 'thou shalt not kill'.[88] St Augustine aimed to counteract the romantic narrative of the Stoics by discouraging self-murder as a moral imperative and Aquinas reinforced the fundamental principles of the Divine's right to give and take life. In the interim of both philosophical works a number of Catholic Councils at Orleans (533), Braga (541), Auxerre (*c.*561–605) and Toledo (693) deliberated suicide and attempted suicide from a theological perspective. Each produced canons about how, and if, the body of a suicide victim should receive rites or whether they should be buried on consecrated ground. Eventually these canons took root in Roman and common law practices. In her study of canon law with respect to suicide in England, Charlotte Wright traces the first resolution to the Council of Hereford in 672 which denied normal funerals and burials to suicides.[89] An ecclesiastical prohibition on suicide was first formally adopted in 673 and it permeated other jurisdictions thereafter. Early evidence of the criminalisation of suicide in England can be traced to a thirteenth-century Latin manuscript translated as Bracton's *On the Laws*, which accounted for circumstances leading to suicide case law and distinguished between sane and insane actions.[90] Brehon law, an ancient code, prevailed in Ireland at that time and it made no specific mention of suicide compensation or reparations for it, as was customary for other homicides.[91] Inevitably, as W.N. Osborough posits, canon law influenced Brehon law because very often the same person administered ecclesiastical court and Brehon law judgements.[92]

According to MacDonald, from 1600 to 1800 in England religious and popular beliefs both gave way to and 'were gradually eclipsed by medical and philosophical ideas that exculpated it' but there was still a strong appetite for posthumous punishment.[93] Further to this he found that after the Reformation the English Protestant preachers evoked the spectre of the devil as tempter to denounce suicide.[94] This religious zeal was not replicated to the same extent in Ireland, where the Book of Common Prayer was adopted following the Act of Uniformity in

---

[88] Alexander Murray, *Suicide in the Middle Ages: Volume 2: The Curse on Self-Murder* (Oxford, 2011).
[89] Charlotte Wright, 'The English Canon Law relating to suicide victims', *Ecclesiastical Law Society*, 19 (2017), pp. 193–211 at 198.
[90] Margaret Pabst Battin, *The Ethics of Suicide: Historical Sources* (Oxford, 2015), p. 220.
[91] Richard E. Cherry, 'The Eric fines of ancient Irish law', *Journal of the Statistical and Social Inquiry Society of Ireland*, Vol. VIII, Part LXII (1884), pp. 544–51.
[92] W.N. Osborough, 'Roman law in Ireland', *Irish Jurist*, 25/27 (1990/1992), pp. 212–68 at 291.
[93] Michael MacDonald, 'The secularization of suicide in England 1660–1800', *Past & Present*, 111 (1986), pp. 50–100 at 52.
[94] MacDonald, 'The secularization of suicide in England', p. 55.

1666. The order for the burial of the dead stated explicitly that it was 'not to be used for any that die unbaptized, or excommunicate, or have laid violent hands upon themselves'.[95] But, as Wright contends, it made no provision for those of unsound mind who could not be held responsible for their actions. In the overlap between common and Brehon law the application of this dictate very much depended on social class and how the law was observed. During the seventeenth century, as R.A. Houston observes, the English settler laws co-existed with Brehon law and the former was not applied to the Irish.[96] It is for such reasons that in Gaelic Ireland common law was slower to gain traction, particularly with respect to the confiscation of property.

From the forfeiture act of 1639 until 1870, when a propertied person committed suicide they were guilty of treason which was a felony and, as with all felonies, his or her estate could be seized by the Crown.[97] Clodagh Tait argues that suicides were regarded as 'bad deaths' in early modern Ireland and considered an affront to both God and Crown. With the overlap of Brehon and common law evidence of how the forfeiture of goods and chattels was applied in the early modern period is scant, but Tait gives a few examples.[98] In the modern period there were some high-profile cases, like that of that of Lord Castlereagh in 1822, but coronial courts were used to great effect to circumnavigate the penalty of forfeiture for treason and felony until it was abolished in England, Wales, and Ireland in 1870 (it did not apply to Scotland).[99]

Even in England, as David Cannadine contends, it was difficult to implement the civil, criminal, and ecclesiastical sanctions for suicide. With legislative and ecclesiastical reform the Church of England's control over burial grounds was gradually eroded.[100] It could be argued that neither forfeiture nor burial implications took root in Ireland. A case in point is that of United Irishman Theobold Wolfe Tone, who was tried for high treason for his part in the 1798 rebellion and sentenced to death—he denied the authorities justice by committing suicide. Marian Elliott described it as 'a godsend' as his execution had such potential to ignite further unrest.[101] His coroner's inquest decreed that he died from

[95] 'The book of common-prayer, and administration of the sacraments, and other rites & ceremonies of the Church, according to the use of the Church of Ireland; together with the Psalter or Psalms of David, pointed as they are to be sung or said in churches. And the form and manner of making, ordaining, and consecrating of bishops, priests, & deacons Date: 1680' (TCD, http://gateway.proquest.com. proxy.lib.ul.ie/openurl?ctx_ver=Z39.88–2003&res_id=xri:eebo&rft_id=xri:eebo:image:31220:159).

[96] R.A Houston, 'People, space, and law in late medieval and early modern Britain and Ireland', *Past & Present*, 230:1 (2016), pp. 47–89 at 52.

[97] Forfeiture Act (Ireland) 1639 (15 Chas.1) c. 3 s. 2; Forfeiture Act 1870 (33 & 34 Vic.) c. 23. Section 1 specified *félo de se* and section 33 outlined jurisdictions.

[98] Clodagh Tait, *Death, Burial and Commemoration in Ireland, 1550–1650* (Basingstoke, 2002), pp. 19–22.

[99] Patrick Maume, 'The Head Pacificator and Captain Rock: sedition, suicide and Honest Tom Steele', in Kyle Hughes and Donald MacRaild (eds), *Crime, Violence and the Irish in the Nineteenth Century* (Liverpool, 2017).

[100] David Cannadine, *History in Our Time* (New Haven, 1998), p. 125.

[101] Marianne Elliott, *Wolfe Tone* (Liverpool, 2012), p. 386.

'inflammation of the lungs due to self-murder'.[102] Not only were his remains promptly handed over to his family, they were interred at Bodenstown, within the churchyard walls. Further to this, some of his property—money, clothes and watch—was given to his relatives.[103] Ignominious burial, which had a tentative legal standing, continued until 1823 when an act pertaining specifically to *felo de se* was passed stating the right to burial in a churchyard or other burial ground between the hours of 9 p.m. and midnight and within twenty-four hours of the inquest verdict. It outlawed the practice of roadside burials and staking.[104] The act received scant attention in Ireland—the *Dublin Journal* hardly registered its significance and *Freeman's Journal* noted it in passing terms as follows: 'An act relative to the internment of persons found *felo de se* received the Royal Assent last week: no more persons committing suicide are to be buried at crossroads.'[105]

Separate legislation governed burial law in Ireland. From 1697 with an act banishing 'popish clergy', the Church of Ireland (a separate entity to the Church of England until 1801), was the Established Church until disestablishment under the Irish Church Act of 1869.[106] Burial for Catholics during that time was a highly contentious matter in Ireland as it fell under the remit of the rites of the local Protestant church, which had requisitioned the use of all churchyards and monastery grounds under penal law. Quite apart from suicides, interment on unconsecrated ground was not uncommon for the Irish poor as penal laws severely restricted burials for Catholics and Dissenters. Punitive fines introduced in 1697 for congregations caught in attendance at burials were beyond the means of the ordinary Irish and acted as a powerful deterrent.[107] Catholics had to pay fees to the Established Church for burial rites. Burial fees of £10 were cited by the

---

[102] *Trial of Theobald Wolfe Tone for High Treason, before a Court Martial holden at Dublin on Saturday, November 10th, together with the Proceedings in the Court of King's Bench on Monday, November 12th*: 27 St Tr 613; Elliott, *Wolfe Tone*, p. 386.

[103] Elliott, *Wolfe Tone*, pp. 385–6.

[104] Burial of Suicide Act 1823 (4 Geo 4) c 52: Rites of Christian Burial not to be performed, 1823 c. 52 s II. The act stipulated that 'such Coroner or other Officer shall give Directions for the private Interment of the Remains of such Person *Felo de se*, without any Stake being driven through the Body of such Person, in the Churchyard or other Burial Ground of the Parish or Place in which the Remains of such Person might by the Laws or Custom of *England* be interred if the Verdict of *Felo de se* had not been found against such Person; such Interment to be made within Twenty four Hours from the Finding of the Inquisition, and to take place between the Hours of Nine and Twelve at Night'; Barbara T. Gates, *Victorian Suicide: Mad Crimes and Sad Histories* (Princeton, 1988), p. 6.

[105] *Freeman's Journal*, 21 July 1823; *Dublin Journal*, 28 July 1823. I am grateful to Dr Coleman Dennehy for his advice on how this act applied to Ireland.

[106] An Act for banishing all papists exercising any ecclesiastical jurisdiction, and all regulars of the popish clergy out of this kingdom 1697 (9 Will III) c. 1.

[107] An Act for banishing all papists exercising any ecclesiastical jurisdiction and all regulars of the popish clergy out of this kingdom 1697 (9 Will III) c. 1 s. 6–7: 'No person shall bury any dead in any suppressed monastery, abbey, or convent, upon pain of forfeiting ten pounds, which sum shall be recovered from any person present at the burial, one half to the informer, one half to the minister and church wardens of the parish where such offences shall be committed. Appeal may be made to the next judges of assize or to the justices at the next quarter sessions.'

Catholic Association in 1823 in its deliberation of the then current burial bill.[108] A series of burial acts from 1824 to 1868 pertaining to Ireland only, gradually repealed the restrictions for Dissenters but were not without controversy. Although the 1824 act attempted to ease some grievances, it brought in new regulations that, some Irish MPs argued, degraded Catholic parish priests who had to apply in writing to their Protestant opposite numbers for permission to say prayers at funerals. Furthermore, as Murphy and Murphy have argued, the act was

> a major source of dispute in the bitter sectarian climate of the 1820s and the 1830s. The more extreme element of the Protestant interest manifested a new level of hostility to Catholic funerals in parish churchyards under the control of the Established Church. Catholics, for their part, resented the payment of funeral charges to clergy of the Church of Ireland.[109]

New legislation introduced in 1856 vested power for the management of grounds in burial boards, which went some way towards secularisation and shifting power away from the Church of Ireland.[110] The 1868 act retained some of the controversial elements of the 1824 act, and while the necessity to get permission was dropped, Catholic priests still had to notify the rector in writing of the time they wished to recite prayers.[111] Once the Church of Ireland was disestablished in 1869, the burial grounds formerly under its control were handed over to the Poor Law guardians.[112] Under the 1878 Public Health Act, burial became the remit of sanitary authorities. Very little attention was paid to religion under these acts save the rights to erect monuments if they were approved by respective clergy. According to that act the sanitary authority became the burial board.[113]

The separation of Church and state in England brought major changes to bear on legislation with the Burial Laws Amendment Act 1880, which dealt primarily with the right to burial without Church of England rites and did not apply to Ireland.[114] According to Wiggins, 'the graveyards of England and Wales became the battleground for the final struggle between the Church and

---

[108] The Catholic Association was established by Daniel O'Connell in 1823; *Proceedings of the Catholic Association in Dublin, May 13, 1823 to Feb. 11* (London, 1825), p. 76.

[109] John A. Murphy and Clíona Murphy, 'Burials and bigotry in early nineteenth-century Ireland', *Studia Hibernica*, 33 (2004/5), pp. 125–46 at 125.

[110] Burial Grounds (Ireland) Act, 1856 (19 & 20 Vic.) c. 98.

[111] An Act to amend the Law which regulates the Burials of Persons in Ireland not belonging to the Established Church, 1868 (31 & 32 Vict.) c. 103; The Burial (Ireland) Act, 1888—see (59 & 60 Vict.) c. 14.

[112] Irish Church Act 1869 (32 & 33 Vict.) c. 42, s. 26.1, Burial Grounds (Ireland) Act, 1856 (19 & 20 Vic.), c. 98.

[113] Public Health (Ireland) Act, 1878, c. 52, s. 183. '... for the burial of the members of any particular religious denomination; and each such allotment shall, as the case may require, be consecrated according to the rites and by the proper ministers of the respective religious denominations for which each such allotment is so set apart.'

[114] Burial Laws Amendment Act 1880 (43 & 44 Vic.) c. 41.

the disestablishmentarians.'[115] Legislation introduced in Interments (*felo de se*) Act 1882 relaxed the draconian requirements and removed all remaining obstacles with respect to the burial of suicides in England and Wales, but that was not extended to Ireland either. This underscores the importance of separating the Irish (and Scottish) experience both in law and custom regarding suicide, from the English and Welsh.

Increased anxieties surrounding good deaths gave rise to new beliefs and superstitions surrounding suicides in Ireland. Ignominious roadside burials were by the early modern period accompanied by a set of practices in England and across Europe that included decapitation but were more commonly characterised by driving a stake through the heart. It was believed that this 'anchored the ghost, and burying the corpse at a crossroads confounded the revenant, ensuring that it would not be able to return to the community and inflict harm on the living.'[116] Such practices were not that common or evenly spread across Ireland. In his analysis of eighteenth-century Irish suicide, Kelly found evidence of the prevalence of nocturnal roadside burials and 'strand burial' for those living in maritime areas.[117] There is some evidence of the latter in the National Folklore Collection (NFC). For example:

> This is the story of a stud groom who had charge of a gentleman's horses at Gerrardstown Dunshaughlin. He was extremely jealous of his wife. This morning when he went out to work he chanced to hear some injudicious remark concerning his wife. He rushed back, shot his wife and baby and then himself. No churchyard would take his remains for burial[.] Mrs Reilly remembers seeing the coffin being taken from one to another on a cart and being refused admittance everywhere. At last it was thrown into the sea at Balbriggan. The house of tragedy was demolished by order of the Dunshaughlin priests. The place is said to be haunted since.[118]

The story contains attributes typical of most recollections of suicides in the NFC; the reason for it, the mode of self-murder, the unorthodox burial and the restless soul. The centrality of the priest was a common trope in Irish folklore as an authority on moral issues who acted in strong opposition to the power of the supernatural. Other lore gathered as part of the Schools' Collection in 1937 detail how the ghosts of suicide victims tended to linger near their burial sites and one

---

[115] Burial Laws Amendment Act 1880 (43 & 44 Vic.) c. 41 s. 1; Interments (Felo de se) Act 1882 (45 & 46 Vic.) c. 19; Deborah Wiggins, 'The Burial Act of 1880, The Liberation Society and George Osborne Morgan', *Parliamentary History*, 15:2 (1996), pp. 173–89 at 173.

[116] Sarah Tarlow and Emma Battell Lowman, *Harnessing the Power of the Criminal Corpse* (Basingstoke, 2018), p. 101.

[117] James Kelly, 'Suicide in eighteenth-century Ireland', in James Kelly and Mary Ann Lyons (eds), *Death and Dying in Ireland, Britain and Europe* (Dublin, 2011), pp. 95–142.

[118] NFC, *The Schools' Collection*, Volume 0687, p. 165.

accounts for a very unusual coronial jury rider in Kilkenny that recommended driving a stake through the heart of a suicide victim, but it was ignored. Implicit in this story is that the customs in rural Ireland differed to, or indeed explicitly rejected those of Britain and the continent. The respondent noted how:

> Within living memory there was a suicide in a house in Dereen, belonging to Mr. Thompson and the jury at the inquest added a rider to the verdict that the body be taken to the nearest cross roads and a hazel stick driven through the body and buried but this injunction was not carried out. All suicides were buried at cross-roads on olden times – in this district anyway. [119]

Suicides had legacy impacts for families who had to bear the perceived stigmata of mental health problems in the lineage. The matter of burial took some time to resolve because of the way the law over the centuries permeated the everyday and the definite Catholic stance about denying rights to burial on consecrated ground; this in turn had an impact on coroners' juries—verdicts and riders that were often vague and illusive in tone and intent. In the Catholic tradition, suicides were then and continue to be officially precluded from religious ceremonies but some priests, aided by coronial court verdicts, exercised compassion.

Suicide Figures

Coroners' verdicts were given in writing and verbatim to the local registrar, which in turn should have been transcribed precisely by the registrar. The verdicts were later used to underpin cause of suspicious death in the aggregate returns of the Registrar General. The nosology supplied to registrars in 1864 considered the term suicide vague and the coronial court verdicts, as we shall shortly see, were far from transparent.[120] Determining the relationship between the various datasets is therefore complicated and it seems some degree of translation occurred on the part of the registrar. In 1900 the Registrar General returned 118 deaths by suicide nationally, eighty-four of which were male, occurring primarily after the age of 35.[121] The figures are not broken down by county but a provincial dispersion is given: thirty-three suicides occurred in Leinster and twenty-two involved men. According to the 1901 ARRG there were 127 suicides: 101 were of men, twenty-four occurred in Leinster, and six of the twenty-six female cases recorded

---

[119] NFC, *The Schools' Collection*, Volume 0854, pp. 129–30—efforts to correlate this to a coroner's case has proven fruitless.

[120] *Statistical Nosology*, p. 50.

[121] Of the thirty-four female cases, four were in the earlier age cohorts (15–20 age bracket) but an even distribution as follows 15–1, 20–4, 25–4, 35–8, 45–4, 55–8, 65–2, 75–0, 85–3: *Thirty-seventh detailed annual report of the Registrar-General* [Cd. 697], pp. 20, 142–3.

nationally were located there too.[122] Attempted suicide returns were given under class VI of the criminal statistics.[123] In 1900, there were 103 indictments for attempted suicide, of which thirty were tried summarily in Dublin.[124] The following year the corresponding figures rose to 128 and fifty-six, respectively.[125]

In their reassessment of the Dublin City coronial records from 1900 to 1904, Brugha and Walsh contend that there was a fair degree of underreporting. They calculated that 1,412 inquests occurred in that timeframe. They revisited the records with four criteria for determining suicides, as follows:

> First, those for which the coroner had returned a suicide verdict. Second, those for which the coroner had not returned a suicide verdict for reasons, social as well as legal, not evident from the record, but in whose case we believed that the death was suicidal because the evidence in the record showed that the deceased understood the fatal consequences of his self-destructive action and intended that consequence. Third, those cases in which we were satisfied the death was accidental. Fourth, those in which we regarded the outcome as 'undetermined'; that is, where the circumstances and the manner of death were highly suspicious of suicide but because of insufficient evidence in the inquest report we could not be absolutely sure of the intention of the deceased.[126]

It is not clear if by 'inquest records' they mean original reports, morgue registers or the coroner's registers. Their figures of four returns of suicide in 1900 and seven each in 1901 and 1902 do not tally with mine, nor is it clear how they interrogated the records or indeed if they examined the original reports as opposed to the registers, but their second classification of suicide by virtue of supporting evidence finds much fruitful expression in the inquest reports and in the newspaper reporting.[127] It is not possible to say with any degree of certainty which of the twenty-one cases (see Table 4.3) I discuss here were subsequently classified as a death by suicide in the ARRG—of these, thirteen were men. I selected the cases based on the evidence provided, or if the DMP report mentioned suicide, for example, that of the unknown woman found drowned. Six cases were deemed to have occurred while of unsound mind, four while temporarily insane, and seven

---

[122] *Thirty-eighth detailed annual report of the Registrar-General (Ireland)* [Cd. 1225], pp. 144, 152.

[123] David Johnson, ' Trial by Jury in Ireland, 1860–1914', *Journal of Legal History*, 17:3 (1996), pp. 270–93 at 273.

[124] *Judicial statistics, Ireland, 1900* [Cd. 725, 682], pp. 13, 104.

[125] *Judicial statistics, Ireland, 1901* [Cd. 1208, 1187], pp. 13, 82.

[126] Traoloc Brugha and Dermot Walsh, 'Suicide past and present: the temporal constancy of underreporting', *The British Journal of Psychiatry*, 132 (1978), pp. 177–9.

[127] *Thirty-eighth detailed annual report of the Registrar-General (Ireland)* [Cd. 1225], p. 159. The ARRGs note five suicide deaths in 1901 for Dublin and a further seven for Dublin County Borough. Brugha and Walsh's re-categorisation of the records differs somewhat from mine, and in the absence of their detailed methodology I cannot untangle this further.

Table 4.3 Cases of alleged suicide

	Surname	Forename	Sex	Age	Occupation	Date of inquest	Cause	Classification
1	Unknown woman [1]		F	About 30		26-Apr-00	Drowned	DMP suspicion
2	Cowley[2]	Margaret	F	19	Servant	30-Aug-00	Drowned herself	Unsound mind
3	Lee[3]	James	M	28	Herd	13-Oct-00	Died from shock following injuries	Unsound mind
4	Leonard[4]	Anne	F	35	not given	06-Nov-00	Shock and exhaustion resulting from wounds self inflicted	Dangerous Lunatic
5	Matthews[5]	Robert	M	24	Van driver	05-Jan-01	Poisoning by some coal tar preparation	Undetermined
6	Cronan[6]	Jas	M	63	Boot maker	09-Jan-01	Injury to the medulla oblongata caused by a bullet	Temporary insanity
7	Moriarty[7]	Ellen	F	72	Not given	04-Mar-01	From shock result of immersion in the water at Dollymount	Undetermined
8	Hennessy[8]	Mary	F	15	NA	18-Mar-01	Found drowned in the Royal Canal	Undetermined
9	Hodgins[9]	George	M	39	H-car driver	27-Mar-01	Died from asphyxia the result of immersion in the River Liffey	Undetermined
10	Gorey[10]	Mary	F	33	Single and a Servant	01-Apr-01	Cannonisation of the uterine veins after her confinement	Undetermined, poisoning mentioned
11	Holen [11]	Edward	M	31	Piano tuner	19-Apr-01	Died from compression of the brain	Undetermined
12	Moran[12]	Martin	M	20	Single brass turner	17-Jun-01	Asphyxia caused by immersion in the river Liffey	Undetermined
13	Treacy[13]	John	M	26	Single Labourer	17-Jun-01	Died from immersion in the River Liffey	Unsound mind
14	Flanagan[14]	Bridget	F	50	NA	19-Jul-01	Haemorrhage	Unsound mind
15	Burke[15]	John	M	80	Widower and ex-hotel keeper	30-Jul-01	Died from shock consequent on the injuries self inflicted	Unsound mind
16	O'Neill[16]	Michael	M	€5	Widower and watchman	06-Sep-01	Septic anuerism resulting from self inflicted wounds of the neck	Temporarily insane
17	Higgins[17]	John	M	60	Single labourer	30-Oct-01	Asphyxia the result of immersion in the River Liffey	Unsound mind

Continued

Table 4.3 *Continued*

	Surname	Forename	Sex	Age	Occupation	Date of inquest	Cause	Classification
18	Flood[18]	Evelyn	F	52	Married	12-Dec-01	Asphyxia the result of immersion in the Grand Canal	Undetermined
19	Hunter[19]	William	M	18	Single soldier	29-Mar-02	Asphyxia caused by hanging himself	Temporary insanity
20	Ryan[20]	Michael	M	30	Single coachman	29-Apr-02	Haemorrhage caused by the cutting of the blood vessels of the neck	Temporary insanity
21	Nevin[21]	Thomas	M	28	Single plater	20-Mar-02	Syncope following disease of the aortic valves	DMP suspected poisoning

Sources:

[1] NAI/1900/7 Inquest on the body of an unknown woman 26 April 1900.
[2] NAI/1900/102 Inquest on the body of Margaret Cowley.
[3] NAI/1900/137 Inquest on the body of James Lee, *Irish Examiner*, 29 November 1900.
[4] NAI/1900/153 Inquest on the body of Anne Leonard.
[5] NAI/1901/6 Inquest on the body of Robert Matthews.
[6] NAI/1901/9 Inquest on the body of Jas Cronan.
[7] NAI/1901/67 Inquest on the body of Ellen Moriarty.
[8] NAI/1901/76 Inquest on the body of Mary Hennessy.
[9] NAI/1901/89 Inquest on the body of George Hodgins.
[10] NAI/1901/96 Inquest on the body of Mary Gorey.
[11] NAI/1901/115 Inquest on the body of Edward Holen.
[12] NAI/1901/162 Inquest on the body of Martin Moran.
[13] NAI/1901/163 Inquest on the body of John Treacy.
[14] Munster Express, 27 July 1901, headline 'Sad suicide in Dublin', 'suffering from nervousness for some time past'. *Evening Herald*, 12 December 1901; *Irish Daily Independent*, 13 December 1901.
[15] NAI/1901/197 Inquest on the body of John Burke.
[16] NAI/1901/235 Inquest on the body of Michael O'Neill.
[17] NAI/1901/276 Inquest on the body of John Higgins.
[18] NAI/1901/308 Inquest on the body of Evelyn Flood.
[19] NAI/1902/50 Inquest on the body of William Hunter.
[20] NAI/1902/77 Inquest on the body of Michael Ryan.
[21] NAI/1902/47 Inquest on the body of Thomas Nevin.

were passed off as accidents, or what Brugha and Walsh term 'undetermined' (one mentioned poison) although they exhibited all the characteristics of deliberate actions. There were three cases that mentioned poison: one, that of Mary Gorey, who admitted to taking poison and mutilating the body of her infant (discussed earlier), was completely unclear and returned a verdict of 'canonisation of the uterine veins' (see Table 4.1). Coronial court inquiries and their verdicts were of critical importance to bereaved families and this had a very strong bearing on the ways in which jurors classified deaths arising from self-murder. Eye-witness testimony of unusual behaviour characteristic of suicidal intent was routinely dismissed out of hand and, in the case of drowning for instance, were often returned as 'having no evidence of how the body got in the water'.

Included in this tally of twenty-one are seven cases where there is clear evidence of mitigating circumstances or a set of behaviours consistent with suicidal intent but did not yield verdicts to that effect. Take the case of Evelyn Flood (called Good in newspaper articles) who was sent to Dublin from Hull in England, for 'a change of air'; she was stopping with Mrs O'Connor of 40 Grosvenor Square as a paying guest from 31 October until her death in early December. During that time she was under the care of Dr Goulding, 16 Rathmines Road, and as she was suffering from nervousness and general breakdown, she was effectively on suicide watch. On 25 November she was brought to the Richmond Asylum—Nurse Woodhouse of 20 Rathmines Road took charge of her from then until 9 December and on that date Nurse Massy took charge; the following day she escaped. A search party commenced and the matter was reported to police. She was observed in the act of trying to commit self-murder by drowning. Efforts were made to save her but the absence of a lifebuoy made efforts defunct. The verdict returned made little of the fact that she was labouring under serious mental illness and instead encouraged the authorities to have better provisioning of life-saving equipment on the canal.

> Asphyxia the result of immersion in the Grand Canal at Parnell Bridge on the 10th Inst. And we consider the conduct of Constables Patrick Rooney 193A & John Clarke 58A also James White most praiseworthy. And we consider the authorities having charge of this district should place life buoys for the protection of the public on bridges.[128]

Ellen Moriarty was 72 years of age and living at 38 Mountjoy Square at the Irish Distressed Ladies Home described as a home for 'reduced Catholic ladies' when she decided to take her own life at Dollymount Strand.[129] She had been unwell for a few weeks and, although she was practically destitute, it transpired that she

---

[128] NAI/1901/308 inquest dated 12 December 1901; *Belfast Newsletter*, 12 December 1901.
[129] *Kerry Sentinel*, 6 March 1901.

created a will the day before. Moriarty took a cab to the seaside and when asked by the driver of the H-car if she would be in need of a return journey—she replied no. Witnesses watched her alight from the cab, walk straight across the road and 'disappear over the wall'. A young woman who observed the entire episode alerted her brothers immediately.[130] They pulled her from the water and, together with a police constable, attempted to revive her but their efforts were in vain. The newspapers described it as 'A mysterious occurrence at Dollymount'.[131] The jury deemed the whole affair an accident and added a veneer of verisimilitude to its reasoning by advising 'And we wish to add that this place is very badly protected there being no life buoy or rope and we consider that same should be at once procured'.[132] Her cause of death was registered as 'shock the result of accidental immersion in the water at Dollymount'.[133]

Less than a fortnight later, 15-year-old Mary Hennessy's drowning in the Royal Canal elicited yet another public safety warning by way of jury rider to the local authorities: 'we wish to add the authorities in charge of the canal should have the place better lighted'. Her death was also deemed accidental and the DMP report stated that the section of the canal on which she was found was 'very dark and decidedly dangerous as there is no lamp between Clarke's Bridge and the Public Library'. It may well have been entirely accidental but her father's evidence raised questions about her state of mind. He deposed that 'She was in poor health lately suffering from melancholia at intervals especially at the period of menstruation, and at those periods showed weakness of the mind and was treated for said complaint about a month ago by Dr Crinion of Amiens St.'[134] It was also revealed that Mary Hennessy had recently moved from Dundalk, where she had lived with her grandfather, to Dublin and was dreadfully unhappy. Her death was registered as a drowning and the status of accident was removed.[135] A few weeks later, Edward Holen's father testified that he had suicidal tendencies and was 'not of sound mind for the last two years'. Holen was a piano tuner who was working as a window cleaner and plying his trade at a hotel at 86 Marlboro Street, when he jumped from an upper-floor window sill. Witnesses who were passing by noticed his unusual behaviour and ran into the hotel to raise the alarm but it was too late. Holen jumped/fell forty feet—first a doctor and priest were called, and then an ambulance brought him to Jervis Street Hospital where he died the following day. The verdict was that his fall causing brain compression was accidental, and his

---

[130] *Evening Herald*, 9 August 1901. Thomas Longmire received a certificate from the Royal Humane Society for his attempt to save Ellen Moriarty.

[131] *Kerry Evening Post*, 6 March 1901.

[132] NAI/1901/67 Inquest on the body of Ellen Moriarty, 4 March 1901.

[133] See https://civilrecords.irishgenealogy.ie/churchrecords/images/deaths_returns/deaths_1901/05737/4619607.pdf (accessed 7 June 2020).

[134] NAI/1901/76 Inquest on the body of Mary Hennessy, 18 March 1901.

[135] See https://civilrecords.irishgenealogy.ie/churchrecords/images/deaths_returns/deaths_1901/05737/4619636.pdf (accessed 7 June 2020).

death was registered accordingly.[136] Financial ruin prompted H-car driver George Hodgins to take to the River Liffey. He was ill, of no fixed abode, and had lost his job in January. Passers-by spotted him in the river and threw him a lifebuoy, which he made no effort to catch. His topcoat was found on the steps of the quay wall at Batchelor's Walk close to O'Connell Bridge but further to the verdict of 'Died from asphyxia the result of immersion in the River Liffey', the jury claimed 'and we have no evidence to how deceased got into the water'—his death was registered as accidental.[137] Placement of clothing on watersides was considered a tell-tale sign by the police in some cases. For example, the unknown woman who was found drowned in the canal in April 1900 was described in the DMP report as 'believe it to be a case of suicide as a woman's hat supposed to be hers was found on the bank adjacent…about 30 years of age…shabby appearance'.[138]

Whether drowning, the result of having jumped into the Royal or Grand Canals or the River Liffey, was determined to be suicide or accidental hinged to a large degree on whether or not alcohol was involved. A juxtaposition of the deaths of Martin Moran, aged 20, and John Treacy, aged 26, illustrates this point. Both happened within twenty-four hours of one another in mid-June 1901. Moran worked as a brass turner for the Midland Railway Company and was seen leaving the Workmen's Library Broadstone at 9.30 p.m. 'perfectly sober'.[139] Shortly after that Bridget Byrne, a charwoman from 25 Coombe, observed him stripping off his clothes down to his trousers, shirt, and socks—he left a 'coat, vest, cap, boots, collar and tie' neatly on the bank, and jumped in; it was summertime so there would have been good levels of natural light and no issues with visibility were mentioned.[140] His actions were not an alcohol-fuelled misjudgement like that of Denis McGuirk, who decided after consuming a lot of drink to go for a swim and subsequently drowned four days later.[141] Bridget Byrne raised the alarm in Moran's case and the police dragged the river immediately. His father, who identified the body, testified that he was perfectly sober and to his knowledge 'there was no trouble in the house with my son'. James Lynch, who was the doorman at the Workmen Institute stated in evidence that 'He walked perfectly straight and I believe he was perfectly sober'.[142] The verdict in Moran's case was 'Asphyxia caused by immersion in the river Liffey and we have no evidence to show how

---

[136] NAI/1901/115 Inquest on the body of Edward Holen, 19 April 1901; https://civilrecords. irishgenealogy.ie/churchrecords/images/deaths_returns/deaths_1901/05729/4616657.pdf (accessed 7 June 2020).
[137] NAI/1901/89 Inquest on the body of George Hodgins, 27 March 1901; https://civilrecords. irishgenealogy.ie/churchrecords/images/deaths_returns/deaths_1901/05738/4619687.pdf (accessed 7 June 2020).
[138] NAI/1900/7 Inquest on the body of an unknown woman dated 26 April 1900.
[139] References to 'railway benevolent institution' in *Evening Herald*, 9 February 1892 and Broadstone Institute in *Evening Herald*, 18 December 1907.
[140] NAI/1901/162 Inquest on the body of Martin Moran, DMP Report dated 16 June 1901, Constable Cornelius Kiernan 26D.
[141] NAI/1901/166 Inquest on the body of Denis McGuirk, 20 June 1901.
[142] NAI/1901/162 Evidence of James Lynch dated 17 June 1901.

the body got into the water.' Bridget Byrne bore witness to his deliberate actions but the court spared his family the verdict of death by suicide. His 'immersion' was registered erroneously as having occurred in the Royal Canal and was the last of the seven cases in the 'undetermined' category, which had evidence of intent to self-harm.[143]

Contrary to the Moran and Moriarty cases, Treacy's involved alcohol and Stephen Sweeney testified that the deceased was in his licensed premises (1 Bolton Street[144]) on the night he died: 'he was sober...I cannot say how many drinks he had. There were no angry words.'[145] In other words, he had not had any kind of altercation with anyone in his company. His friend Patrick Wynne testified that he had had three drinks and was quite sober when he left at 10.45 p.m. Witnesses stated that he climbed up on the wall on Ormond Quay and went into the water. Mrs Eliza Mezzitti testified that she saw Treacy climb up on the wall and watched him 'fall over the wall'.[146] In contrast with the other cases of drowning where there was 'no evidence', his alcohol consumption cast him into the unsound mind category. The verdict was that he 'Died from immersion in the River Liffey on Saturday night having jumped in while of unsound mind' and this cause of death was registered verbatim.[147] On his person were 'two love letters bearing the name Jack Treacy, 7 Bolton St.' and a photo of two women.[148] Suspected cases of suicide in the city's waterways were treated with great sensitivity by the coroner's court.[149] John Higgins's case was also one where people watched as he jumped into the River Liffey at Wellington Quay—gallant rescue efforts were made but to no avail. There was no evidence of alcohol consumption but the jury returned the verdict of 'Asphyxia the result of immersion in the river Liffey on Monday Night the 28th Inst said act being done while of unsound mind.' It was duly recorded as such by the registrar Dr Porter Newell.[150]

Letters were also found on Margaret Cowley's person describing her loss of honour and good moral standing owing to accusations of 'keeping company with a married man'. The police report stated that it was 'in consequence of the above letters it is supposed she committed suicide'.[151] The 19-year-old servant was

---

[143] See https://civilrecords.irishgenealogy.ie/churchrecords/images/deaths_returns/deaths_1901/ 05729/4616706.pdf (accessed 7 June 2020).

[144] Listed as E. & F. Sweeney, Wine and spirit merchants: *Thom's Directory, 1901*, p. 1368.

[145] NAI/1901/163 Inquest on the body of John Treacy, report dated 17 June 1901.

[146] NAI/1901/163 Evidence dated 17 June 1901.

[147] See https://civilrecords.irishgenealogy.ie/churchrecords/images/deaths_returns/deaths_1901/ 05729/4616667.pdf (accessed 7 June 2020).

[148] NAI/1901/163 Inquest on the body of John Treacy, DMP Report dated 16 June 1901, William Gordon, Station Sergeant.

[149] Georgina Laragy, 'Suicide and insanity in post-Famine Ireland', in Catherine Cox and Maria Luddy (eds), *Cultures of Care in Irish Medical History, 1750–1970* (Basingstoke, 2010), pp. 79–91.

[150] See https://civilrecords.irishgenealogy.ie/churchrecords/images/deaths_returns/deaths_1901/ 05712/4611499.pdf (accessed 7 June 2020).

[151] NAI/1900/102 DMP report on the case of Margaret Cowley, signed by Cornelius Kiernan 26C, 29 August 1900. Report stated she was 26; father identified her as 19.

accused by her employer Mrs Batty of improper behaviour and was 'dismissed' from her job six weeks prior to her death for 'stopping out at night'. Letters expressing her anguish were found on her person. To her sister she wrote:

> My dear sister, I am leaving this world judged wrongfully by that women and my father who believes her talk and called me names she said words to take my character from me, she has even told you Bridge something that I never said... I was told I was keeping a married man's company, but that is another lie, I knew him as a friend and him the same with me... The only one I blame for this is Mrs Batty God forgive her again again [*sic*, page turn] I say it she has a vile tongue... Good bye Molly mind yourself and remember me to all the old friends from your loving sister Maggie.

Her father, with whom she was living following her dismissal, 'remonstrated her for attending a dancing academy at Gt Brunswick St' in the company of Jack Daly, a married man. Mr Cowley followed his daughter on the morning of 28 August to her meeting with Daly and once he approached them, she ran away. Margaret Cowley went to the home of Mrs Annie Dignam, a sympathetic neighbour, where she recounted her dilemma and threatened to 'take the water and drown herself'. Dignam told her not to go through with it and later recalled that she did not take her seriously. Following her father's telling off, and with a mere 1*s*. ½*d*. in her pocket, it seems that she despaired. She threw herself into the Royal Canal that evening at 9 p.m. and the immediate rescue efforts of three passers-by were in vain. The canal was immediately dragged and she was found quickly but pronounced dead on arrival at the Mater Hospital. Both the *Irish Daily Independent* and the *Evening Herald* reported her death under the headline of 'Sad Suicide in the Royal Canal'.[152] The jury stated that it occurred 'while of unsound mind', which was recorded in her death registration.[153] For young women, allegations of moral impropriety could do irreparable reputational damage. The second letter found on her person was addressed to her aunt. She wrote: 'It is hard to leave this world but it is not better than to live with a broken heart.' The jury added a rider to restore her reputation by stating that 'there was no foundation for the allegations made by Mrs Batty'.[154] There were other suspicious cases of drowning that I have not included here as there was no witness statements as to typical reasons for suicide like financial embarrassment, loss in love, or general depression. I am not alleging that all drownings were attempts of suicide but there can be no doubt other than the Dublin waterways were commonly used for such purposes.[155]

[152] *Evening Herald*, 30 August 1900; *Irish Daily Independent*, 31 August 1900.
[153] See https://civilrecords.irishgenealogy.ie/churchrecords/images/deaths_returns/deaths_1900/05753/4625058.pdf (accessed 7 June 2020).
[154] NAI/1900/102 Inquest on the body of Margaret Cowley, 29 August 1900.
[155] *Belfast Newsletter*, 4 January 1902; NAI/1902/2 Inquest on body of James Duff, 2 January 1902. Registered cause of death was the same as the coroner's court verdict: https://civilrecords.irishgenealogy.

Drowning accounted for a sizeable percentage of suicides in Australia and New Zealand, where, as in Ireland, several were returned as open verdicts.[156]

There were three potential suicide cases that involved poison: the first, that of Mary Gorey, discussed earlier in relation to the mutilated body of her child, and the second, that of Matthew Roberts from 30 Lower Kevin Street. Roberts worked at the Daily Independent Company, St Andrew's Lane, and John Devlin who was in charge of the yard gave evidence that he noticed the deceased acting in a strange manner for about nine months. Suffering from paranoia, according to his wife Mary, 'he believed police & others were watching him'. On the day he died, he went to his cousin's house at 2 Dodder Bank, Donnybrook, and complained of feeling unwell (he did not go to work that day) and wanting to see a priest. His cousin John Matthews stayed with him for most of the day because he was worried about him. He said he seemed better after seeing the priest so he left him feeding the horses in Trinity Buildings. He was found at 5.20 p.m. unconscious at the stables, and was brought at once to hospital. The verdict was unclear and stated how he died from 'Poisoning by some coal tar preparation and we had no evidence to show how same was administered.'[157] In the third case, the verdict of 'syncope following disease of the aortic valves' was returned for 28-year-old Thomas Nevin but the DMP report indicated that it 'looks like a case of suicide as a phial was found near the body with the remains of some brownish fluid in it'. He lodged at 25 John Dillon Street with Mary O'Meara and left at 7.30 a.m. as usual to go to work. He was found by men walking across the North Bull between 4 p.m. and 5 p.m. that day.[158]

The remaining eight cases used more violent means involving instruments like razors, ropes, and a gun. Robert Bigly, Michael Ryan, Michael O'Neill, Anne Leonard, Bridget Flanagan, and John Burke all opted for cutting major arteries and haemorrhage. In cases of self-inflicted wounds the coroner's jury nearly always returned the verdict of 'temporary insanity'.[159] Originally from County Roscommon, Robert Bigly was a retired RIC head constable who, by the 1901 census, was living in Cabra Park, Glasnevin, with his wife, brother and five children. Using the name A. Begley, he checked into a cheap hotel and slit his own throat with a razor on Christmas Day 1901. He had been at the hotel since

ie/churchrecords/images/deaths_returns/deaths_1902/05704/4608768.pdf (accessed 7 June 2020). Another case that was treated as potentially suspicious was that of 70-year-old labourer James Duff whom the *Belfast Newsletter* described, as a 'teetotaller for sixteen years'. Duff was missing for a few days prior to the discovery of his body and was found drowned in the Grand Canal in January 1902—the jury added 'we have no evidence to show how the deceased entered the water'.

[156] John C. Weaver, *Sadly Troubled History: The Meanings of Suicide in the Modern Age* (Montreal, 2009), pp 113–17.

[157] NAI/1901/6 Inquest on the body of Robert Matthews, 1 January 1901. Industrial risks of poisoning were recognised by the authorities and may have been an issue in this case.

[158] NAI/1902/47 Inquest on the body of Thomas Nevin, 20 March 1902.

[159] Georgina Laragy, 'Locating investigations into suicidal deaths in urban Ireland, 1901–1915', in Georgina Laragy, Olwen Purdue, and Jonathan Jeffery Wright (eds), *Urban Spaces in Nineteenth-Century Ireland* (Liverpool, 2018), pp. 144–61.

16 December; an insurance policy dated 2 October 1891 on the life of Robert Bigley of the RIC Barracks, Glenbeigh, County Kerry was found in the hotel lavatory. Hotel staff noticed he did not answer his door and called the DMP. His brother Joseph came from Athlone to identify his remains—his death was not subsequently registered.[160] Similarly, Michael Ryan came from Loughrea in County Galway to Dublin to commit suicide three weeks after being fired from his job with Mr Dolphin, Turol, Loughrea, 'for intemperate habits'. Three days after his arrival he was seen cutting his throat at Rutland Square West by DMP Constable Brady 24B who ran over and took razor from him and had him conveyed by cab to Jervis Street Hospital—he died twenty minutes after admission.[161] Ryan's suicide was recorded as occurring while 'temporarily insane'.[162] Michael O'Neill was also seen slashing his own throat with a razor in the hall of 30 Francis Street—he lived alone at 68 Braithwaite Street; he had called to see a relative at 22 Upper Bridge Street and was probably on his way home when he entered the open hall and committed the act. He had been suffering from melancholy according to co-resident Mrs Kearney. In her evidence she implied that he exhibited signs of paranoia too; she recalled how he asked her 'if the detectives were after him'. The verdict and death registration was 'Septic aneurism resulting from self-inflicted wounds of the neck while temporarily insane.'[163]

Former hotel-keeper John Burke's case was described as extraordinary in the *Irish Daily Independent*. He had been committed to the 'lunatic department' at the NDU and had written to his niece-in-law Fanny Spaight asking for darning materials and a knife for the purposes of cutting his finger nails. A neighbour, John Nolan, dropped the items to him and thus they did not attract the attention of the workhouse authorities as it might have had they arrived by post. Spaight went to visit him at NDU on 27 July and noticed that he had blood on his hands, which he claimed came from a harmless cut on his finger. He asked her to open the knife but she was unable and asked a fellow inmate to oblige. Once it was open, he sent her out of the room and proceeded to cut his throat. On her return she raised the alarm. He died from his wounds and registrar Dr J.A. McFarland documented his unsound mind in the official cause of death.[164] Both she and Nolan were admonished by the coroner for their poor judgement in providing a deadly weapon to a mentally ill man, but no criminal charges were brought against them.[165]

---

[160] *Kerry Weekly Reporter*, 4 January 1902. NAI/1901/321 Inquest on the body of Robert Bigley, 26 December 1901. See http://www.census.nationalarchives.ie/reels/nai003679954/ Bigley household in 1901 (accessed 13 March 2022).

[161] NAI/1902/77 Inquest on the body of Michael Ryan, 29 April 1902.

[162] See https://civilrecords.irishgenealogy.ie/churchrecords/images/deaths_returns/deaths_1902/05696/4605708.pdf (accessed 8 June 2020).

[163] NAI/1901/235 Inquest on the body of Michael O'Neill, 6 September 1901: https://civilrecords.irishgenealogy.ie/churchrecords/images/deaths_returns/deaths_1901/05720/4614036.pdf (accessed 8 June 2020).

[164] See https://civilrecords.irishgenealogy.ie/churchrecords/images/deaths_returns/deaths_1901/05719/4613907.pdf (accessed 7 June 2020).

[165] *Irish Daily Independent*, 31 July 1901.

Serious mental health problems and possible 'religious mania' beleaguered Anne Leonard, who was considered a dangerous lunatic and a 'Sad case of dementia'.[166] Her husband noticed she had been 'strange in her manner' for a few days and on 2 November he went for a priest as she had requested. Two women, Anastasia Byrne and Ms Kinsella, stayed with her while he was gone—they noticed that she was tearing at something under the bed clothes; they got hold of her hands which were covered in blood. They had tried to restrain her. She claimed she was about to give birth to the son of God. DMP Constable Gilchrist was brought to the scene and, as she had sustained very serious injuries, he brought her to the Coombe Hospital. In the interests of safety, hers and other post-surgical patients, she was transferred by Gilchrist to SDU lunatic department for a night. Weakened and in no fit state, she had to attend the police court the following morning on dangerous lunatic charges. She was left waiting there for three hours prior to her hearing—afterwards she was sent to the Richmond Asylum where she died three days later 'from acute mania'.[167] Her death registration noted the shock and exhaustion from her self-inflicted wounds but her husband protested, citing the delays and mishandling of the entire affair.[168] In a similar fashion Bridget Flanagan was suffering from mental health problems. She had twice been a patient at the Mater Hospital suffering from debility and was acting strangely—she had asked a neighbour, Bernard Banks of 128 Church Street, if he would cut her daughter's (Christina, aged 10) throat. In an attempt to contain the matter at home, her husband and daughters were on suicide watch. On the morning of her death she got up at 3 a.m. and paced the floor for two hours. Her husband testified that immediately prior to her self-inflicted fatal wounding she said 'I may as well cut my throat as anyone else when you won't do it.' Using a razor, she cut her throat between 5 a.m. and 6 a.m.—her daughter Christina wrapped a towel around her wound and ran for assistance.[169] A constable happened to be on the beat nearby; he procured an ambulance, she was rushed to the Meath Hospital and was pronounced dead on arrival.[170] Her inquest verdict and death registration noted her 'unsound mind'.[171]

When bootmaker James Cronan shot himself in the head his wife claimed that it was an accident, that he was in fine fettle in the weeks prior to his death and had consumed no alcohol on the night in question. His friend and customer for twenty-five years Sir Thorney Stoker contended that this was untrue and that he

---

[166] *Freeman's Journal*, 7 November 1900.

[167] NAI/1900/153 Inquest on the body of Anne Leonard, 6 November 1900; *Evening Herald*, 6 November 1900; *Freeman's Journal*, 7 November 1900.

[168] See https://civilrecords.irishgenealogy.ie/churchrecords/images/deaths_returns/deaths_1900/05746/4622546.pdf (accessed 7 June 2020).

[169] See http://www.census.nationalarchives.ie/reels/nai003720612/ (accessed 11 November 2021); *Evening Herald*, 19 July 1901.

[170] *Munster Express*, 27 July 1901: 'Sad suicide in Dublin: Labourer's wife cuts her throat'.

[171] See https://civilrecords.irishgenealogy.ie/churchrecords/images/deaths_returns/deaths_1901/05720/4614024.pdf (accessed 7 June 2020).

had warned his family of what he observed was a definite change in character over a few weeks. The gun was an old but functioning family heirloom and the jury was unconvinced that the death was an accidental discharge. It was not reported in the newspapers but it was entered into evidence that his diary entry of 8 January stated: 'The day I married you my days of enjoyment were over.' Mrs Cronan confirmed that it was the deceased's handwriting and that 'he might have wrote it while they were at dinner'.[172] The verdict and subsequent death registration for Joseph Cronan noted the 'bullet wound to the medulla oblongata self inflicted'.[173]

William Hunter, an 18-year-old Private in the Northumberland Fusiliers 4th Battalion hanged himself with 'his braces in the water closet of Richmond Barracks whilst temporarily insane'. He had only been part of the regiment for two months and his suicide arose from deep embarrassment and bullying on the part of his commanding officer (CO) Captain Braithwaite. Hunter, according to the newspapers, had suffered 'an affection of the kidney' and it gave rise to two bed-wetting incidents. His CO punished him by confining him to his barracks for ten days and fining him the cost of the bedding. Braithwaite admitted in the course of his testimony that bed-wetting incidents were usually associated with excessive alcohol consumption and punished as 'a very disgraceful offence'. Hunter had been to the see the regimental doctor Purcell Harford on the morning of his death, complaining of urinary incontinence and was prescribed 'the usual treatment'. Clearly his incontinence was not as a result of heavy drinking and the jury added the rider: 'And we consider it would have been more discreet for the commanding officer at the outset to get the Doctor's opinion instead of punishing the deceased for what was merely a defect of nature and not a crime in any sense of the law.'[174]

Following his attempted suicide, James Lee was compos mentis enough to readily admit the fact that he threw himself in front of an oncoming train:

> I threw myself under the train this morning about 9.30am. The train was going to Dublin. The place where I did it is about a mile this side of Butterstown. It was a passenger train. The driver pulled up. I was taken to Butterstown railway station on a truck. Drs Daly & Dillon of Butterstown saw me and sent me here in the Union Ambulance two men came with me I dashed in front of the train and my head got cut.[175]

---

[172] *Irish Daily Independent*, 10 January 1901, suicide of Mr Cronin: NAI/1901/10 inquest report.

[173] See https://civilrecords.irishgenealogy.ie/churchrecords/images/deaths_returns/deaths_1901/05738/4619898.pdf (accessed 7 June 2020).

[174] NAI/1902/50 Inquest on the body of William Hunter, 29 March 1902; *Freeman's Journal*, 31 March 1902.

[175] NAI/1900/137 Inquest on the body of James Lee; *Irish Examiner*, 29 November 1900.

In fact the train had not only hit his head—it passed over his legs and caused serious injuries from which he did not recover. Alcohol abuse gave rise to his problems and he deposed 'I have been drinking heavily for some time. I was not drunk this morning, I was in some difficulty of late. I neglected my business more or less.' The jury found that he died from 'shock following injuries received... having thrown himself upon the line in front of the train while of unsound mind'. His death registration in No 1 North City by Dr J.H. McAuley omitted his state of mind and simply recorded 'run over by a train shock'.[176]

Reconciling the verdicts with the official statistics for suicide is not entirely possible as this section has shown. We can take for granted that the inclusion of 'unsound mind' and 'temporary insanity' were euphemisms to describe suicide. Of the cases discussed here only ten verdicts cite mental health problems and we can assume that these were categorised as suicide for cause of death, but the first five cases of Moriarty, Hennessey, Holen, Hodgins, and Moran arguably belong in the unsound mind category too. Of the twenty-one cases, we know from a census-matching exercise that ten professed as Roman Catholic, so there might have been burial implications for them under the Code of Canon Law 1240, which might explain why open verdicts were returned and why registrars exercised their discretion.[177]

An analysis of the inquests shows that some degree of moral arbitration occurred on the part of the coroners' courts and again in the translation that occurred in the death registration process, as in the case of James Lee. The finding of temporary insanity or actions while of unsound mind was, as Houston contends, 'no more a respectable medical judgement than it was a tenable legal one, for doctors were selective rather than indiscriminate in their association of madness with suicide and few saw any necessary association between suicide and mental ill-health'.[178] But it provided not only surviving relatives with an ease of conscience—it also gave licence to Roman Catholic priests to permit burial on hallowed ground. The coroners' courts were increasingly dominated by Roman Catholics by the close of the nineteenth century. Dr Louis Byrne was Roman Catholic and many of his subjects and jurors were co-religionists.

---

[176] See https://civilrecords.irishgenealogy.ie/churchrecords/images/deaths_returns/deaths_1900/05746/4622494.pdf (accessed 7 June 2020).

[177] Reverend Joseph N. Perry, 'The right of ecclesiastical burial', *The Catholic Lawyer*, 28:4 (1983), pp. 315–35 at 323. 'The expression deliberato consilio in Canon 1240, section 1, 30 of the 1917 Code delineated a clear line between culpable and inculpable suicide. It is unclear which principles or concepts in the Code serve as the basis for the Church's position on deliberate suicide. The increasing realization that there were frequently mitigating circumstances and factors surrounding an act of suicide, not to mention a presumption against one's mental stability at the time of the act, directly limited the frequency of the imposition of denial'.

[178] R.A. Houston, 'Explanations for death by suicide in Northern Britain during the long eighteenth century', *History of Psychiatry*, 23:1 (2012), pp. 52–64 at 61.

Interpersonal Violence

Levels of interpersonal violence resulting in death ranged in severity from unprovoked common assault to premeditated and wilful murder. The criteria for inclusion in this final subset of twenty-nine deaths (Figure 4.2) was whether or not there was evidence of an assault in the DMP report to the coroner's court or if criminal proceedings were subsequently taken against the perpetrator. Of the fatalities discussed here, twenty-six arose from some form of personal assault, two were of premeditated murder where the victims had their throats cut, and there was a case of hanging arising from one of the murders. Rather than discussing each of the twenty-eight (excluding the hanging) cases individually, I approach this section thematically by focusing on the two primary classifications that naturally emerge—domestic violence and assaults occurring in public. Location of death arising from interpersonal violence was a highly gendered matter, and women were more likely to suffer violence in their homes than men. Eleven of the fourteen females in this sample died as a result of domestic violence, all of which involved alcohol consumption on the part of the deceased or the perpetrator. Alcohol, and often its excessive consumption, was common to twenty-one of the twenty-nine cases. There were two cases of men being killed in domestic contexts, but public brawling was the primary risk factor for men (ten in total and nine involving alcohol). Most of these cases were spontaneous and do not conform to the type of 'recreational violence' that Carolyn Conley has outlined.[179] Nor do they neatly fit the categories that Richard McMahon identified in his study of

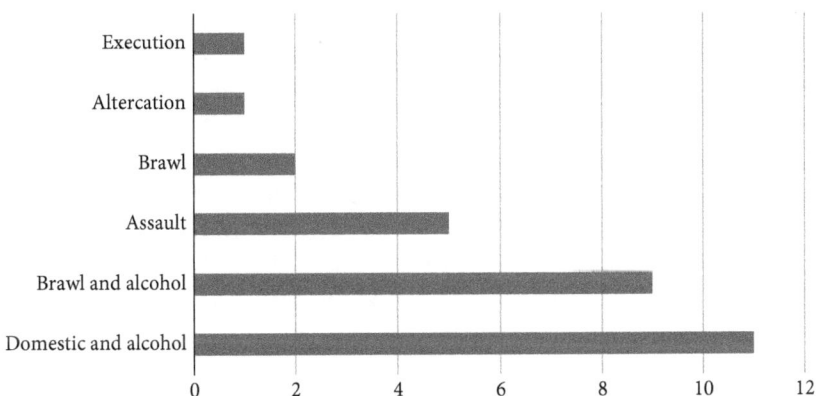

Figure 4.2 Cause of violent death
Source: NAI/Dataset 1900–2.

[179] Carolyn Conley, 'The agreeable recreation of fighting', *Journal of Social History*, 33:1 (1999), pp. 57–72.

homicide in pre-Famine Ireland, save perhaps his miscellaneous category, as most lack a clear motive.[180] Very few of these cases proceeded to the criminal courts.

This section focuses on the degree to which social norms dictated judicial proceedings and what these cases can tell us about thresholds of violence in Irish society. I have identified some patterns in the legal proceedings that accrued from these coroner's cases, definite evidence of discretionary justice, and what I am terming vernacular justice. By this I mean situations whereby the community meted out its own forms of justice or, for instance, refused to cooperate with police investigations and were simply complicit by silence on events. There are cases where witnesses were slow to come forward for fear of community rejection or reprisal. The chapter concludes with a discussion of two deaths of women in the Coombe area of Dublin, which was an established and close-knit working-class community and, as we shall later see, both cases contain evidence of extra-legal mechanisms used to maintain social control.

Domestic Violence: 'I said to the "chiseller" if you come here I'll break your face'

There are two instances of children getting caught in the crosshairs of marital disputes—the first was in utero. After Sarah Bennet was assaulted by her husband Christopher at 2 a.m. on 29 October 1901, he was charged with assault 'by striking her a box on the face knocked her down and striking her a blow with the heel of his boot on the head cutting and injuring her'. The case would hardly have come to the attention of the coroner's court had she not received surgical treatment at Richmond Hospital and subsequently suffered the loss of her prematurely born baby on 1 November. Dr Anderson of the Rotunda believed that her early labour was because of the assault. It also emerged that her husband previously assaulted her two years' prior.[181] He was sentenced by Mr Wall at the Northern Police Court to one calendar month at Mountjoy prison for the assault on his wife on 29 October, but there were no further charges.[182] Because the child lived for an hour the unnamed male infant's death was registered.[183] The second case was that of Joseph McCabe, aged 12, whose father came in drunk and, according to his mother's recollection (recorded in the first person by the court clerk),

---

[180] McMahon, *Homicide in Pre-Famine Ireland*, pp. 193–6.

[181] NAI/1901/280 Inquest on the body of infant Bennet, 2 November 1901.

[182] NAI, PRIS 1/43/02, General register of convicted male prisoners, Mountjoy, no. 3660, Christopher Bennet. I am very grateful to Natalie Milne, Archivist, NAI for her advice on archival convention for these data.

[183] See https://civilrecords.irishgenealogy.ie/churchrecords/images/deaths_returns/deaths_1901/05712/4611390.pdf (accessed 6 August 2021).

pulled myself and deceased out of bed he knocked me down and kicked me about the body he then put myself and deceased out. When deceased was standing outside leaning on the window stool – his father who was inside took the poker up and said to me get away out of that you cow. He made a blow with the poker at me he through [sic] it through the window and it struck the deceased on the side of the head knocking him down I went to him at once and took him in a cab to Jervis Street Hospital where he was detained.[184]

The child died the following morning as a result of the wounds he sustained—the verdict found 'Fracture of skull & compression of brain caused by a missile thrown by his father at 11 Quinn's Cottages, whilst in a state of excitement.'[185] In the subsequent death registration his father's assault was not mentioned.[186]

As it concerned the case of an innocent child wanting to protect his mother from his brutal father it received due consideration from the police and the judiciary. From her work on English working-class autobiographies, Griffin explains that 'corporal punishment was everywhere', and Dublin was no exception.[187] Men could beat their wives and physically discipline their children behind closed doors but once it spilled out into public spaces or resulted in a death they were held accountable in an era when the fervour of child protection was in its heyday.[188] John McCabe was brought before the City of Dublin Commission on 16 October 1900. Witnesses included Ellen Gorman, Edward Galvin, DMP constables John Carroll 2C and Peter Corbally 17C, and Dr John Begley. Ellen Gorman lived next door, where she also kept a shop. The disturbance was so great that she went to rescue Mrs McCabe and her child and assisted them from the hall of the cottage out onto the street. Gorman made a telling comment about the thresholds of domestic abuse she was willing to ignore: 'I never heard deft. [defendant] use threat towards his wife + child. They often quarrelled as man and wife.'[189] Edward Galvin, who happened to be in the area, heard Mrs McCabe roaring for help after the child was struck down and he went with her to Jervis Street Hospital.[190] The following day Mr McCabe was apprehended in a public house, Delaney's on North Strand, and after initially denying his identity he was arrested on the charge of murdering his son. He was asked if he wanted to make a comment or statement to which he replied 'No, not in a public house'—once outside he said, 'It was an

---

[184] NAI/1900/124 Inquest on the body of Joseph McCabe, 2 October 1900.

[185] NAI/1900/124 Inquest on the body of Joseph McCabe, 2 October 1900.

[186] See https://civilrecords.irishgenealogy.ie/churchrecords/images/deaths_returns/deaths_1900/05746/4622515.pdf.

[187] Emma Griffin, 'The emotions of motherhood: love culture, and poverty in Victorian Britain', *The American Historical Review*, 123:1 (2018), pp. 60–85 at 72–3.

[188] Joanne Bailey, '"I dye [sic] by inches"', pp. 273–94.

[189] NAI, Dublin Crown Files at Commission, 16 October 1900, Ellen Gorman evidence dated 9 October 1900.

[190] NAI, Dublin Crown Files at Commission, 16 October 1900, Edward Galvin evidence dated 9 October 1900.

accident I am sorry for the boy.'[191] DMP officer John Carroll recorded the fact that he was very drunk. At Summerhill station John McCabe made the following voluntary statement:

> Its [sic] an accident…Just this way it occurred I said to the "chiseller" if you come here I'll break your face. I had a few words with the woman. She was boozed. She is drinking this last six weeks. There was no supper + I going to work all night. Only for her I would not have thrown it at the poor child. I idolized him although he would not go to school. I don't care if I'm hung. May God bless my son for what I'm after doing on him.

DMP constable Peter Corbally swore that when he made that deposition the effects of the drink had worn off. Despite his full and heartfelt confession, when the case came before Justice Gibson, John McCabe pleaded not guilty. The *Irish Examiner* described the case as 'A Father's Crime in Dublin: a light sentence'. Echoes of the 'doctrine of provocation' as a mitigating factor in cases of spousal abuse and murder, which Martin Wiener uncovered in English cases and Georgina Rychner found in colonial Victoria, also prevailed in the Irish courts.[192] McCabe's defence centred on the fact that his actions were consequent to his wife's neglect of her duties: he came home at 10 p.m., found the fire out and no food prepared. His wife, Sergeant Carroll argued, was a good woman who kept a clean and neat home and had to go out to work to supplement their income. He said that John McCabe was given to heavy bouts of drinking, had assaulted her the previous week, and he had seen no evidence to support the claim that she drank. The besmirching of a woman's character was easily achieved with loose allegations about alcohol consumption, which is why the DMP officer set the record straight in this instance. The jury wasted no time in finding him guilty but Justice Gibson revealed his own difficulties in passing sentence as follows:

> persons like the prisoner should not be allowed to wreak their wickedness upon defenceless women and children. Their women and children should be protected from drunken scoundrelism, but his lordship could not shut his eyes to the fact that in punishing the prisoner, he was to a certain extent, punishing his wife. His lordship was not certain that in the long run she might be happier and

---

[191] NAI, Dublin Crown Files at Commission, 16 October 1900, John Carroll SS 2C evidence dated 2 October 1900.

[192] Georgina Rychner, 'Defences to intimate partner homicide: historicising the relationship between provocation and temporary insanity in Victoria, Australia', *Law & History: Journal of the Australian and New Zealand Law and History Society*, 8:1 (2021), pp. 106–33. Many thanks to Georgina for generously sharing this excellent piece. Martin J. Wiener, *Men of Blood: Violence, Manliness, and Criminal Justice in Victorian England* (Cambridge, 2012).

more comfortable if she were thrown on her own unsupported resources with her children, and if the prisoner were gone away from her life.[193]

On balance, Gibson thought it best to sentence him to twelve months' hard labour and not to penal servitude, but warned of no mercy if he came before him again. By the time the census was taken in March 1901, a mere five months later, he was out of custody—the return showed that the McCabes were still living at Quinn's Lane (by that time at number 9) with their five surviving children who ranged in age from 17 down to 2 years. Mary Anne was described as a charwoman and he identified as a domestic servant/gardener. The income of their oldest son John, aged 17, and Thomas, aged 15, as vanman and grocer's messenger, respectively, undoubtedly contributed to their ability to maintain their home while the bread-winner was serving his time.[194] Returned as a widow in 1911, Mary Anne still resided at 9 Quinn's Lane—she had nine children during her twenty-nine-year marriage, five of whom were living; her eldest is not accounted for but four other children mentioned in the 1901 census still lived with her in 1911.[195]

Twelve-year-old Timothy O'Brien had the unenviable task of having to testify to his mother Elizabeth's brutal attack at the hands of his father at their tenement home 193.1 Great Britain Street. The assault happened between 6 p.m. and 7 p.m. on 13 November 1901, and it was likely witnessed by her two younger children Michael, aged 8, and Edward, aged 3. Richard O'Brien came home drunk and pushed her down on her back and went out to pawn a pair of new boots. He was even more inebriated when he came back and he laid into her again, with kicks and blows. He broke several ribs. The assault was so vicious that a neighbour, Eugene Gardland, and another unnamed young man intervened and he assaulted them too. Dr O'Sullivan tended to Elizabeth about five or six times and on 22 November, when her condition deteriorated, Dr Harvey brought the attack to the attention of the DMP who started an investigation. By then the visible wounds on her face had healed somewhat, but traces of the bruising about her body were still there. O'Brien was charged at the Northern Police Court with her wilful murder when she died the following day.[196] The jury returned the verdict of death from pneumonia and did not add a rider. The outcome was that O'Brien was sentenced to six calendar months for assault, which he served at Mountjoy prison.[197]

[193] *Irish Examiner*, 19 October 1900.
[194] See http://www.census.nationalarchives.ie/reels/nai003812221/, McCabe family Quinn Lane, 1901 (accessed 13 June 2020).
[195] http://www.census.nationalarchives.ie/reels/nai000208658/, McCabe family Quinn Lane, 1911 (accessed 13 June 2020).
[196] NAI/1901/295 Inquest on the body of Elizabeth O'Brien, 25 November 1901—died from pluera pneumonia; *Evening Herald*, 25 November 1901. http://www.census.nationalarchives.ie/reels/nai003692072/ O'Brien household, 1901 (accessed 13 March 2022)
[197] NAI, PRIS 1/43/02, General register of convicted male prisoners, Mountjoy, no. 3995. Michael Richard O'Brien.

At the more extreme end of financial and domestic abuse was the case of Margaret Graham, who was 34 years of age. Her husband Richard was seen kicking her in the side by Kathleen Ellis of 15 Charlemont Place, on the hall door steps of their nearby residence. She testified that a week prior to that attack Margaret Graham came to her house seeking protection as she feared for her life. Ellis questioned her as to why she was in such danger and Graham explained a multiplicity of reasons—they had fertility problems for which she had undergone a procedure with Dr Moore Madden and after nine years of marriage they had not been able to have a family.[198] They quarrelled over money too and he was angry that she had not signed over her ownership of her house on the South Circular Road to him. Graham was estranged from her family because she had 'turned with her husband' from Roman Catholicism and 'now she could go nowhere'. Ellis testified, 'I never saw her drunk but Shane seen drink on her'.[199] Margaret's brother, William Desmond, was indifferent to her well-being and maintained a relationship with her husband. He testified that she was a drinker who had been in treatment a few times in the Maison de Sante and at the Richmond Asylum. In a signed statement he recounted an event one afternoon four weeks prior to her death whereby she was allegedly drunk in bed. Richard Graham pulled her out of bed and kicked her three times in an attempt to retrieve a pawn ticket from her pocket. So normalised was the abuse that William Desmond did not intervene and said 'I did not mind at the time'. Following the 25 November attack she was brought to the Adelaide Hospital by Kathleen Ellis and was treated by Dr Millar, who found her 'nervous and excited with bruises in different parts of the body'.[200] Although there was significant evidence of marks of violence on her body, Dr Byrne stated that her brother's testimony confirmed she was a dipsomaniac. He encouraged that the verdict include some indication of her husband's ill-treatment but, according to the newspaper coverage, the jury did not agree. The coroner asked the foreman to clarify if the husband's ill treatment caused her death and he responded 'Oh no'. Dr Byrne's opinion held sway and the following verdict was returned: 'Cardiac syncope following congestion of the lungs and we consider the husband ill-treated her.' Richard Graham had legal representation at the inquest and it seems that no charges were brought against him.[201]

---

[198] See https://civilrecords.irishgenealogy.ie/churchrecords/images/marriage_returns/marriages_1892/10652/5880771.pdf (accessed 12 November 2021).

[199] NAI/1901/301 Inquest on the body of Margaret Graham report, 3 December 1901.

[200] *Freeman's Journal*, 4 December 1901.

[201] *Evening Herald*, 3 December 1901. Graham remarried in 1906 and by 1911 was living at 17 SCR (possibly the contested house Margaret owned) with his wife Sarah and his three step-children, named Price: https://civilrecords.irishgenealogy.ie/churchrecords/images/marriage_returns/marriages_1906/10115/5680649.pdf and http://www.census.nationalarchives.ie/reels/nai000194575/ (both accessed 12 November 2021).

Unless there were signs and eye-witness testimony to extreme violence the police could not do much in terms of prosecution—turning state's witness carried longer-term social risks and even when they did come forward their own integrity was called into question. On 5 September 1901 Bridget McDonnell fell from a height of 10 feet 6 inches through an open window and landed heavily on the 'flags' of the footpath below. She was immediately conveyed to Mercer's Hospital and did not recover consciousness—she died the following day. She lived at no 1 Digges Street Lower in the drawing room with her husband and two children. They had been quarrelling the previous day and night. Between 2 p.m. and 3 p.m. on 5 September he was seen by a 9-year-old neighbour's child named Mary Kenna hitting her a 'box (punch) in the face on the lobby of the house and pushing her through the window'. Her parents came upon Bridget McDonnell's body on the footpath and raised the alarm. Station Sergeant Thomas Cullen documented how the DMP responded straight away and interviewed Mr McDonnell at the hospital—he claimed she fell out the window and was not pushed.[202] He added that she had 'threatened to throw herself out of a window before'. Dr Thomas P. McKell believed that her cause of death was coma due to head fracture. The coroner's jury returned 'Coma caused by fracture of the skull we have no sufficient grounds on the evidence submitted to us to attach guilt to anyone.'[203]

Nonetheless, Patrick McDonnell was brought before the October sitting of the City of Dublin Commission for the manslaughter of his wife Bridget on 5 September 1901. On the ill-fated day, his cousin Jane Dillon visited the house at 1 Digges Street Lower at 1.30 p.m. and she went upstairs on Bridget McDonnell's invitation to the top front room occupied by Essie Kenna. She testified how the victim was 'very full of drink' and her husband had followed them upstairs. Dillon remained in the room while McDonnell went back downstairs to the front drawing room. She heard the couple argue in the lobby about a key. Essie Kenna was alerted to a problem when she heard a child crying and calling 'Mammie Mammie'—she watched as he tried to grasp his wife as she fell out the window—'she was gone out the window, all but her feet. I roared "she's dead" I roared "police"... I saw the husband grabbing for the woman's feet as if to try and save her.'[204]

Eliza McBirney the occupant of the front parlour which was beneath the McDonnells' room described hearing a woman scream and qualified by saying it was 'a scream of fright'. It was followed by a thud outside. She also heard Mrs Kenna say 'oh you murderer you've thrown her through the window. I saw you + I'll swear against you.' Bridget McDonnell had been living there for about five

---

[202] NAI, Dublin Crown Files at Commission, *The King v Patrick McDonnell*; evidence of Thomas Cull, DMP, dated 6 September.

[203] NAI/1901/233 Inquest on the body of Bridget McDonnell, 6 September 1901.

[204] NAI, Dublin Crown Files at Commission, *The King v Patrick McDonnell*; evidence of Essie Kenna, dated 6 September.

weeks and during that time she befriended McBirney who had no choice but to bear witness to the highly abusive and violent relationship. The night before the incident there was a loud quarrel and Bridget specifically called out to her for help. Mary Clancy testified that McBirney, with whom she shared a room, went up at 2 a.m.[205] McBirney came to her defence and pretended she had a policemen with her, but he locked the door and threatened her to mind her own business. Retreating, she said to him how 'he would not beat a man as he was beating that woman...I had heard them quarrelling during the last 3 weeks'.[206]

Dublin Corporation cleaner Peter Whelan recalled that he met Mr McDonnell in the yard on the morning of the incident and 'bid him the time of day' to which he replied 'I'm mad, they've driven me mad'. He later overheard the quarrel and McDonnell say 'give it to me –give me it out or I'll be hung for you'.[207] Ellen Delaney bore witness to his physically abusive and threatening nature too; he stormed into her living space in the back drawing room looking for his 'missus' at 1 p.m. on the ill-fated day. She reckoned he was very drunk and agitated, and she later heard him in angry voice say to his wife ' "go into your room and mind your two children"...I heard Mrs McDonnell say "don't murder me", she appeared to be frightened so far as I know.' Allegations of drinking against female witnesses operated in the favour of defence teams, and with great predictability, Mr Eustace Johnson called Ellen Delaney's character into question by asking if she was a drinker: 'I am not a teetotaller –neither one way or the other. I have never had a drink with her.' She testified that she had seen the child Kenna in the hallway.[208] Her husband partially corroborated the details but clarified that he had hearing problems' he noted how McDonnell, on barging into his home, 'excused himself to me'.[209]

Francis McCourt was fixing his front door lock when Mr McDonnell barged in looking for his wife; she was not there and he left but returned a few minutes later looking again, this time saying 'that his w____ of a wife should be there'. Recognising that he was drunk, McCourt warned him to be careful going down the stairs—he also watched him trying to shoulder through the door of another empty residence on his corridor looking for her. He went down a flight of stairs and met his wife coming against him. An angry verbal exchange occurred and McCourt witnessed him 'slapping her across the face several times'—he later

---

[205] NAI, Dublin Crown Files at Commission, *The King v Patrick McDonnell*; evidence of Mary Clancy, dated 13 September.

[206] NAI, Dublin Crown Files at Commission, *The King v Patrick McDonnell*; evidence of Jane McBirney, dated 13 September; *The Irish Times*, 18 October 1901.

[207] NAI, Dublin Crown Files at Commission, *The King v Patrick McDonnell*; evidence of Peter Whelan, dated 13 September.

[208] NAI, Dublin Crown Files at Commission, *The King v Patrick McDonnell*; evidence of Ellen Delaney, dated 13 September.

[209] NAI, Dublin Crown Files at Commission, *The King v Patrick McDonnell*; evidence of Thomas Delaney, dated 13 September.

clarified to the court that it was with an open hand. At that point, Bridget McDonnell threatened her husband with the police which made matters worse. McCourt watched McDonnell slap her repeatedly and 'catching hold of the woman throwing her out of the window. I fell back in my own room in a weakness when I seen it done. The window of the lobby was open – the bottom portion was open. There was nothing to save her.' The quarrel was over the key to the room and McCourt did not regain consciousness until the ambulance arrived. Eustace Johnston also attempted to discredit the witness and asked him if he had been drinking that day. Of 5 September he said, 'I hadn't a glass of porter in me – no more than I have now – that's none.' He clarified to the court that he had not given evidence at the coroner's court but that his 'conscience was pricking me when I saw no one was giving evidence'.[210] This provides an indication of the level of community complicity in silence, an understood code that pervaded inner city Dublin life. Stepping out of line by complaining about a neighbour carried enormous risk of reprisal if the law did not punish or censure behaviour or if the perpetrators held a grudge. Lord Chief Justice Baron sentenced McDonnell to ten years' penal servitude.[211] According to the register he was admitted to Mountjoy convict prison on 18 October.[212]

Silence, and community complicity in it, served to create a strong barrier between extra-judicial and judicial means. On 2 July at 11.30 p.m. a drunken Christopher O'Connor entered Bridget Treacy's house to order his wife 'up to bed'. As they were returning to their home, the quarrel continued—Treacy intervened and physically assaulted him.[213] According to Mary O'Connor's testimony, Treacy rolled up her skirt and her sleeve and said 'I dare you to hit me' and proceeded to run at him. While both of them fell on the street, he hit his head off the kerbstone and she 'caught him by the waistcoat and banged him on the ground two or three times'. She used such force that she tore the waistcoat off him, and it was produced in evidence by Sergeant Rutledge 13A. Treacy ran at him again as he tried to escape. Margaret Meagher rushed to help him and keep his attacker away—she brought him indoors and washed his face. He sustained head injuries in the fracas and initially refused to attend medical care, perhaps because of the humiliation associated with being found to be a wife abuser and the slur that might be cast on his masculinity because he was physically brought into line by a woman while he was drunk.[214] He later became weak and Meagher called for his

---

[210] NAI, Dublin Crown Files at Commission, *The King v Patrick McDonnell*; evidence of Francis McCourt, dated 18 September.

[211] *Evening Herald*, 17 October 1901.

[212] NAI, PRIS 1/43/02, General register of convicted male prisoners, Mountjoy, no. 3525. Patrick McDonnell.

[213] Only two women named Bridget Treacy were returned in the 1901 census for Dublin http://www.census.nationalarchives.ie/reels/nai003818627/ (26-year-old draper's assistant)' http://www.census.nationalarchives.ie/reels/nai003706117/ (28-year-old children's nurse/domestic).

[214] NAI/1900/60 Inquest held on the body of Christopher O'Connor, reports dated 7 July 1900.

mother-in-law and sister-in-law, Catherine Graham. They brought him to Dr Steevens' Hospital where his wounds were dressed—on the way home he fell to his knees thrice. Catherine Graham noted in her testimony that her hearing was not good but she recalled that he said he would 'never forgive the girl'. Margaret Meagher testified that he threatened Treacy, saying 'for nobody to do anything to her [meaning Bridget Treacy] that he would take her life himself and that he knew he would never get over it'. He died a few days later and on 7 July the coroner's jury returned the verdict of 'coma and exhaustion, following delirium the result of the injuries received to his nose and forehead'. Although James Mahon of 3 Eccles Street testified that Treacy 'had done the injuries', she was not brought before the courts. The newspapers reported that his accidental death was as a result of a fall on the street and made no mention of Treacy's role.[215]

Matricide and patricide featured irregularly in the coroners' courts and only one instance of each can be found in this sample—both involved heavy drinking. Elizabeth Payne was attacked by her son and subsequently died: 'she had drink on her at the time of the occurrence. Her son also… They were in the habit of quarrelling frequently.' He beat her viciously both within and outside their room at 40 Jervis Street. When neighbour Anna Maria Teeling tried to intervene she was assaulted in the process—Martin Payne pushed her out the door and shut it; she watched through the keyhole as he kicked his mother, who was described as delicate, in the head. After his rage subsided, 50-year-old Elizabeth Payne managed to stagger outside—she was woozy from the effects of the beating and he was heard shouting: 'To hell with her. Let her die there.' Teeling and another neighbour, Mrs Manning, rescued her and brought her to Jervis Street where she died the following morning.[216] Martin Payne was subsequently charged with her murder.[217] The verdict found that she died owing to 'Compression of the brain caused by injuries inflicted by her son Martin Payne.' He was brought before the August Commission where his previous fourteen offences of drunkenness were discussed. That he was drunk while conducting the fatal assault worked in his favour and ensured a manslaughter rather than a murder charge. He was sentenced to five years' penal servitude and was admitted to Mountjoy convict prison on 4 August 1900.[218] By contrast, when Mortimer Oldfield was brought before the City of Dublin Commission, 8 April 1902, on a manslaughter charge he was described as 'a respectable looking young man' and found not guilty.[219] On 7 March, Robert Oldfield died at 5 Hollybrook Park, Hollybrook Road, Clontarf, after an argument

[215] *Freeman's Journal*, 9 July 1900.
[216] NAI/1900/75 Inquest held on the body of Elizabeth Payne, 23 July 1900; *Irish Daily Independent*, 23 July 1900.
[217] *Kerry Weekly Reporter*, 28 July 1900; *Irish Daily Independent*, 24 July 1900.
[218] *Freeman's Journal*, 4 August 1900; NAI, PRIS 1/43/01 General register of convicted male prisoners, Mountjoy, no. 2525. Martin Payne was transferred to convict division 4 August 1900 for a 5 year sentence.
[219] *Evening Herald*, 8 April 1902.

with his son Mortimer Oldfield about the family finances. The incident took place at about midnight. A lodger named Mr Henry Taaffe claimed that he heard but did not see Mortimer landing the blows and he went to separate the struggling men. After he had pulled them apart Robert Oldfield used his boot to strike his son in the face, which reinitiated the tussle. Although he was under the influence of drink, Mortimer went to get a doctor for his victim and this action stood him in good stead later.[220] The gendered elements of both cases deserve mention: whereas a fight between father and son was not considered to be out of the ordinary, Martin Payne's actions were considered 'gross and unnatural'.[221] Foul play was in evidence in the case of Mary Anne Burke, who was thrown through the window of her home by her nephew Edward Fagan and his wife Bridget. Witnesses heard quarrelling going on and stated that Bridget Fagan was drunk. Margaret Byrne of 35 Royal Canal Bank heard Mary Anne Burke state 'if his mother was alive you would not say that' and she said 'out you go'. They were both subsequently arrested and brought before the Dublin Commission on assault charges.[222] Bridget Fagan was sentenced to twelve months while a charge of *nolle prosequi* (we shall no longer prosecute) was entered against her husband because he 'had returned from Ladysmith, and that the evidence would not sustain the charge upon which he had been sent forward'. His military service in the South African war was used to excuse and rationalise his behaviour and exempted him from punishment.[223]

There are a few instances of homicide in this sample concerning couples in 'tally' arrangements, where they were unmarried but lived as if they were.[224] When Frances Glynn who was described as a 'hotel keeper' died from 'Disease of the heart, liver and kidneys' at 44 Lower Ormond Quay she had been separated from her husband for over eighteen months. But she had taken up with a William Drea, a 42-year-old civil service pensioner, who 'lived with her and assisted her in the management of the hotel'. One newspaper described their relationship as 'of an irregular character'.[225] Several witnesses accounted for the fact that Drea repeatedly assaulted her over a four-month period prior to her death. The jury added a rider to state 'and we consider the conduct of Wm Drea accelerated her death'.[226] James John Murray testified that between 8 a.m. and 9 a.m. on 16 March William Drea sent Lizzie Fox out to get some brandy for him. Before she left she heard Drea order a man named Ward 'out of the house'—when she returned with

---

[220] *Evening Herald*, 8 April 1902.

[221] *Freeman's Journal*, 4 August 1900.

[222] NAI/1900/73 Inquest on the body of Mary Anne Burke; *Freeman's Journal*, 20 July 1900.

[223] *Irish Daily Independent*, 4 August 1900; NAI, PRIS 1/46/01, General register of female remand prisoners, Mountjoy, no. 192. Bridget Fagan.

[224] Ginger Frost, *Living In Sin: Cohabiting as Husband and Wife in Nineteenth-Century England* (Manchester, 2013).

[225] *Nationalist and Leinster Times*, 23 March 1901.

[226] NAI/1901/77 Inquest on the body of Frances Glynn, 18 March 1901.

the brandy she witnessed a brutal assault on Mrs Glynn where he beat her about the head and face first with a clenched fist and then with his open hand. During this beating Glynn was clad in a nightdress and her head hit the ground and the wall. As he beat her, he questioned her: 'Who is this man you are bringing in here?' to which she did not, or possibly could not, respond. Bridget Holahan who was present was crying and pleaded with him to stop 'or you will be sorry for it'.[227] Lizzie Fox claimed in her evidence that she had not witnessed an assault but had heard him threaten her: 'I heard Mr Drea say he would take Mrs Glynn life if she would not give him money. That was on Tuesday last 12th inst. I am a fortnight in the place'.[228] Bridget Hanrahan, who lived at 44 Lower Ormond Quay, witnessed the assault the previous Saturday that Murray accounted for—further to this she said she saw him 'strike her with a chair on Monday last the 11th inst'. Josephine Murray corroborated the accounts of the horrendous abuse that Mrs Glynn had suffered at the hands of Drea for four months prior to her death. She too saw Mrs Glynn with a bloody nose on 14 March and Drea with blood on his sleeves. William Murray saw Drea beating her 'on many occasions' but between 6 p.m. and 7 p.m. on Tuesday 12 March he witnessed an assault in the kitchen 'by boxing her in the face and neck also kicked her in the leg'. On 16 March, between 8 a.m. and 9 a.m., witnesses to the attack and its aftermath warned Drea to get a doctor, which he did not do, and Glynn died. Sergeant John Carroll 2C Store Street went to the house on 16 March at 1 p.m. Glynn was lying on 'a bed tick in the kitchen near the fire place. There were marks of violence on the arms, legs and face'. At that point Drea was in bed fully clothed in another room—he had blood on his sleeves and was charged with her wilful murder on 17 March 1901. When Drea was woken up by the arresting DMP officer he said, 'Poor Mrs Glynn is dead', she 'died off suddenly'. So confident was he in his right to physically assault her with impunity that his response to the arrest was 'he would clear himself at the inquest'. Apart from all the fresh bruising about the limbs, the injuries of the scalp and face were a few days old and contiguous with the accounts of the beatings over the previous few days. Alas, the post-mortem found significant enlargement of the liver and extensive kidney disease, which Dr Oulton argued were sufficient to cause death naturally but would 'naturally be hastened by any violence'. Drea had viciously and repeatedly assaulted Mrs Glynn and was brought before Mr Wall at the Northern Police Court on 21 March.[229] He was 'returned for trial on a reduced charge of manslaughter'.[230] He was found guilty of assault and Justice Barton sentenced him to twelve months.[231]

[227] NAI/1901/77 Inquest on the body of Frances Glynn, 18 March 1901.
[228] NAI/1901/77 Inquest on the body of Frances Glynn, 18 March 1901, testimony of Elizabeth Fox, 25 Townsend Street.
[229] Freeman's Journal, 22 March 1901.
[230] Freeman's Journal, 22 March 1901; Evening Herald, 6 April 1901, p. 5.
[231] Belfast Newsletter, 12 April 1901; NAI, PRIS 1/43/02, General register of convicted male prisoners, Mountjoy, no. 1046. He is referred to as John and not William Drea in the prison records.

The horrific murder of 33-year-old widow Mary Duffy sparked outrage because of the heightened levels of violence. She died from 'haemorrhage caused by wounds inflicted on her throat by George Pepper on the 15 December 1900 in the back parlour of the house 36 Coombe' (Map 4.1 and Figures 4.3 and 4.4).[232] Mary Enright, who described herself as the proprietress, had let the room to Pepper for 1s. 'for himself and his wife'—she stated that she had never seen him before but '[I] knew the deceased was an unfortunate'.[233] The veneer of respectability conferred by marital status, although clearly fabricated and known to both parties to be a fabrication, was an important element of the exchange, as Enright's business could be tarnished as a house of ill repute and Duffy's modesty was also at stake. Duffy and Pepper took this room late on 14 December—it was shared with two other couples and partitioned by curtains. Descriptions of such living arrangements were not routinely captured and according to DMP Inspector Andrew McDonald the room contained three large beds and measured 16 feet by 14 feet.[234] The following morning Pepper got up and went to O'Connor's Public House, 95 Coombe, at 7.30 a.m. (Map 4.1).[235] Joseph O'Connor testified that Pepper drank a glass of whisky, bought a bottle of porter to take away and commented that he was sober.[236] Pepper returned to the room afterwards with his bottle of porter and summarily proceeded to attack Duffy. One of his co-lodgers, Mrs Margaret Fitzpatrick, awoke when she heard the deceased saying 'Oh my God what is that', she noticed Pepper standing over Mary Duffy. Mrs Fitzpatrick cried out to Mrs Nolan, who was in the same room 'Mary, Mary Molly is dead'. Nolan, who knew 'Mollie' for the past eighteen months, bravely challenged Pepper by running full force at him and hitting him on the back with her shoe as he hacked at Mary Duffy's throat. She shouted 'Oh you blackguard don't take the woman away in the midst of her sins' (meaning that she had not had the chance to make an act of contrition in the Roman Catholic rite).[237] Mrs Nolan stated in evidence that she fled barefooted from the deranged Pepper and he followed her out onto the street: 'I turned to the left when I got to the Coombe he turned to the right I went back to the house and dressed myself.'[238] Mrs Fitzpatrick alerted Mr Nolan who followed and kept Pepper under surveillance, while she ran to Newmarket Station where she met Constable James Byrne 31A. The 'proprietress' Mrs Enright was returning to the house shortly before 9 a.m. as Pepper 'was rushing out of the hall his hand was all blood and he flung something out of his

---

[232] This building was listed as a 'tenement, 11l', by *Thom's Directory, 1901*, p. 1398.

[233] NAI/1900/195 Inquest on the body of Mary Duffy, 17 December 1900.

[234] NAI/1900/195 statement, dated 17 December 1900.

[235] NAI/1900/195: listed as 'William O'Connor, Tea and wine merchant, 95 Coombe, 18l', *Thom's Directory, 1901*, p. 1398.

[236] NAI/1900/195 statement, dated 17 December 1900.

[237] NAI, Dublin Crown Files at Commission, *Queen v George Pepper*, 5 February 1901, evidence of Mary Nolan, 18 December 1900.

[238] NAI/1900/195 report dated 17 December 1900.

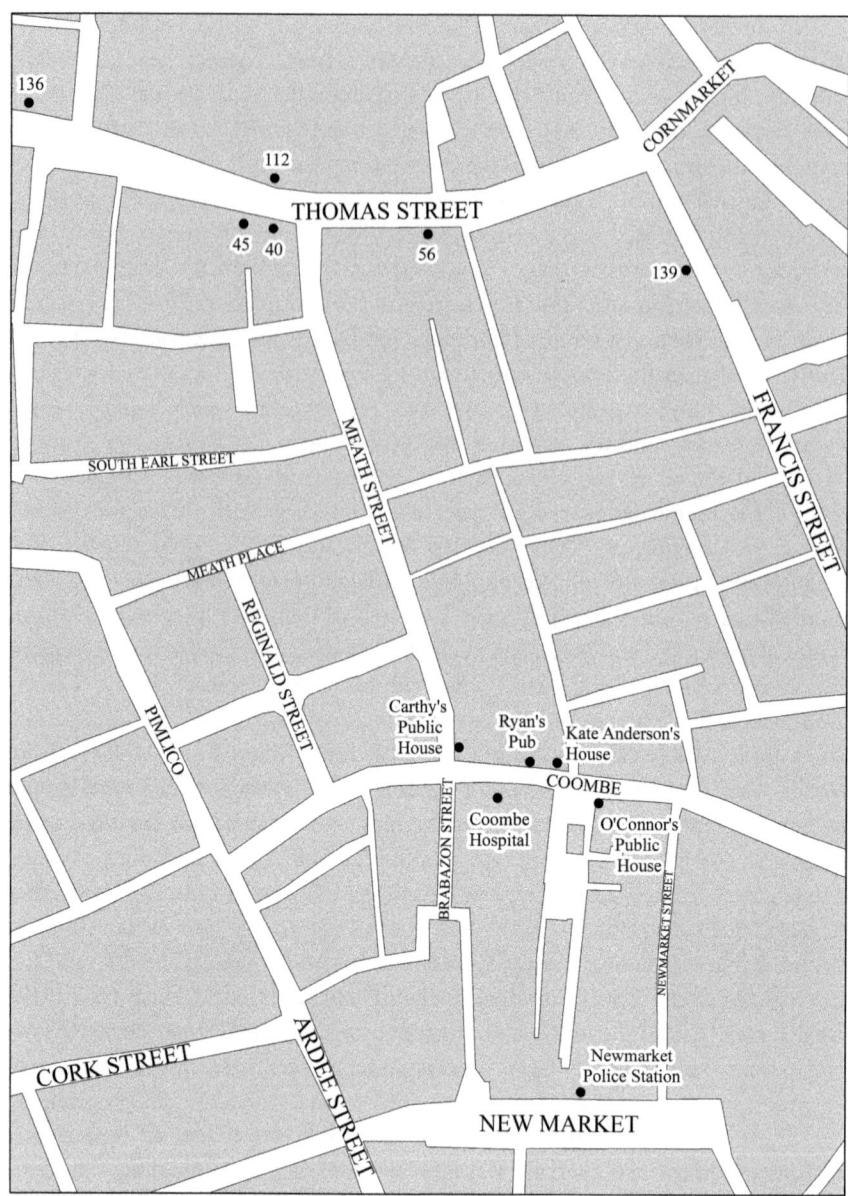

Map 4.1 Key addresses for the Duffy, Anderson, and Mooney cases

Source: NAI/Dataset 1900–2; OSi historic 25-inch basemap © Ordnance Survey Ireland/Government of Ireland Copyright Permit No. MP 006821. Cartography: Dr Rachel Murphy.

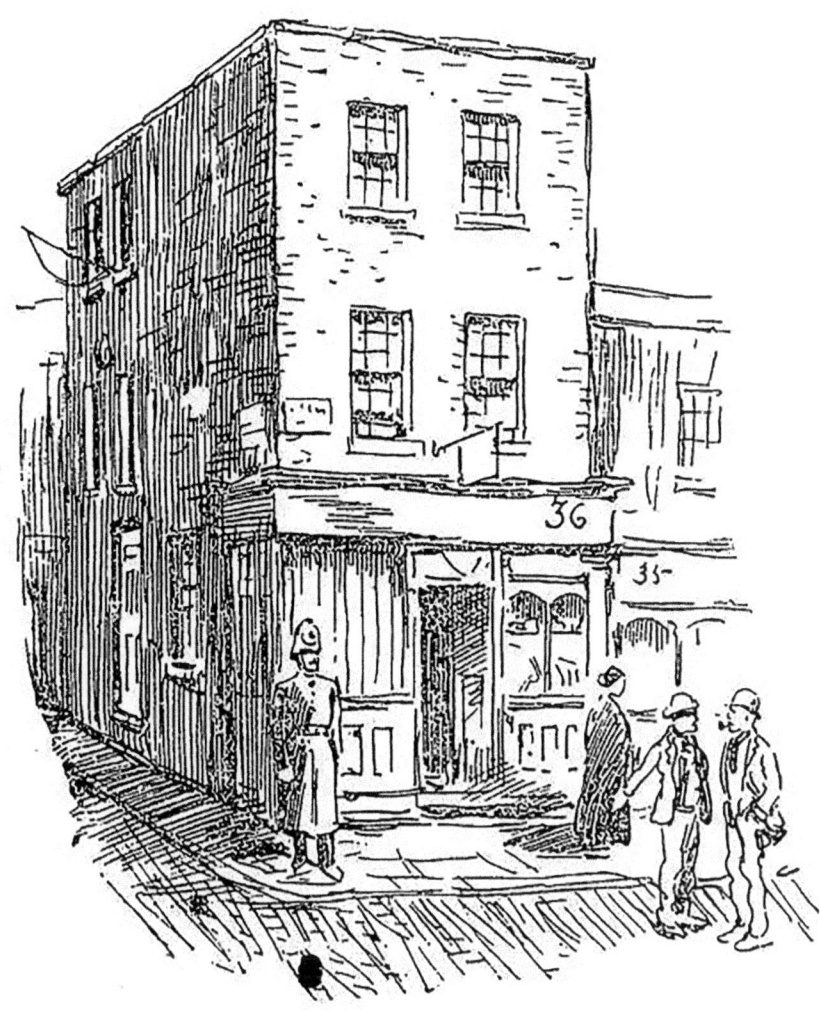

SCENE OF THE MURDER.

Figure 4.3 Scene of the murder
Source: Evening Herald, 8 February 1901.

hand – and I found (razor) case produced on the dresser'. Constable Byrne later found the razor in the bed between Duffy's body and the wall. Enright said she knew the women for about three years and that Duffy had been 'stopping with me for about four months before this occurred'.[239]

---

[239] NAI, Dublin Crown Files at Commission, *Queen v George Pepper*, 5 February 1901, evidence of Mrs Enright, 15 December 1901.

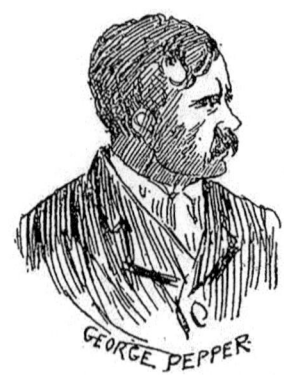

Figure 4.4 George Pepper
Source: Evening Herald, 8 February 1901.

After fleeing the scene, a blood-stained Pepper ordered a whiskey at a nearby public house, Ryan's at 41 Coombe.[240] James Byrne 31A was quick to respond and found Pepper in the water closet in the rear of the pub—he asked 'what are you at' to which Pepper replied 'something for myself'. They vacated the water closet and re-entered the pub; at that point Mrs Nolan had followed and she identified him as follows: 'thats [*sic*] the man that cut the woman's throat hold him'.[241] When arrested for the murder and cautioned, the deranged Pepper retorted 'what is it what do you mean?'.[242] Byrne brought Pepper back to the scene of the crime.

Dr Thomas O'Neill, Assistant Master of the nearby Coombe Hospital, was called to attend the scene on 15 December and within earshot of Pepper he pronounced life extinct. Byrne cautioned him again and stated that he was arresting him on a murder charge—Pepper did not reply. They proceeded to the station and when the eye-witnesses arrived Pepper said 'I admit it all, I did do it, drink was the cause of it.' O'Neill was subsequently ordered to conduct the post-mortem. He described some superficial cuts around Mary Duffy's ears and a first wound that 'started a little in front of the angle of the lower jaw on the left side and ended just on the middle of the neck, it was not very deep'. It was probably one of the smaller cuts that made Duffy cry out, which in turn alerted Mrs Fitzpatrick, who knew Duffy for two months prior.[243] Mr Nolan stated in evidence that he knew Duffy 'from her infancy' but had not seen Pepper prior to the previous night.[244] Patrick

---

[240] Listed as 'P. Ryan, grocer, 41 Coombe, 9l', *Thom's Directory, 1901*, p. 1398.
[241] NAI, Dublin Crown Files at Commission, *Queen v George Pepper*, 5 February 1901. (The King is also stamped on the file, as the Queen had died).
[242] NAI/1900/195 DMP report James Byrne, 31A, Newmarket Station, 17 December 1900.
[243] NAI, Dublin Crown Files at Commission, *Queen v George Pepper*, 5 February 1901, evidence of Mary Fitzpatrick, 18 December 1900.
[244] NAI, Dublin Crown Files at Commission, *Queen v George Pepper*, 5 February 1901, evidence of Michael Nolan, 18 December 1900.

Ryan, the proprietor of 41 Coombe, stated that he had seen Pepper three weeks before.[245] The second wound, which, it seems, all three women witnessed, O'Neill described as being

> of a terrible nature…It commenced one behind and two inches below the left ear it pressed horizontally at first for about two inches, then deep down severing all the structures and nicking the 2nd cervical vertebral bone, amongst the structures severed were the internal carotoid artery + irregular vein upper portion of gullet and windpipe the wound ended about an inch + a half beyond the middle line of the neck on the right side.

Duffy tried to defend herself and there were what modern forensics would call defence wounds of 'deep cuts on thumbs first and fourth fingers on the left hand I found deep cuts on back of thumb fore fingers and wrist'. O'Neill deemed the razor capable of causing the wounds described. Pepper was subsequently charged with murder and was remanded in Kilmainham gaol from 18 December until February, when his case came before the City Commission.[246] Pepper's deposition at the police court was brief: 'All I have to say is that for 3 or 4 week [sic] before that I was taking a lot of drink and I didn't really know what I was doing.'[247]

By coincidence, true bills were found on the same day at the City Commission at Green Street against Pepper and another man named John Toole for an eerily similar crime that occurred two weeks prior to Duffy's murder. Toole was charged with the wilful murder of Lizzie Brennan (alias Lizzie Toole) in a lodging house at 45 Charlemont Street—her throat was also slit.[248] I have written at length about this case elsewhere as John Toole was subsequently brought before the criminal courts and sentenced to death for his crime, and was the first man executed at Mountjoy prison on 7 March 1901, but it is worth briefly recounting some of the details here.[249] Both were problem drinkers and Lizzie's marital status was unclear. Dr Henry W. Oulton in his post-mortem examination of Brennan's body gave clear evidence of the fact that the wound was so deep and requiring such force that it could not have been self-inflicted.[250] The coroner's jury found that while her death was 'from haemorrhage due to the main arteries of the neck being cut',

---

[245] NAI, Dublin Crown Files at Commission, *Queen v George Pepper*, 5 February 1901, evidence of Patrick Ryan, 18 December 1900.

[246] NAI/1900/195 report dated 17 December 1900; NAI, PRIS/1/10/27 Register of remand prisoners, Kilmainham, no.1188. George Pepper.

[247] NAI, Dublin Crown Files at Commission, February 1901, *Queen v George Pepper*, 5 February 1901, evidence of George Pepper, 18 December 1900.

[248] *Irish Daily Independent*, 6 February 1901.

[249] NAI/CRF/1901/T-6 (criminal reference file for John Toole).

[250] NAI/1900/181 report dated 3 December 1900, 'found a deep gash extending across the throat from the angle on the right severing all the structures and large vessels on that side to the spine—the wound extended to the left side where it was not so deep and the vessels were in tact.'

as there was no witness to the crime, it was unsure 'whether they were self inflicted or not'.[251] Toole was a financially ruined H-car driver who had sold up his business a few weeks prior. There was evidence to show that it may have been a murder suicide as he was found with a gash on his throat, which severed when he was executed. But his defence did not make an insanity plea for him—he was sentenced to death and the plea for clemency fell on deaf ears. Pepper, who was previously an inmate at Ennis District Lunatic Asylum, was deemed to be guilty but insane and was 'to be kept in strict custody till the pleasure of the kind be made known'.[252]

Violent Streets

Streets were not just fraught with vehicular dangers—by day there were other insidious threats of bullying in all age cohorts, and by night the excesses of alcohol became more apparent. There were two cases where children were the perpetrators. The first was the case of Elizabeth McKenna, discussed briefly in the Introduction, who was assaulted by another little girl named Dooley but complicit silence on the part of the deceased's parents ensured that inquiries went no further, so it is not included in the tally of twenty-nine here.[253] But on 15 April 1902 a stone-throwing game took a sinister turn. At the rear of North Cumberland Street, John Quigley, aged 14, Patrick Quigley, aged 13, Patrick Kelly, aged 13, James Cullen, aged 10, and Henry Dent, aged 8, were throwing stones and one struck William Talbot on the forehead. He went to his home at 48 Marlborough Street where his sister-in-law tried to urge him to go to hospital, but he refused. A week later he complained of a pain in his head—she went down to him between 10 a.m. and 11 a.m. with a cup of tea and he could not speak. Kelly of 28 North Cumberland Street was charged with unlawfully causing the death. The coroner's jury found: 'Abscess on the brain brought on by a neglected wound caused by the blow of a stone, we have no evidence to prove who threw the stone and we believe it was thrown by boys playing and without malice.'[254] According to DMP Constable James Cunningham the 'boys are constantly on this wall throwing stones several complaints have been made and I have frequently hunted them off it'. They used a side door leading into the laneway to avoid capture. John Quigley testified that it was Patrick Kelly who threw the stone and that he shouted 'Now Kelly the man is all cut'. On 23 April, Kelly was charged by Inspector Lynam for unlawfully causing the death and he was released on bail until his case came before the northern

---

[251] NAI/1900/181 Inquest on the body of Elizabeth Toole, 3 December 1900.
[252] NAI, PRIS/1/10/27 Register of remand prisoners, Kilmainham, no.1188. George Pepper.
[253] NAI/1901/75 Inquest on the body of Elizabeth McKenna, 15 March 1901.
[254] NAI/1902/72 Inquest on the body of William Talbot, 24 April 1902.

division on 1 May. Owing to his mother's intercession, Mr Mahony discharged him with a caution.[255]

Excesses of alcohol not only heightened domestic tensions—it also gave rise to a series of random but serious late-night assaults. Patrick Murray was knocked down in a fracas on Eustace Street by 'John/Joseph Clinton/Clifton/Clifden' of the Rifles Brigade.[256] Mrs Susan Gulliver was standing with Mr and Mrs Clifden and witnessed the entire affair and said that Murray passed by them roughly and rudely, and struck Mrs Clifden on the back with a stick. Mr Clifden asked 'why did you do that?' and Murray responded: 'What are you doing walking with the prostitute for'. Murray was originally able to give testimony. 'Defendant said I called his missus a bad name and struck me and knocked me down. I was knocked quite senseless and don't remember anything afterwards until I found myself in hospital this morning.'[257] He did not return home until Monday and, in the interim, his brother-in-law, Joseph Comerford of 58 John Dillon Street, with whom he lived had reported him missing. He noticed Murray's behaviour becoming erratic two days later and called the DMP—he was arrested on a dangerous lunacy charge and it was while he was in custody that he was seen by Dr Joseph Dallas Pratt who advised that he be immediately conveyed to hospital.[258] He was turned away from Mercer's which was overcrowded and then brought to Jervis Street Hospital where he died. The jury found that cause of death was from 'Fracture of the base of the skull & septic meningitis following a blow received by Joseph Clifden on 23 July.'[259] Clifden was brought before the Southern Police Court on a manslaughter charge and was supposed to appear again on 28 July with proper legal representation. On 30 July Mr Tobias sent him for trial before the August commission—the outcome of this charge is unclear and it seems that no true bill was found against him.[260] An unprovoked attack led to the death of Patrick Hallinan at the hands of Private Edward Palmer, 1st Dragoon Guards.[261] Elizabeth Deane was out walking with her sister on North King Street and they bumped into Palmer; after they had passed one another he turned back and confronted her about 'what she knew about his wife's marriage'. Hallinan, who was passing, made a comment 'Oh don't argue the point with the ladies'—Palmer hit him in the face and he fell down. Hallinan was apparently 'under the influence'

---

[255] NAI/1902/72 Inquest on the body of William Talbott, 24 April 1902; *Freeman's Journal*, 24 April 1902; *Freeman's Journal*, 2 May 1902.

[256] *Freeman's Journal*, 28 July 1900.   [257] *Irish Daily Independent*, 31 July 1900.

[258] *The Medical Directory, 1900*, p. 1674.

[259] NAI/1900/79 Inquest on the body of Patrick Murray, 27 July 1900; *Evening Herald*, 26 July 1900.

[260] *Evening Herald*, 26 July 1900; NAI, PRIS 1/10/26 Register of remand prisoners, Kilmainham, Dublin, no. 676—it seems he was released after a few days; the outcome of this manslaughter charge is unclear; *Irish Daily Independent*, 31 July 1900.

[261] *Irish Daily Independent*, 9 August 1900. Another newspaper reported that he was in the 21st Lancers: *Freeman's Journal*, 9 August 1900.

according to one newspaper account.[262] Palmer was brought before Mr Mahony at the Northern Police Court on 8 August on a murder charge.[263] Unlike the Clifden case, he was brought before the October city commission on a manslaughter charge and pleaded not guilty—the jury found him guilty but with a recommendation to mercy; he was released on his own recognisance.[264] William Tallon's death after taking a fall on Digges Lane later turned into a manslaughter case when a young boy named Joseph Curran came forward to say that he saw how William Cruise 'boxed the old man in the mouth'. William Cruise was charged with manslaughter and sentenced to twelve months with hard labour at the August commission.[265]

A Sunday drinking session ended in calamity for Nicholas Atfield, who had been drinking all evening. He caught the 5 p.m. train from Westland Row to Blackrock where he had four bottles of stout in Blackrock and Kingstown. He returned to Westland Row at 10.46 p.m. and, according to his friend Henry Thorpe, an altercation occurred on the platform with Patrick Canavan. Atfield died the following day at Sir Patrick Dun's Hospital from the head injury he sustained in the fracas. According to DMP constable Thomas Cullen, 6B, Canavan deposed that as he bent down to get his hat Atfield pushed him off the carriage.[266] He also maintained that Atfield followed him down the platform and struck him.[267] In a rather unusual turn of events, Patrick Canavan had legal representation at the coroner's court, James Brady solicitor, and the Dublin, Wicklow and Wexford Railway Company was represented by Mr Keogh. Byrne was careful to add that 'it would be in another Court that Canavan would have to answer for his assault' and that the evidence of one of the railway attendants pointing to Canavan as the man who struck the fatal blow was nothing to do with the coroner's proceedings.[268] Canavan was charged at the Southern Police Court on 21 May with wilful murder and came before the City of Dublin Commission on 4 June 1901 on a murder charge—his sentence was deferred.[269] In opening the proceedings, the Lord Chief Justice raised concerns about the rise in the number of cases associated with drunkenness. Canavan pleaded guilty but T.M. Healy made an appeal to merciful consideration owing to the previous good character of the defendant, who had no prior convictions—sentencing was deferred.[270] The Lord Chief Justice reasoned that 'the assault was as a result of a drunken row, and

---

[262] NAI/1900/91 Inquest on the body of Patrick Hallanin, 8 August 1900; *Evening Herald*, 12 October 1900.
[263] *Irish Daily Independent*, 9 August 1900.   [264] *Evening Herald*, 12 October 1900.
[265] *The Irish Times*, 8 August 1901; NAI/1901/178 Inquest on the body of William Tallon, 3 July 1901.
[266] *Evening Herald*, 14 May 1901.
[267] NAI, Dublin Crown Files at Commission, 4 June 1901, evidence of Thomas Cullen, dated 13 May 1901.
[268] *Evening Herald*, 14 May 1901.   [269] *Evening Herald*, 4 June 1901.
[270] *Freeman's Journal*, 5 June 1901.

accompanied by some provocation'. Canavan was released on bail 'of £10 to come up for sentence on receiving ten days' notice'.[271]

Two cases of violent assaults occurred on board steamers, which caused jurisdictional problems for police and the coroner's inquiries. Both cases were outliers. Michael Kennedy died of septicaemia after suffering multiple stab wounds to the back of the head in an unprovoked and extremely violent attack on board the SS *Handon*. His wife Julia testified that he was attacked by a Spaniard on board the ship while it was at Tilbury Docks, London on 5 February. Kennedy was dragged out of his bunk, kicked, and stabbed with a breadknife in the back of the head and on his hands as he tried to protect himself. Were it not for another crew member, described as a 'donkey man', he believed that he would have been killed. The case was reported to the London police who 'would not take charge owing to the interference of some of those on board the SS *Handon*'. His wife brought him to Jervis Street to get his wounds dressed on 9 February and the following day to the NDU where he was detained a patient and died.[272] No police investigation followed. In the second case John Myers was charged with the murder and indicted for the wilful manslaughter and assault of Kate Fitzgerald (alias Catherine Wilson) at the City of Dublin Commission, April 1902. The incident occurred on 8 March on board the SS *Belfast* that operated between Belfast and Dublin. They were both steerage passengers and were seen boarding in the former port together. Able seaman John Tallant witnessed him viciously beat her with a stick and threaten her at 8.20 p.m.: 'Shut up, you cow or I'll knock your brains out'.[273] Shortly after leaving shore Myers was seen striking her with a clenched hand in the face and she fell down; she got up and he hit her again with his clenched fist on the right cheek. This time when she fell her leg hit off the anchor chain. John McBride witnessed the assault as he was going on shift at 10.45 p.m. and he told Myers 'you oughtn't be carrying on like that, striking the woman'. At 2.30 a.m. he heard another 'yell of a woman' and she was the only one on board. He qualified the fact that it was 'a yell of fear'. He went to look for them and found them in the gully seated opposite the fire—the woman looked unwell and he asked if she had fainted. Myers responded 'Jesus Christ! I don't know'. McBride had his rest and arose again at 7 a.m. when the boat was in Dublin Bay—at that point he noticed a lot of blood on some timber on deck; he then found her lying dead on the starboard side of steerage.[274] Both boarded the SS *Belfast* with drink on them; it was reported at North Wall that her name was Kate Fitzgerald late of 71 Carrick Hill, Belfast and that she was a single servant. She was drinking with

---

[271] *Belfast Newsletter*, 6 June 1901, referred to the victim as Hatfield.

[272] NAI/1902/26 Inquest dated 14 February.

[273] NAI, Dublin Crown Files at Commission, 8 April 1902, *King v John Myers*, manslaughter, evidence of John Tallant, 11 March 1902.

[274] NAI, Dublin Crown Files at Commission, 8 April 1902, *King v John Myers*, manslaughter, evidence of John McBride, 8 March 1902.

Myers before they boarded at Belfast on 7 March—he assaulted her before they got on board and several times after. A few officers testified that she was the only woman on board and heard her screaming 'as if in fear'.[275] Dr Matthew Maughan found extensive bruising on her left thigh—one was 6 in. to 7 in. long and she had another on her hip that he reckoned was caused by being beaten with a stick. Her two eyes were blackened. She also had evidence of ulceration on both legs and he guessed that a varicose vein had burst. The coroner's verdict was that she died of 'haemorrhage due to rupture of a large vein in the leg'.[276] The couple both lived and worked as servants at a lodging house in Carrick Hill for Edward O'Hara.[277] William Birch, the ship's captain, had made an effort at 3 a.m. to resuscitate her using smelling salts—she was then dead and he locked up Myers until he got to the DMP jurisdiction.[278] Myers was a 3rd Battalion Munster Fusilier of no fixed abode.[279] He was found guilty of manslaughter and sentenced to twelve months' hard labour.[280]

Cases of assaults perpetrated by women on other women were not uncommon either. Mary Newman, who lived at 14 Rock Lane East, James Street, complained to Constable Martin Power that a woman named Mrs Graham 'was annoying her'. Her daughter testified that her mother was assaulted between 7 p.m. and 8 p.m. on the night she died and, while the verdict was heart disease, Graham was arrested for disorderly behaviour.[281] Mary Aspall was found in a dying and destitute state by a neighbour Hannah Sheridan, who reported the case to the DMP. Aspall asked to be sent to hospital but not the Union. For women of her social class and means there were few other recourses. When asked to explain her bruises by Dr Powell at NDU, she explained that she was assaulted on Mabbot Street on 2 May 1900 and again on Granby Row by some women. She he had no friends or relatives in Dublin but had in America; she refused to give their addresses.[282] Nobody was prosecuted for the injuries that led to her death.[283]

---

[275] NAI/1902/39 Inquest on the body of Catherine Wilson, 8 March 1902.

[276] NAI, Dublin Crown Files at Commission, 8 April 1902, *King v John Myers*, manslaughter, evidence of Dr Matthew Maughan, 11 March 1902.

[277] NAI, Dublin Crown Files at Commission, 8 April 1902, *King v John Myers*, manslaughter, evidence of Edward O'Hara, 11 March 1902.

[278] NAI, Dublin Crown Files at Commission, 8 April 1902, *King v John Myers*, manslaughter, evidence of William Birch, 11 March 1902.

[279] *Freeman's Journal*, 10 March 1902.   [280] *Freeman's Journal*, 9 April 1902.

[281] NAI/1902/42 Inquest on the body of Mary Newman, 11 March 1902.

[282] NAI/1900/15 Inquest on the body of Mary Aspall, 3 May 1900; *Evening Herald*, 3 May 1900.

[283] NAI/1902/32 Inquest on the body of Margaret Moroney, 28 February 1902. In a similar manner the case of Margaret Moroney, aged 65, and a servant, was categorised as from pneumonia on 27 February 1902 at NDU. She entered the NDU on 20 February at 2.45 p.m. and told the Master she had been assaulted at 104 Church Street by a lodger there named Michael. She admitted to having hit him with a brush and he in return gave her 'a box in the eye'. He absconded and she died a few days later from pleurisy, but as the doctors stated that assault had nothing to do with death, she is not included in the twenty-nine cases discussed here.

Precarious Lives

Vernacular justice operated in parallel to the judiciary. Communities decided who to respect and what respectability was. Furthermore, the decision to conceal or cast out by offering up to the reach of the law rested with communities. Many of these silently understood social dynamics are undocumented, but the final two cases in this discussion scratch at the surface of their history. The cases relate to a mother and daughter, whose low social standing in a tight-knit community, I surmise, contributed to their slow deaths. The beginning of Kate Anderson's demise occurred on 15 October following an assault 'at the Coombe' by William 'Bill' Holmes, a soldier of the 10th Hussars on furlough at 139 Francis Street. He struck her on the right side of the head with a 'clenched hand' and she fell down on the street. At that time, the DMP report documented how 'she felt the drum or brain injured and was in great pain' and when she tried to get on her feet he struck her with his whip. Margaret Kavanagh deposed that she had witnessed the assault from the vantage point of 38 Coombe (where she and Anderson lived) between 11 p.m. and 12 p.m. and had heard crying.[284] Shortly thereafter Anderson began to suffer a discharge from her ear and, although she confided in Mary Anne Lambe about the assault, she asked her friend 'not to let on' (to pretend nothing had happened and to do nothing about it). Two nights later, Anderson was assaulted again in the Coombe area, this time by a woman named Lizzie McEntee, who was in the company of Holmes.[285] McEntee, who was armed with a wrench, attacked Anderson. This time, Mary Anne Lambe was present and intervened as both women were scuffling on the ground. Lambe managed to first take the wrench from the altercation and then she broke up the fight. After that she brought Anderson to the 'Station house' together with the bloodied wrench as evidence. McEntee had already brazenly presented herself at Newmarket Police Station and announced how the woman behind her would be charging her with assault. McEntee was a serial offender who was regularly before the Petty Sessions—she was arrested and sentenced to one month in jail under the name Eliza Cashin in August 1899 for the illicit sale of porter at 24 Golden Lane.[286] In August 1901, when she was arrested for using obscene language, she was then living at 38 Coombe, so it seems these women were well known to one another.[287] Anderson was bleeding from the head wound she sustained from a blow of the wrench so she was sent by the DMP to the Meath Hospital to have it dressed.

---

[284] NAI/1900/146 Inquest on the body of Kate Anderson, DMP report dated 25 October 1900.

[285] *Evening Herald*, 29 October 1900.

[286] NAI, PRIS 1/44/1, General Register of convicted female prisoners, Mountjoy, no. 3732.

[287] NAI, PRIS 1/44/02, General register of convicted female prisoners, Mountjoy, no. 4529. Acquitted on 3 December 1900, produced at police court under the writ of habeas corpus while undergoing sentence. NAI, PRIS 1/46/01 General register of female remand prisoners, Mountjoy, no. 5365, Elizth (O Brien Caslim/Cashin).

When she returned to the 'Station house' McEntee was charged and sentenced to three months and a further month 'in default of bail'.[288] Mary Anne Lambe testified at Anderson's coroner's inquest that McEntee announced that she had just come out of prison after serving six months and that 'she was willing to go back for twelve for her'.[289] Implied in the willingness to serve a twelve-month month sentence was her intent to commit grievous bodily harm or indeed manslaughter, as that was a typical punishment meted out.

On 20 October, dispensary doctor, George Stritch visited Anderson at 38 Coombe (Map 4.1) and gave her an admission order to the SDU hospital. He maintained that there were seven or eight women present who were all under the influence of alcohol. A few months later, on the night of the 1901 census, the building at 38 Coombe had five families, comprising twelve male and fourteen female inhabitants.[290] It is entirely plausible that all of the women who claimed the address of 38 Coombe at the December inquest and in the February commission had moved on. It is possible that they were sub-renting part of some of the above household rooms but none of these women of little trace are recorded in the census. Furthermore, there is strong evidence of witness intimidation and gender-based violence in the locale, where women were kept in line by bully-boy tactics and pervasive low-level threats of physical violence. Kate was married to Albert Anderson, a private in the Oxford Regiment, in 1895 before she reached the age of majority—she was described as 'under age' in the records.[291] She had previously served seven days in Mountjoy prison for larceny in January 1900, where her maiden name was used and her husband's name is recorded, but he was not mentioned at her inquest at all.[292]

Anderson eventually presented at the SDU hospital on 25 October 'quite incoherent' according to Resident Surgeon Dr George F. McNamara, but the dye had been cast and, by then, she had what he described as 'a large abscess'. The incidents were subsequently described in a *Freeman's Journal* article as 'Low life in Dublin Revelations of a Slum Area'.[293] The article revealed that although the inquest was scheduled for 1 p.m., and after waiting thirty minutes for a sufficient minimum number to arrive, Dr Byrne had 'to call the jurors summoned on fines'.

[288] NAI/1900/146 Inquest on the body of Kate Anderson, Statement signed by Thomas Calahan, 91A Newmarket Street, 27 October.

[289] NAI/1900/146 report dated 27 October 1900.

[290] William Sutton and family 38.1 (niece and nephew, aged 12 and 7, named Malone); Bridget Byrne & family, husband Michael, name incorrectly spelled Brien 38.2, three children; Annie Marshall 38.3 (household of six); Mary Byrne in 38.4 (six in household), John Murphy 38.5 (household of four): http://www.census.nationalarchives.ie/pages/1901/Dublin/Merchants_Quay/Coombe/ (accessed 26 November 2021).

[291] See https://civilrecords.irishgenealogy.ie/churchrecords/images/marriage_returns/marriages_1895/10536/5837591.pdf (accessed 8 August 2021).

[292] NAI, PRIS 1/44/01 General register of convicted female prisoners, Mountjoy, no. 57, Kate Anderson. She was sentenced on 3 January 1900.

[293] *Freeman's Journal*, 29 October 1900.

Indeed, one juror had sent a 16-year-old boy in his stead.[294] The intensely local nature of the series of events becomes apparent when the locations of jurors, doctors, and institutions are mapped (Map 4.1). On 27 October 1900, Anderson's coroner's inquest was held at the SDU mortuary. Three of the jurors were from addresses delineated on Thomas Street; others were from Meath Street, doors away from Carthy's public house, which is central to her mother's case. Much of Kate Anderson's death remains a mystery as to why Bill Holmes and Lizzie McEntee attacked her—perhaps it was a love tryst but it is most certainly lost to history. McEntee went out armed and with premeditation—she hit Anderson on the head and drew blood. Were it not for the actions of Mary Anne Lambe in wresting the weapon out of her hand it could possibly have been a murder case from the outset. The jury found that she had 'Disease of mastoid bone and cerebral abscess, and we have no evidence as to how said abscess was caused but we believe that said assaults committed by Bill Holmes and Elizabeth McEntee accelerated her death.'[295] Her cause of death was registered as being from a disease of the mastoid bone from 'information received'.[296] McEntee was sentenced to three months for her assault on 29 October 1900.[297] According to the 1901 census, a 26-year-old Elizabeth McEntee was 'houseless' at 3 Wood Quay.[298]

With McEntee in prison the case should have come to a natural conclusion in the police court were it not for the fact that Holmes conducted another brutal assault on Mary Hayden, who was a witness in the Anderson case and lived with her at 38 Coombe—this time he pushed his victim to the ground and kicked her.[299] It seems he liked to have women do his bidding and his accomplice on that occasion was Catherine O'Rourke who bit the poor woman on the nose. Holmes and McEntee were brought before the commission of Oyer and Terminer on 3 December 1900. Despite evidence of repeated prior assaults on women, his sentence was initially deferred for the assault on Anderson but he was handed down eighteen months' hard labour following the second assault on Hayden. The deferred sentence of six months was reinstated and ran concurrently.[300]

Following her return from giving evidence in her daughter Kate Anderson's case, Mary Anne Mooney decided to go with Mary Anne Lambe into Carthy's public house at 48 Meath Street between 7 p.m. and 8 p.m.[301] The latter went to the bar and called for two 'halves' of whiskey and when she turned around she

---

[294] *Freeman's Journal*, 29 October 1900.

[295] NAI/1900/146 report dated 27 October 1900.

[296] See https://civilrecords.irishgenealogy.ie/churchrecords/images/deaths_returns/deaths_1900/05746/4622623.pdf (accessed 8 August 2021).

[297] *Evening Herald*, 29 October 1900, p. 4.

[298] See http://census.nationalarchives.ie/reels/nai003791148/ (accessed 14 December 2019).

[299] *The Irish Times*, 4 December 1900.

[300] *Freeman's Journal*, 4 December 1900; NAI, PRIS 1/43/01 General register of convicted male prisoners, Mountjoy, no. 4024, William Holmes.

[301] Carthy's registered in the census as a public house: http://census.nationalarchives.ie/reels/nai003715566/.

found Mooney was on the floor. Mary Hayden testified that Lambe asked 'who done that?' It was clearly a tense environment aggravated by the presence of a raft of witnesses from the courthouse that day. Someone shouted out that John Brogan was after hitting Mooney. Lambe confronted him for striking an old woman like that and Brogan threatened her at that point: 'go away you old w____ or I'll give you the same'.[302] Whore was considered such a slur in the early twentieth century that it was rarely spelled out in full in the court documents. As Julia Laite has astutely observed, 'it is fundamentally important to recognize the distinctions between doing prostitution and being a prostitute, and, of course, the difference between being a prostitute and being called one.'[303]

Brogan declared with no fear of repercussion that he had struck Mooney. A newspaper account of the ensuing court case revealed that Mooney, who had been under police protection, had approached Brogan who was also drinking in Carty's and twice he asked her to go away but she persisted. Brogan asked the foreman to have her removed from the pub but before he had the opportunity to do so, the assault occurred. Mary Hayden of 37 New Row saw Brogan 'give deceased a box under the chin and deceased fell on the ground unconscious'. Although the records are very patchy, it is highly likely that she was the same Mary Hayden that was assaulted by Bill Homes and Catherine O'Rourke.[304] In the coroner's court, Hayden said to a juror: 'I heard Brogan say that the "deceased was an old prostitute reared nothing but prostitutes"'. He also said that it was no wonder two of her daughters were dead. On 4 December, Brogan was brought before the police court on a manslaughter charge but the presiding Mr Byrne changed it to murder.[305] As it transpired, Brogan, who was a repeat petty offender, who was 'many a time' before the police court, was not charged with murder. Instead, he was brought before the courts on 11 February on a manslaughter charge.

Mary Hayden testified at the City of Dublin Commission on 3 December that she saw Brogan shake Mooney, 'box' her in the throat, and knock her to the ground. He called on the foreman of the establishment to take Mrs Mooney out before she would 'lose her pocket or her purse'. Thomas Hayden, her husband, deposed that he heard Brogan say that she was 'Along with a lagger, and drinking with laggers'.[306] Lagger in popular parlance meant someone who grassed to the police or turned state's witness. To become a lagger in a tight-knit community was dangerous business. Equally dangerous was to side with the wrong person and probably why Thomas Hayden tried to mitigate risk by saying in court that Brogan was 'a decent man'.[307] Bridget McGawley, another daughter of the deceased

[302] NAI, Dublin Crown Files at Commission, February 1901, Case of *King v John Brogan*, 5 February 1901.
[303] Julia Laite, *Common Prostitutes and Ordinary Citizens: Commercial Sex in London, 1885–1960* (London, 2011), p. 26.
[304] *Irish Daily Independent*, 4 December 1900.   [305] *Skibbereen Eagle*, 8 December 1900.
[306] *Irish Daily Independent*, 5 December 1900.
[307] NAI, Dublin Crown Files at Commission, *King v John Brogan*, 5 February 1901, 3 December testimony of Thomas Hayden.

also resident at 38 Coombe, claimed that she had known Brogan for several years and that, while she was not present on the fateful night she had heard him three or four months prior to that threaten her mother, that 'he'd never leave the world 'till he left her a corpse.'[308] She further stated that her mother was 'in perfect health on the day of the assault'. Mary Brennan said that he threatened Mrs Lambe: 'that he would do the same to her and she also was a prostitute'. It is interesting to note that there is no trace of Bridget McGawley in the 1901 census. The 'foreman of the shop' Micheal Kiernan (described in the census as a 30-year-old assistant to John Carthy the head of household)[309] was entirely unsympathetic— he lifted the barely conscious Mrs Mooney off the floor and put her outside the door; he advised Mrs Lambe to leave with her. Neither help nor water was offered to Mrs Mooney. Lambe brought her home with the assistance of some children and left her lying on the floor at 38 Coombe while she went for Fr O'Brien, Francis Street, who came at once, but on their return Mooney was pronounced dead. Lambe brought her back to 38 Coombe Street which (as Map 4.1 shows) was a stone's throw from the Coombe hospital but no doctor was called for a few hours. Dr Louis Byrne remarked: 'It is the most extraordinary thing I ever heard, that this woman was not brought to the Coombe hospital which was just on the other side of the road.' It was nearer to the pub than the house Mooney died in. Mary Anne Lambe's first inclination was to go for 'the priest at once…I lost no time in going for the priest.' The coroner's jury found that 'Cardiac failure accelerated by the blow received from John Brogan in the house 48 Meath St on the 3rd December 1900.' Again, most of the jurors were drawn from a short radius within the Coombe area despite the fact that the inquest took place at the mortuary of the city morgue in the city centre. In evidence in the case against Brogan, Dr Dallas Pratt stated that Mrs Mooney was a 'frail delicate-looking woman' with a weak and small heart and the attack she had suffered would have accelerated her death.[310]

Mr Healy, Brogan's counsel, stated how the 'unhappy transaction occurred in a public house and there had been previous dispute between the parties'. Healy contended that the accused was 'in no sense a man of bad character', had 'a large family' and was in the employment of Messrs Arnott and Company.[311] Despite his previous conviction for assaulting a woman in 1888 'and he got a month for a false charge', the Crown was happy to accept his plea of guilty for common assault of Mooney who was described as the 'unfortunate deceased'. He was convicted and Mr Bryne sentenced him to a year of hard labour.[312]

[308] NAI, Dublin Crown Files at Commission, *King v John Brogan*, 5 February 1901, 3 December testimony of Bridget Ganley.
[309] See http://census.nationalarchives.ie/reels/nai003715670/ (accessed 15 December 2019), residents of 48 Meath Street.
[310] NAI, Dublin Crown Files at Commission, February 1901, *King v John Brogan*, 5 February 1901, evidence of Dr Joseph Dallas Pratt.
[311] *Thom's Irish Almanac 1900* (Dublin, 1900), p. 1705. A wholesale and retail drapers, carpet, curtain and general warehousemen, upholsterers, and cabinet makers, 11–15 Henry Street.
[312] *Evening Herald*, 11 February 1901.

Conclusion

This chapter has covered some of the more violent deaths in the sample and has exemplified the ways in which vernacular and formal justice systems co-existed. In tracing how infanticide, suicide, and cases of interpersonal violence moved between both systems it has shown that the law was indeed an ass and was highly localised in its implementation and interpretation.

Physical violence was common and an accepted part of life in early twentieth-century Dublin. It erupted in public spaces in spontaneous ways but the nature of domestic violence was different—it was omnipresent for some women and children living with brutal men. Men were permitted to beat their wives and physically discipline their children so long as it was not too severe. Much of the history of domestic violence is lost as so few cases were reported and, when they were, it was so easy to argue provocation or to cast aspersions of bad character on wives whose public profile did not equal that of their 'breadwinner' husbands. Within the male breadwinner model another rationale for light sentences could also be found. The judge in the case of Joseph McCabe recognised his father's monstrous nature but grappled with the financial dire straits the family would have been left in, in his absence.

Like all other major cities, Dublin streetscapes had an undeniable air of menace. It was a tough place to eke out a living, especially for vulnerable women. Women who drank and had associations with sex work like Brown and Hanlon were granted no concessions while the likes of John Brogan was seen to be justified in his actions because he was a family man with a job, and his victim was considered 'low life'. Quite apart from the invisible layers of biopower there existed informal layers of social control. Tragic cases like that of Kate Anderson and her mother Mary Anne Mooney exemplify forms of 'vernacular justice'. Both were physically assaulted in public spaces to bring them into alignment with the wishes of dominant men in their community—those who stood by the women suffered intimidation and ostracisation according to inferences made in the evidence presented. Mooney was under DMP protection and another woman who was a witness linked to both cases was physically attacked by Bill Homes. Both Anderson and Mooney died as a result of wounds they sustained in beatings and neither case found justice, either in extra-judicial or in judicial terms. I show and argue that the social fabric and the judiciary were highly selective in the women it chose to champion and defend, and Anderson and Mooney, both drinkers and 'dealers', with vaguely described marital arrangements were to contemporary sensibilities the wrong kind of women.

Conclusion

Meticulously kept and methodical, what remains of Dr Byrne's records are a hugely important source for historians of all hues, yet they have been subject to limited scholarly investigation.[1] The attributes of Dublin city inquests embody inherent ironies: while they provide highly detailed accounts of the final movements of their subjects, what is most striking is their capacity to recount the everyday in a commercially busy but over-crowded inner city with a largely impoverished resident population. Experiences of an overly bureaucratic and regimented system did little to encourage poor people to engage. In order to avail themselves of free medical care, the poor had to negotiate with Poor Law relieving officers to get tickets for the dispensary doctor's services. DMP constables took active roles in cases where they had been the first port of call and marshalled people to the correct course of action. Those who resisted, ignored, avoided, or were simply unaware of, the reach of biopower during their life, were subjected to an intensely medico-legal process on the occasion of death. The original inquest reports show how important coroners' courts were in terms of medical jurisprudence and Irish social life. By arranging them thematically and adopting the analytical frameworks of blame, gender, and power in all its manifestations I contend that it is possible to develop understandings of how life was experienced by the city's poorest people. These frameworks offer ways of interpreting the dynamics of the social inequalities of health in early twentieth-century Dublin. The coronial court system acted as an important nexus of medico-legal discourses that ranged from the paid expert medical witness to the vernacular. Riders were where middle-class men cast their opinions on the circumstances leading to death and, in cases that involved criminality, these held significant weight especially if they were reported in the newspapers.

The Dublin City coroner's court evolved in a separate way to the rest of the country, and was dominated by medical men. Within a short timeframe, Dr Louis A. Byrne established himself as a steady, consummate medical professional who provided an efficient service—he served as coroner to the City of Dublin from 1900 to 1932. Under his tenure the court rarely became a source of controversy, even during the revolutionary era 1916–21, although at times martial law

---

[1] Breathnach, 'Infant life protection and medico-legal literacy', pp 781–98; Breathnach and O'Halpin, 'Scripting blame: Irish coroners' courts and unnamed infant dead, 1916–32', pp. 210–28; Breathnach and O'Halpin, 'Registered "unknown" infant fatalities', pp. 70–88.

Ordinary Lives, Death, and Social Class: Dublin City Coroner's Court, 1876–1902. Ciara Breathnach, Oxford University Press. © Ciara Breathnach 2022. DOI: 10.1093/oso/9780198865780.003.0006

was periodically imposed and civil courts were replaced by inferior military 'Inquiries in Lieu of Inquests'.[2] Even when other doctors, who were perceived as being complicit in the imperial project were subject to intimidation, Byrne was held as an honest broker and was not adversely impacted in any way, especially during the Republican hunger striking campaign of 1917.[3] In general terms, and in the period I focus on, the court operated in close collaboration with the DMP and the local medical community, and they were rarely at odds with one another. The coroner's court had an unusual legal status—it was categorically a court of record and was bound by the rule of evidence but it retained some of the powers of a judicial court. It was where suicide and some cases of infanticide reached conclusion, and, as in the case of John Brogan for the manslaughter of Mary Anne Mooney, the coroner could place prisoners on remand for trial at the next Oyer and Terminer or City Commission.[4] Dr Byrne was always careful to ensure that those without legal representation did not implicate themselves in ways that could be used against them in future criminal proceedings as the DMP was always present. Solicitors for the tram and railway companies regularly used the coroner's court to question witnesses, to get statements on the record, and sway juries in their verdicts and riders.

Blame, as Mary Douglas argues, was based on an intensely localised interpretation of legislation.[5] This reinforces King's ideas surrounding the core and the periphery in both interpretations and perceptions of the law, and it is very interesting how degrees of othering from ethnic and nativist perspectives accrued from it.[6] The frameworks of gender and class are central to my analysis because those identities and how they were formed in the Dublin tenements had a long history of rejection and neglect in terms of Irish nationalism. Indeed, cultural nationalist organisations like the GAA and the Gaelic League sharpened these divides. In Dublin, different forms of masculinity held sway—the thousands of Irish men who served in the South African wars and the DMP were the antithesis of the anti-colonialism that was inherent to 'Gaelic masculinity'. Their wives and widows were equally derided for accepting the shilling of the Crown forces. Later termed the 'separation women', they were othered within an othering of lower

---

[2] Ciara Breathnach and Eunan O'Halpin, 'Sexual assault and fatal violence against women during the Irish War of Independence, 1919–1921: Kate Maher's murder in context', *Medical Humanities*, 48: (2022), pp. 94–103.

[3] Dr Byrne presided over the inquest of Thomas Ashe who died as a result of a botched force-feeding exercise in September 1917. Irish republican propagandists seized the opportunity to publish the proceedings at a time when medical doctors were themselves targets for assisting or facilitating the British Crown forces: NAI/CSO/RP/1918/2000; William Murphy, *Political Imprisonment and the Irish, 1912–1921* (Oxford, 2014).

[4] Criminal Law (Ireland) Act, 1828 (9 Geo. IV) c. 54. Section 6 remained in place until the Coroner's Act 1962.

[5] Douglas, *Blame and Risk*.

[6] Peter King, *Crime and Law in England 1750–1850: Remaking Justice from the Margins* (Cambridge, 2006), p. 2.

working-class life in urban Dublin.[7] This othering continued in the early decades of the Free State, when, for example, the government turned to rural Ireland to find idealised forms of Irishness. The Irish Folklore Commission was instrumental in the choreography of Irish gender identities. It was interested in the ordinary and the everyday but in a very self-aware context of a rapidly changing world and fading traditions, and it was highly selective in its mandate. Its focus was on rural Ireland where women rarely frequented pubs and the gendered spheres of work and social life were routinely separate, mainly for practical reasons. The regressive social policies of the Free State were underpinned by conservative and patriarchal ideologies and the national narrative focused disproportionately on the family and the body of the mother. Again, it was again a highly selective process—single mothers and what I term 'weak families' were very vulnerable to biopower and in some cases subject to vile treatment, as successive Irish government Commissions of Investigation into historical abuse have shown.[8]

This book has focused on the subjects of the coroner's court and has aimed to tell a history from below with records mainly taken from above. It contends that as a genre, coronial court records contain authentic voices of the poor, particularly in cases of violent death discussed in Chapter 4 and indeed in cases of those who were killed 'outside', which form the basis of Chapter 3. In both case types, witness statements tended to be longer and both the DMP and court reports used less by way of paraphrase. In such instances, the 'rhetorical flourish' of working-class Dublin is captured in the unmistakeable turns of phrase, idioms and, to a lesser extent, swear words. Direct speech is denoted in the DMP reports and in the court records by inverted commas, which are carefully applied in the more controversial cases. That was the Dublin of O'Casey's childhood that later inspired his Dublin Trillium and the setting of 'The Plough and the Stars', devoid of the religiosity that marred its debut in the changed and aspiring Free State Ireland of 1926.[9] By setting the play in a tenement O'Casey eschewed the 'synecdoche' cottage setting of the West of Ireland that had come to dominate the Abbey Theatre productions.[10] In so doing he reminded audiences of elements of Irish life that were deliberately ignored. Drawing attention to systemic poverty, sub-standard and limited domestic space, violence, and prostitution did not fit with the vision of Ireland that the Free State wished to project. But to ignore those elements of

---

[7] Fionnuala Walsh, *Irish Women and the Great War* (Cambridge, 2020); Janis Lomas, 'Delicate duties': issues of class and respectability in government policy towards the wives and widows of British soldiers in the era of the great war', *Women's History Review*, 9:1 (2000), pp. 123–47.

[8] Although flawed in many ways the Final Report of the Commission of Inquiry into Mother and Baby Homes provides an overview of appalling treatment of single mothers at the hand of the State and its instruments. https://www.gov.ie/en/publication/d4b3d-final-report-of-the-commission-of-investigation-into-mother-and-baby-homes/ (accessed 1 June 2021).

[9] O'Keefe and Ryan, 'At the world's end', p. 21.

[10] Amanda Clarke, '"Keepin' a home together": Performing Domestic Security in Sean O'Casey's "The Plough and the Stars"', *The Canadian Journal of Irish Studies*, 38:1–2 (2014), pp. 208–27.

Irish social life also meant that a large part of the urban population continued to live very precarious lives until the relative prosperity of the 1960s.

An overarching aim of this research was to show who from class, gender, life cycle, and socio-economic perspectives were among the city's most vulnerable dwellers at the beginning of the twentieth century. It also aimed to provide a context to their often unexpected deaths and to provide understandings as to why they died without medical attention or in suspicious circumstances, as the case might be. The lines between the various rungs of the lower orders were fluid, and it was easy to slip between them—few had the buffer zones of savings, insurance policies, pensions, or trade union membership for tough times. Most of the cases discussed here concern those living in a makeshift, hand to mouth economy. Intergenerational disadvantage is evident in the dataset used here, meaning that systemic social inequalities placed upward mobility beyond the capacity of ordinary individuals, especially for those born and raised in Dublin. Inward migrants from elsewhere could fake credentials or indeed their lineage and, because of prevailing stereotypes, they often found it easier to find employment.

Usually it was the coronial court system that first processed the sudden deaths of Dublin's most vulnerable citizens, the near complete absence of the middling and upper classes demonstrates its medico-legal positioning as a primary recourse when poor working-class people died. Its natural constituency, as this study has shown, was at the lower end of the social spectrum, that is, the precarious classes who were most likely to die suddenly without medical supervision or in suspicious circumstances. To understand cause of death this book has foregrounded the importance of outlining the everyday lives of the subjects of the Dublin coroner's court. The cause of the majority of sudden deaths was linked inextricably to oppressive features of the home, work, and built environments that shaped their daily lives. While some died through personal neglect of chronic ill-health, the majority died because of the social determinants of health they had little control over. Overcrowded, substandard housing and miserable living standards both directly and indirectly caused over half of the deaths in this sample. By dividing their working-class world into domestic spaces and the world outside the front door this book has shown the perils these ordinary and very vulnerable people faced.

By using a combination of microhistory, prosopography, and medico-legal and social history approaches, this study has provided a thematic reading of the cases coming before Dr Louis A. Byrne over a two-year period. As explained in the Introduction, a random sampling approach could not be employed over his thirty-two-year career because of the patchy nature of the surviving records. My study of original inquest reports is based on 611 consecutive cases and does not aspire to a statistical representation of overall trends in sudden or suspicious deaths. The value of wrapping this sample around the 1901 census is clear, and the absence of the women, for example at 38 Coombe in the Anderson and Mooney cases, speaks volumes about the potential true extent of household occupancy in the tenements. It points to even higher levels of overcrowding than was officially known, which is indicative of fear of surveillance, officialdom, and biopower. It is a pity that the same type of study could not be conducted with respect to the 1911 census to provide longue durée and longitudinal perspectives, but only sixteen full inquest reports survive from 1910 to 1912. Using the register in tandem with newspapers could yield further returns in future studies but as this study has shown, coverage of cases is too inconsistent to support a uniform methodology. The Irish press was fickle in its reporting—if a sensational murder occurred then newspaper columns were dominated by it and other cases were cast aside. Coverage of cases was short, and in abbreviating the record it often omitted names or published completely inaccurate information. Social class dictated content too, as some elements of working-class Dublin life were at odds with early twentieth-century political ideologies of nationalism and unionism. For reasons I explored throughout the book, I chose to work systematically from the original inquest reports to other sources rather than trying to establish and resolve the complicated relationship between the coroner's register and potential newspaper articles.[11]

By creating a robust dataset of continuous records it was possible to ascertain patterns in how blame was allocated and how social class, gender, and power differentials operated in tandem to produce riders that were all too often biased against the very poor. In using a gender framework to understand power dynamics, the positioning of deaths inside and outside domestic spaces naturally emerged. Prosopography proved to be a very important methodological device to group cases of similar causation together to see how gender combined with class and respectability to influence verdicts and riders. It is a very useful approach to developing understandings of the lived experience of people who otherwise leave a faint or indeed no impression on the historical record. For many of those who died prior to census night 1901, their deaths are very often the only official records of their lives; like, for example, John Healy. More vulnerable still were children like 4-year-old Catherine McLoughlin, who died after her clothes caught fire in May 1901, but she does not feature in the census.[12]

Subjects of the Dublin City coroner's court were akin to what Emma Griffin describes as 'lower-class groups scraping along a very coarse material edge'.[13] For most of those coming before Byrne's court the divisions of public and private were fluid—if we consider the fact that room doors were rarely locked and the front doors of buildings remained open then the physical parameters of tenement life included the streetscape, especially for children. I opted to use the front door

---

[11] Sexual violence is not mentioned at all in these coronial data—topics such as rape were considered indelicate and rarely received coverage in the newspapers, which were highly selective in their coverage of criminal court cases.

[12] NAI/1901/130 Inquest on the body of Catherine McLoughlin, report dated 10 May 1901.

[13] Emma Griffin, 'The emotions of motherhood: love culture, and poverty in Victorian Britain', *The American Historical Review*, 123:1 (2018), pp. 60–85 at 82.

of the building to divide cases into those occurring inside and outside because the risks associated with domestic and non-domestic spaces differed greatly and, in ideological terms, doorways were important thresholds for family life. The space between a tenement room and the front door was considered a partial extension of domestic space and was where smaller children played. Room doors afforded a degree of privacy, albeit sometimes in adverse forms. Behind doors, health deteriorated and, for some, it was where neglect and abuse occurred. In a city of high infant mortality, few cases raised eyebrows or public attention unless there was evidence of foul play, alcohol abuse, or of low moral standards, and the same can be said of older persons dying of cardiac or lung disease. Outsiders rarely interfered with domestic situations—problems had to spill onto the street or reveal themselves as public before various modes of surveillance and censure could mobilise, at community and more formal biopower and governmental levels. Moreover, the street as a neutral space offered mothers a veneer of support and protection if things went awry. The two years under review happen to be ones where the full impact of the technological innovation of electric trams was having a greater influence on the space available to other vehicular traffic and pedestrians alike.

DMP officers were the primary foot soldiers of biopower—very little escaped their notice and they must have tolerated high levels of neglect, injustice, illicit alcohol sales, prostitution, and vice. Sometimes it was easier for them to ignore matters that the system did not have enough capacity to contend with. O'Keefe and Ryan posit that brothels were permitted to operate in plain sight because the bridewell and local prison system did not have enough cells.[14] Furthermore, DMP officers lived in tenements themselves—even those living in second-class housing like the Wall family who had three children at 111.1 Clonliffe Road kept three lodgers in their three-roomed abode, to make ends meet.[15] Lower ranking policemen and DFB officers were but a rung or so above some of the most vulnerable people in these data. The personal neglect of health problems was a pervasive problem and there were a number of deaths of serving DMP officers per annum from pulmonary tuberculosis. Reticence on the part of ordinary people to engage with biopower instruments and fear of its foot soldiers (be they dispensary doctors, acting in the normal course of duties or in a civil registration capacity, or a DMP officer gathering census information), is one of this study's main findings. It reveals that there was a whole cohort of people who existed outside of formal surveillance mechanisms—perhaps some were captured in institutional records like workhouses and prisons, but it is unlikely that they were all incarcerated on census night. A more likely story is that this cohort were occupying sub-let rooms or parts of beds within rooms in the range of informal practices that exacerbated the city's housing problem. The discovery of dead bodies in sheds, roofless houses,

---

[14]   O'Keefe and Ryan, 'At the world's end', p. 27.

[15]   See http://www.census.nationalarchives.ie/reels/nai003747553/ (accessed 10 August 2021).

and doorways shows that despite the proliferation of cheap lodging houses, homelessness was a real problem in the city. There are a few cases of serious mental health problems and addiction being managed in domestic settings—a few resulted in suicide.

When the commission on working class housing reported in 1914, it described the tenements as 'exceedingly old structures' that were 'more or less in an advanced state of decay'.[16] The nature of tenement buildings were inadequate—their plumbing, cooking, and sanitary arrangements were not designed for multiple-family occupancy. Their denigration into slums was the first in a host of risks and dangers to working-class family lives. The very architecture of tenement rooms provided the first set of problems for mothers and children. Tenement rooms were physically treacherous spaces for children and ones where mothers and guardians were fully responsible. The limited cooking space in erstwhile bedrooms, and the lack of space to safely place pots off the boil away from small children, meant that mothers could not turn their backs even for split seconds. Motherhood came under intense and unfair scrutiny in all child deaths for root causes that were simply beyond their control. The censure of Mrs Woodcock, discussed in Chapter 2, whose husband slept while their daughter Isabella's clothing went up in flames, was a deeply unfair assessment of her as a mother. There was no evidence to support her husband's allegations of past neglect or intemperance. He was clearly a menacing presence, which was noticed by the DMP officer and evidenced by the reluctance of a neighbour to enter the same room as him. Social convention positioned his word as having more gravitas than hers and the mere mention of alcohol cast her into unfavourable light.[17]

Respect and respectability was hard earned. It was easily snatched away at community level, and there was no margin for error for inner-city mothers, especially those who were unmarried. Irrespective of income, married women and widows were afforded a certain degree of social status but to maintain that respectability a strong record of good living was requisite. Married women with steady homes were clearly identified as such in DMP reports. Even if they were irresponsible in, for example, leaving children in the care of other children, all aspects of reporting and questioning was usually sympathetic. If there was any imputation of intemperance or vice then verdicts and riders could and did take a very different course.

Blame, loosely rooted in the law, was meted out via jury riders, and if they were published in the newspapers they could cause shame. These socially conditioned opinions were highly sensitive to class and moral codes. Of the 611 cases, 162 were of children aged under 12. Apart from the case of Joseph McCabe, who was

---

[16] *Report of the departmental committee appointed by the Local Government Board for Ireland to inquire into the housing conditions of the working classes in the city of Dublin* [Cd. 7273].
[17] NAI/1901/48 Inquest on the body of Isabella Woodcock, 20 February 1901.

struck by an object thrown by his father, the majority of the child deaths discussed in Chapter 3 were associated with, or blamed on, mothers. With respect to the sixty-nine infants aged under 1 year, alcohol consumption by mothers was a particular focus in all types of cases from accident to neglect. For reasons explained in Chapter 2, in working-class and in underemployed areas of Dublin, alcohol addiction was a significant problem.[18]

Conspicuous alcohol consumption was a central issue in the coroner's court even if it was not supported by statistical evidence in per capita consumption levels as Ferriter has argued.[19] Some of the cases involving women at public houses were of those who had their own cash income streams as hawkers or dealers. The average income and expenditure estimates gathered by Lumsden and Cameron show that there was no room for luxury items. Within limited household budgets, to afford money for drink, other sacrifices were made, in clothing through pawning, or in doing without the basic necessities of food and domestic comforts. Many of the mothers in the sample used here were a far cry from Lumsden's relatively more comfortable Guinness' housewives. In her study of autobiographical writing Emma Griffin 'found no configurations anywhere that permitted mothers to spend the housekeeping money on drink, or to neglect or abandon their children. Yet in a significant minority of families, these unscripted behaviors occurred.'[20] Study of the coronial court records has uncovered the social realities of those who plumbed the lowest depths of Irish social inequality for gendered and class reasons. Other than having access to cash income, there is nothing to suggest that money used for drink was somehow extra. Some of Dublin's most vulnerable people can be found in these data for reasons that they had no agency over, primarily structural poverty and patriarchal control over resources and space. Perhaps because I am dealing with othered cohorts, these unscripted behaviours find repeat expression in the coronial court record. In the working-class areas of Dublin City that are the focus here, alcohol abuse and the illicit sale of alcohol were common and tolerated features of social life—the poor were vilified for its consumption but the powerful brewers, distillers, and vintners were rarely taken to task or held accountable by the authorities in any meaningful way. The DMP tried to govern by consensus not by coercion and it turned a blind eye unless it had to make necessary interventions. Their efforts were dwarfed by the real issue which, as explained in Chapter 2, was the power brokerage of the

---

[18] Claire Langhamer, 'A public house is for all classes, men and women alike': women, leisure and drink in Second World War England', *Women's History Review*, 12:3 (2003), pp. 423–43 at 431.

[19] Diarmaid Ferriter, 'Drink and society in twentieth-century Ireland', *Proceedings of the Royal Irish Academy: Archaeology, Culture, History, Literature*, 115C, Food and Drink in Ireland (2015), pp. 349–69 at 352; Ferriter, *A Nation of Extremes*.

[20] Emma Griffin, 'The emotions of motherhood: love culture, and poverty in Victorian Britain', *The American Historical Review*, 123(1) (2018), pp. 60–85 at 81.

industry. While some spirit grocers were being prosecuted for breaking licensing laws, in some courts others handed out licences with abandon.

Beyond the front door the prioritisation of progress over public safety took hold. About fifteen fatalities as a result of being 'knocked down' involving horses, trams, and trains occurred every year. Drivers were usually arrested at the scene or shortly thereafter, and great attention was paid to whether or not alcohol was involved in the case of either the driver or the deceased. Chapter 3 has argued that in this period of tram expansion not only were people at risk of the direct associated dangers, they suffered indirect adverse impacts too. The relentless pace of modernity was stacked against the very poor who could barely afford to engage yet their lives were inexorably impacted by it. The uneasy shift from horsepower to modern forms of transportation altered the hierarchy of road users and placed new expectations on pedestrians. Smaller streets undoubtedly had heavier traffic flow as a result of the space taken up by the tram lines. The cause of pedestrian fatalities mirrors the patchwork state of Dublin's layered transportation systems and the continued reliance on horsepower. Children were more likely to be knocked down outside their own door, which was an important place for them to play as their mothers tried to conduct chores. Accidents, bullying, and moral hazards abounded, but outside the door responsibility for child welfare was more communal in nature. Mothers were rarely censured or pursued to criminal courts for cases involving children that occurred outside.

It is not surprising within the male breadwinner model that men were the most at-risk group in the workplace. Female occupational hazards were slower moving mortality threats, for example, pulmonary tuberculosis which was so prevalent in overcrowded factory settings or simply the physical demands placed on their bodies from overwork, undernourishment, repeat pregnancies, the mental anxieties of motherhood in poverty, and the very tough lives they lived. It is for such reasons that Greta Jones argues that the death rate from phthisis was higher among teenaged and early adult women working in the Belfast textile factories.[21] Only a handful of female cases in the Dublin coronial data can be categorised as happening at work, but arguably there are others that could be reclassified from the domestic criteria—all three were engaged in outwork in their homes. For example, two deaths by burning of elderly rag-pickers, Elizabeth Keating and Mary Walsh, in October/November 1900 who could not escape their inflammable work-related surrounds and Francis (sic) Floyd who died while making match-boxes.[22] Most of the 109 people who died at work were of casually employed men in unskilled and low paid jobs. Given the limited nature of industry and the weak

[21] Greta Jones, 'Captain of all these men of death': The History of Tuberculosis in Nineteenth- and Twentieth-Century Ireland (Leiden, 2001), p. 74; Report of the Belfast Health Commission to the Local Government Board (Ireland) vol. XXXI (1908) [Cd. 4128], p. 17.
[22] NAI/1900/27 Inquest on the body of Francis Floyd, 24 May 1900; NAI/1900/151 Inquest on Mary Walsh, 2 November 1900; NAI/1900/136 Inquest on Elizabeth Keating, 12 October 1900.

positioning of precariously employed workers it is no surprise that they were most likely to work for smaller and less safety-aware employers. The loss of a breadwinner was devastating at a time when pensions were uncommon. How Dublin families were compensated is difficult to ascertain; much rested on the degree to which workplaces constituted factories within the meaning of the Factory Acts. Twelve cases involved tram and rail workers, and they were more than likely compensated. Widows of men who died in construction accidents had an uphill battle, and if it could be proven, as in the case of Peter Quinn, that workers were negligible in any way then they stood no chance.[23] Dockworkers and seafaring jobs account for twenty-six of the workplace fatalities, of which fourteen drowned. Descriptions of how they died indicated that they were unable to swim, which was again a class issue that had an impact on young men who used the city's waterways to cool off in July and August. Working-class men did not have access to swimming lessons or water sports like the middle classes did. Like road traffic deaths, those by drowning are equally emblematic of displacement; for example, the scarcity of children's play areas combined with boredom and youthful male bravado inevitably ended in tragedy during the warm summer months. Gendered attitudes towards physical exercise almost certainly increased the numbers of young men dying in the waterways. Prevailing modesty standards would have precluded young women from undressing in public and the gendered nature of the allocation of household chores, as well as care of younger siblings, left young girls with little leisure time.

Historically, cities were gendered spaces that militated against poor women and even if late Victorian-era Dublin embraced technological change and modernity it was not a socially progressive city.[24] Patrick Joyce asserts that to understand cities it is important to see the 'ordering' and 'patterning' in temporal and material terms.[25] The records of the coronial court show that municipal ordering most definitely did not consider the impact of technological advance on the poor. The embodied experience of life for working-class people was shaped and negotiated by a city that was designed primarily to meet the needs of upper-class men, who could escape to the suburbs on a daily basis. There is also a stark contrast between streetscapes by day, engendered with maternalised bodies like those in Figure 1.2 of Coles Lane, some selling wares, and their unruly and unwashed children, and the city by night. Respectable poor women did not venture out too late after dark and if they did, they had purpose, were chaperoned, or in safe company. If not, then they ran the risk of reputational ruin. Women were officially defined in proximity to male kin (daughter/sister/wife of), which meant that those without such adult relatives were extremely vulnerable to official and unofficial

[23] NAI/1900/186 Inquest on the body of Patrick Quinn, 6 December 1900.
[24] Judith Butler, 'Bodies in alliance and the politics of the street': http://eipcp.net/transversal/1011/butler/en (accessed 7 August 2018).
[25] Joyce, *The Rule of Freedom*, p. 11.

legal, moral, and social codes, particularly if they were perceived as belligerent. 'Stopping out at night' coupled with alleged liaisons between single servant Margaret Cowley and Jack Daly, a married man, caused her to lose her job. She subsequently lost the respect of her father, and was isolated from her aunt and sister to whom she wrote impassioned letters seeking to clear her name. The loss of her moral reputation led her to commit suicide while of unsound mind.[26]

When violence was witnessed by policemen, as happened in a few cases, there were inevitable and obvious consequences. Infanticide was more prevalent among single mothers who often could not afford to feed another mouth and were faced with the unthinkable. Whether or not named women were permitted to 'get away with it' depended on their prior character and their likelihood of 'reoffending'. Respectability was of great importance in such cases and the same can be said of suicides. Blatant evidence of self murder could not be ignored but in some drowning cases evidence was quietly elided especially if the deceased was regarded as respectable. Indicators of respectability could include evidence of sobriety of the deceased and whether surviving family members were upstanding members of society.

Chapter 4 dealt with some of the more controversial cases in the sample and has shown how useful it is to use the coroner's cases as the first point of departure for the study of thresholds for the toleration of anti-social or violent behaviour. Communities withstood and ignored certain degrees of violence or criminality before it was reported to the authorities. Moreover, it shows there were very high levels of discretionary justice at play. In cases of suspicious/violent death a number had prior indicators of potential for serious and fatal assault. For example, the case of William Drea, who repeatedly beat Frances Glynn for three months prior to her death: none of the witnesses who gave lengthy statements of dreadful attacks saw fit to report them. They were employees of the victim, which placed them in an unenviable position. Just four of the thirteen alleged infanticide cases progressed to the criminal courts, and only two yielded prosecutions, one of which was a mere nineteen days on the reduced charge of neglect.

Chapter 4 has shown that gender-based violence was a normalised and barely hidden facet of Irish social life. Inextricably linked to most of these cases was evidence of alcohol consumption, a drinking session, or alcoholism. Public houses were often central to the narrative, either as the site of interpersonal violence, or in facilitating the alcohol consumption that begot the tragedy. Women who were repeatedly beaten, and the brave children who stood between them and the perpetrator, saw no justice unless judges were strong-minded enough to see cases through to imprisonment or execution. While the state readily intervened and interfered on matters of fit/unfit motherhood, which was routinely conflated with poverty, it has historically drawn the line at keeping women safe in their homes or

---

[26] NAI/1900/102 Inquest on the body of Margaret Cowley, 29 August 1900.

providing legal recourse or financial support when there were physical, emotional, and financial threats from a male breadwinner. The cases discussed in the concluding section reveal much about the construction and performativity of gender in early twentieth-century Dublin. What characterises most of these cases is the level of tolerance of the appalling conduct of what Kearns terms 'hard men', which in a highly patriarchal society left poor women even more vulnerable.

Another striking element of this study is that ordinary women showed extraordinary bravery. They were first responders to many incidents—without hesitation they quenched flames, they rescued, and they picked up unrelated small children and ran to dispensaries and hospitals; they gave testimony against local bullies; and they protected and looked out for other women in violent domestic settings, to their own great personal risk. For example, Bridget Treacy physically tackled the violent Christopher O'Connor who was repeatedly abusive to her friend, his wife.[27] While men received plaudits for their 'pluck' and 'zeal' in coronial court riders, the efforts of women, who were equally brave, were never once acknowledged. Their valour was expected and completely taken for granted.

Communities decided who to defend, protect, offer up, and ignore in their hours of need and these decisions were pragmatically taken. Few would risk their own tentative claims to community belonging to defend lost causes of 'unfortunates'. At all stages, from the discovery of a body to DMP reporting, in a coroner's decision to proceed to full inquest, expert medical testimony, eye-witness statements, verdict and rider, both the law and vernacular and 'discretionary justice' arising from understandings of the law, were in operation.

Those who came before Dr Byrne's court were unquestionably the most vulnerable, forgotten, rarely documented citizens—they existed on the margins and common to several cases was their evasion of biopower surveillance for the life course prior to their inquests.

Until recently, the history of the Dublin City coroner's court has been obscured by its own seamless blending into the fabric of metropolitan life and indeed other important research agendas in the history of medical, legal, urban, and social history. It was part of a close-knit and vital surveillance network that was often resisted by the city's residents. Although sometimes the deaths coming before Dr Byrne's court were extremely violent and the evidence it gathered was integral to the criminal cases that followed, its normal cadence was of a more mundane nature. The function of the court was to record who, and how they died, and most deaths were simply sudden. This book has aimed to bring the history and the records of this fascinating institution to the fore and to elucidate the degree to which death was very much part of the everyday of ordinary Dublin lives.

---

[27] NAI/1900/60 Inquest on the body of Christopher O'Connor, 7 July 1900.

Bibliography

1. Acts

Vagabonds Act, 1530 (22 Hen. VIII), c. 12.

An Act to Prevent the Destroying and Murthering of Bastard Children, 1623 (21 Ja. 1), c. 27.

Forfeiture Act (Ireland), 1639 (15 Chas.1), c. 3. 2.

An Act for banishing all papists exercising any ecclesiastical jurisdiction and all regulars of the popish clergy, 1697 (9 Will III), c. 1.

Malicious shooting or Stabbing Act, 1803 (43 Geo. 3), c. 58 'Lord Ellenborough's Act'.

Burial of Suicide Act, 1823 (4 Geo. 4), c. 52.

Criminal Law (Ireland) Act, 1828 (9 Geo. IV), c. 54.

Coroners (Ireland) Act, 1846 (9 & 10 Vic.), c. 37.

Fatal Accidents Act, 1846 (9 & 10 Vic.), c. 62.

An Act for the better Prevention and Punishment of aggravated Assaults upon Women and Children, and for preventing Delay and Expense in the Administration of certain Parts of the Criminal Law, 1853 (16 &17 Vic.), c. 30.

Dublin Carriage Act, 1853 (16 & 17 Vic.), c. cxii.

Burial Grounds (Ireland) Act, 1856 (19 & 20 Vic), c. 98.

Medical Act, 1858 (21 & 22 Vic.), c. 90.

Refreshment Houses (Ireland) Act, 1860 (23 & 24 Vic.), c. 107.

The Borough Coroners (Ireland) Act 1860 (23 & 24 Vic.), c. lxxiv.

Tramways (Ireland) Act, 1860 (23 & 24 Vic.), c. clii.

Dublin Corporation Waterworks Act, 1861 (24 & 25 Vic.), c. clxxii.

Offences Against the Person Act, 1861 (24 & 25 Vic.), c. 100.

Tramways (Ireland) Act, 1861 (23 & 24 Vic.), c. 102.

Dublin Corporation Fire Brigade Act, 1862 (25 & 26 Vic.), c.cxxxviii.

An Act for the Registration of Births and Deaths in Ireland, 1863 (26 & 27 Vic.), c. 11.

Sanitary Act, 1866 (28 & 29 Vic.), c. 90.

An Act to amend the Law which regulates the Burials of Persons in Ireland not belonging to the Established Church, 1868 (31 & 32 Vic.), c. 103.

Norwich Union Life Insurance Society Act, 1868, c. cxlviii.

Irish Church Act, 1869 (32 & 33 Vic.), c. 42.

Orphan and Deserted Children (Ireland) Act, 1869 (32 & 33 Vic.), c. 25.

Forfeiture Act, 1870 (33 & 34 Vic.), c. 23.

Dublin Tramways Act, 1871 (34 & 35 Vic.), c. lxxxviii.

Juries Act (Ireland), 1871 (34 & 35 Vic.), c. 65.

Summary Jurisdiction (Ireland) Amendment Act, 1871 (34 & 35 Vic.), c. 76.

Infant Life Protection Act, 1872 (35 & 36 Vic.), c. 38.

Licensing (Ireland) Act, 1874 (37 & 38 Vic.), c. 69.

Dublin Traffic Act, 1875 (38 & 39 Vic.), c. cxcv.

Employers and Workmen Act, 1875 (56 & 57 Vic.), c. 54.

Coroners (Dublin) Act, 1876, c. xciii.

Pauper Children (Ireland) Act, 1876 (39 & 40 Vic.), c. 38.

Saint Stephen's Green (Dublin) Act, 1877 (40 & 41 Vic.), c. cxxxiv.
Petty Sessions Clerks and Fines (Ireland) Act, 1878 (21 & 22 Vic.), c. 100.
Public Health (Ireland) Act, 1878, c. 52.
The Sale of Liquors on Sunday (Ireland) Act, 1878 (41 & 42 Vic.), c. 72.
Burial Laws Amendment Act, 1880 (43 & 44 Vic.), c. 41.
Employers' Liability Act, 1880 (43 & 44 Vic.), c. 42.
Coroners (Ireland) Act, 1881 (44 & 45 Vic.), c. 35.
Interments (Felo de se) Act, 1882 (45 & 46 Vic.), c. 19.
Scottish Widows' Fund and Life Assurance Society's Act, 1882, c. lxxv.
Tramways and Public Companies (Ireland) Act 1883 (46 & 47 Vic.), c. 43.
Guardianship of Infants Act, 1886 (49 & 50 Vic.), c. 27.
Married Women (Maintenance in case of Desertion) Act, 1886 (49 & 50 Vic.), c. 52.
The Intoxicating Liquors (Sale to Children) Act, 1886 (49 & 50 Vic.), c. 56.
The Burial (Ireland) Act, 1888 (59 & 60 Vic.), c. 14.
An Act for the Prevention of Cruelty to, and better Protection of, Children, 1889 (52 & 53 Vic.), c. 44.
Dublin Southern District Tramways, 1893 (56 & 57 Vic.), c. ccxx.
Fatal Accidents Inquiry (Scotland) Act, 1895 (58 & 59 Vic.), c. 36.
Dublin United Tramways Act, 1896 (59 & 60 Vic.), c. ccxxii.
Dublin United Tramways (Electrical Power) Act 1897 (60 & 61 Vic.), c. ccxxxvi.
Infant Life Protection Act, 1897 (60 & 61 Vic.), c. 57.
Workmen's Compensation Act, 1897 (60 & 61 Vic.) c. 37.
Dublin Improvement (Bull Alley Area) Act, 1899 (62 & 63 Vic.), c. xi.
Dublin Corporation Act, 1900 (63 & 64 Vic.), c. cclxiv.
Tramways (Ireland) Act, 1900 (63 & 64 Vic.), c. 60.
Intoxicating Liquors (Sale to Children) Act, 1901 (1 Edw. 7), c. 27.
Intoxicating Liquors (Ireland) Act, 1906 (6 Edw. 7), c. 39.
Local Government (Dublin) Act, 1930.
Criminal Law (Suicide) Act, 1993, no. 11.

2. House of Commons Parliamentary Papers

Census of Ireland for the year 1861. Enumeration abstracts, showing, by provinces, counties, cities, boroughs, and towns, 1861 [2865].
Coroners (Ireland). Copy of a memorial addressed to the Lord Lieutenant by the coroners of Ireland, requesting that a measure on their behalf may be brought before Parliament early in the present session, 1871 [86].
Report of Chief Com. of Police for Dublin Metropolis on Dublin Tramways Bill, May 1873 [189].
Royal Com. to inquire into Sewerage and Drainage of City of Dublin. Report, Minutes of Evidence, Appendix, Index, 1879–80 [C.2605].
Criminal and judicial statistics. 1880. Ireland. Part I. Police—criminal proceedings—prisons. Part II. Civil proceedings in central and larger and smaller district courts, 1881 [C.3028].
First report of Her Majesty's commissioners for inquiring into the housing of the working classes, 1884–85 [C.4402 C.4402-I C.4402-II].
Third report of Her Majesty's commissioners for inquiring into the housing of the working classes Ireland, 1884–85 [C.4402].

Royal Commission on Irish Public Works. Second report of the Royal Commission on Irish Public Works, 1888 [C.5264 C.5264-I].

Criminal and judicial statistics, Ireland, 1891 [C.6782].

Statistical Tables of Dublin Metropolitan Police, 1894 [C.7734].

Thirty-first detailed annual report of the Registrar-General (Ireland), containing a general abstract of the numbers of marriages, births, and deaths registered in Ireland during the year 1894 [C. 7800].

Return of Judicial Statistics of Ireland, 1895 [C.8616].

Report from the Select Committee on petroleum; together with the proceedings of the committee, minutes of evidence, appendix, and index, 1896 [xii.i].

Commission on horse breeding, Ireland. Reports by the commissioners appointed to inquire into the house breeding industry in Ireland, 1898 [C.8651 C.8652].

Royal Com. on Liquor Licensing Laws: Statistics relating to Number of Licensed Premises in Great Britain and Ireland, 1898 [C.8696].

Dangerous Trades Committee. Final report of the Departmental Committee appointed to inquire into and report upon certain miscellaneous dangerous trades (1899) [C.9509].

Annual Report of the Chief Inspector of Factories and Workshops, for 1900 (Factories—Shops—Workshops: Annual Report) [Cd. 668].

Annual report of the Local Government Board For Ireland, for the year ended March, 1900 [Cd.338].

Judicial statistics, Ireland, 1900. Part I.—Criminal statistics [Cd. 725, 682].

Report of the committee appointed by the Local Government Board for Ireland to inquire into the public health of the city of Dublin, 1900 [Cd.243 Cd.244].

Royal Com. to inquire into Causes of Accidents, Fatal and Non-fatal, to Servants of Railway Companies and Truck-Owners. Report, Minutes of Evidence, Appendices, 1900 [Cd.41 Cd.42].

Statistical tables of the Dublin Metropolitan Police for the year 1900 [Cd. 615].

Supplement to the thirty-seventh report of the Registrar-General of Marriages, Births, and Deaths, in Ireland, containing decennial summaries of the returns of marriages, births, deaths, and causes of death in Ireland, for the years 1891–1900 [Cd. 2089].

Thirty-seventh detailed annual report of the Registrar-General (Ireland), containing a general abstract of the numbers of marriages, births, and deaths registered in Ireland during the year 1900 [Cd. 697].

Workmen's compensation. Statistics of proceedings under the Workmen's Compensation Act, 1897, and the Employers' Liability Act, 1880, during the year 1900 [Cd. 816].

Census of Ireland, 1901. Part I [Cd. 847].

Census of Ireland, 1901. Part II. General report with illustrative maps and diagrams, tables, and appendix [Cd. 1190].

Dublin Metropolitan Police. Evidence taken before the Committee of Inquiry, 1901 [Cd. 1095].

Dublin Metropolitan Police. Report of the Committee of Inquiry, 1901 [Cd. 1088].

Judicial statistics, Ireland, 1901 [Cd. 1208, 1187].

Local government (Ireland) officials. Return to an order of the Honourable the House of Commons, dated 14th March, 1901 [331], no page or table number. Image 177 of 322 on Proquest.

Railway accidents. Returns of accidents and casualties as reported to the Board of Trade by the several railway companies in the United Kingdom During the three months ending 31st March 1901, in pursuance of the Regulation of Railways Act (1871), 34 & 35 Vict. cap. 78; together with reports of the inspecting officers, assistant inspecting officers, and sub-inspectors of the Railway Department to the Board of Trade, upon certain accidents which were inquired into [Cd. 774].

Statistical tables of the Dublin Metropolitan Police for the year 1901 [Cd. 1166].

Thirty-eighth detailed annual report of the Registrar-General (Ireland) 1901 [Cd. 1225].

Twenty-ninth Annual Report of the Local Government Board for Ireland, for the year ending 31st March 1901 [Cd. 1259].

Workmen's compensation. Statistics of proceedings under the Workmen's Compensation Acts, 1897 and 1900, and the Employers' Liability Act, 1880, during the year 1901 [Cd. 1210].

Street-Trading Children Committee (Ireland). Report of the Inter-Departmental Committee on the Employment of Children During School Age, especially in street trading in the large centres of population in Ireland, appointed by His Excellency the Lord Lieutenant of Ireland. Together with minutes of evidence and appendices (1902) [Cd. 1144].

Report from the Select Committee on Infant Life Protection. Together with the proceedings of the committee, minutes of evidence, and appendix. 1908 (99).

Report of the Belfast Health Commission to the Local Government Board (Ireland) vol. XXXI (1908) [Cd. 4128].

Report of the departmental committee appointed by the Local Government Board for Ireland to inquire into the housing conditions of the working classes in the city of Dublin, 1914 [Cd. 7273].

Royal Irish Constabulary and Dublin Metropolitan Police. Report of the Committee of Inquiry, 1914 [Cd. 7421].

3. Newspapers

Belfast Newsletter.
Evening Herald.
Freeman's Journal.
Irish Daily Independent.
Irish Examiner.
Irish Times.
Kerry Sentinel.
Kerry Weekly Reporter.
Nationalist and Leinster Times.
Munster Express.
Skibbereen Eagle.

4. Archives and Manuscripts

(i) Royal College of Physicians Archive
Kirkpatrick Index.

(ii) Dublin City Library & Archive
Minutes of the Municipal Council of the City of Dublin, 1900–1902.
Dublin Corporation Printed Reports (Dublin City Library & Archive), Volumes I–III, 1900.
Dublin City Archives, Dublin City Council/History/Ambulance Service/R1/01/03.
Annual Reports of the Chief of the Dublin Corporation Fire Brigade Department, 1900–1913.

(iii) National Archives of Ireland

Chief Secretary's Office Registered Papers.
Dublin City Coroner's Registers.
Dublin City Morgue Registers.
Dublin Crown Files at Commission.
General Prison Board, Penal Files, Criminal Reference Files and Prison Registers.
Mountjoy Female Prison Register (available on ancestry.com).
Mountjoy Prison Registers male and female (available on ancestry.com).
Petty Sessions Registers.
Workmen's Compensation Act, Dublin, Book Awards & Applications 1898–1904.
South Dublin and North Dublin Poor Law Union, workhouse admission and discharge records.

(iv) Guinness Archive, Diageo Ireland

GDB/CO04.11/0001.05, Annual Reports.

5. Websites

Amalgamated Society of Railway Servants, register dated 1898–9, MSS.127/AS/2/3/8 on findmypast.co.uk.
Ancestry.com
Nationalarchives.ie.
Irishgenealogy.ie.

6. Secondary Reading

Aalen, F.H.A., *The Iveagh Trust: The First Hundred Years, 1890–1990* (Dublin, 1990).
Abrams, Lynn, *Myth and Materiality in a Woman's World: Shetland, 1800–2000* (Manchester, 2005).
Adelman, Juliana, *Civilised by Beasts: Animals and Urban Change in Nineteenth-Century Dublin* (Manchester, 2020).
Anderson, Olive, *Suicide in Victorian and Edwardian England* (Oxford, 1987).
Andrews, Ann, *Newspapers and Newsmakers: The Dublin Nationalist Press in the Mid-nineteenth Century* (Oxford, 2014).
Anon., 'Burns and scalds', *Scientific American*, 38:25 (1878), p. 387.
Anon., 'The treatment of inebriates', *Charity Organisation Review*, 10:57 (1901), pp. 151–4.
Arnott, Margaret L., 'Infant death, child care and the state: the baby-farming scandal and the first infant life protection legislation of 1872', *Continuity and Change*, 9:2 (1994), pp. 271–311.
Bailey, Joanne, '"I dye [*sic*] by Inches": locating wife beating in the concept of a privatization of marriage and violence in eighteenth-century England', *Social History*, 31:3 (2006), pp. 273–94.
Bailey, Victor, *This Rash Act: Suicide Across the Life Cycle in the Victorian City* (Redwood City, 1998).
Banerjee, Sikata, *Muscular Nationalism: Gender, Violence, and Empire in India and Ireland, 1914–2004* (New York, 2012).
Barclay, Katie, 'Singing and lower-class masculinity in the Dublin Magistrate's Court, 1800–1845', *Journal of Social History* 47:3 (2014), pp. 746–68.

Barclay, Katie, *Men on Trial: Performing Emotion, Embodiment and Identity in Ireland, 1800–45* (Manchester, 2019).

Barron, Fergus, *Swimming for a Century* (Dublin, 1993).

Battin, Margaret Pabst, *The Ethics of Suicide: Historical Sources* (Oxford, 2015).

Beatty, Aidan, *Masculinity and Power in Irish Nationalism, 1884–1938* (Basingstoke, 2016).

Begiato, Joanne, *Manliness in Britain, 1760–1900: Bodies, Emotion, and Material Culture* (Manchester, 2020).

Bennett, Charlotte, '"Help to win the war" or "Ireland above all"?: remobilisation, politics, and elite boys' education in Ireland, 1917–18', *Irish Historical Studies*, 44:166 (2020), pp. 326–48.

Bielenberg, Andy, 'Entrepreneurship, power and public opinion in Ireland: the career of William Martin Murphy', *Irish Economic and Social History*, xxvii (2000), pp. 25–43.

Bielenberg, Andy, 'Late Victorian elite formation and philanthropy: the making of Edward Guinness', *Studia Hibernica*, 32 (2002/3), pp. 133–54.

Borsay, Peter, 'Sounding the town', *Urban History*, 29:1 (2002), pp. 92–102.

Boyd, Gary A., *Dublin, 1745–1922: Hospitals, Spectacle and Vice* (Dublin, 2006).

Boylan, Anne M., 'Claiming Visibility: Women in Public/Public Women in the United States, 1865–1910', in Janet Floyd, Alison Eastman, and R.J. Ellis (eds), *Becoming Visible: Women in View in Late Nineteenth-Century America* (Amsterdam, 2010), pp. 17–40.

Brady, Joseph and Ruth McManus, 'Dublin's twentieth-century social housing policies: tenure, "reserved areas" and housing type', *Planning Perspectives*, 35:6 (2019), pp. 1005–103.

Breathnach, Ciara, 'Medical officers, bodies, gender and weight fluctuation in Irish convict prisons, 1877–95', *Medical History*, 58:1 (2014), pp. 67–86.

Breathnach, Ciara and Eunan O'Halpin, 'Scripting blame: Irish coroners' courts and unnamed infant dead, 1916–32', *Social History*, 39:2 (2014), pp. 210–28.

Breathnach, Ciara, '... it would be preposterous to bring a Protestant here': religion, provincial politics and district nurses in Ireland, 1890–1904', in Donnacha Seán Lucey and Virginia Crossman (eds), *Healthcare in Ireland and Britain 1850–1970: Voluntary, Regional and Comparative Perspectives* (London, 2015), pp. 161–80.

Breathnach, Ciara and Elaine Farrell, '"Indelible characters": tattoos, power and the late nineteenth-century Irish convict body', *Cultural and Social History*, 12:2 (2015), pp. 235–54.

Breathnach, Ciara, 'Infant life protection and medico-legal literacy in early twentieth-century Dublin', *Women's History Review*, 26:6 (2017), pp. 781–98.

Breathnach, Ciara, 'The triumph of proximity: the impact of district nursing schemes in 1890s' rural Ireland', *Nursing History Review*, 26 (2018), pp. 68–82.

Breathnach, Ciara and Laurence M. Geary, 'Crime and punishment: Whiteboyism and the law in late nineteenth-century Ireland', in Don McRaild and Kyle Hughes (eds), *Crime in C19th Ireland* (Liverpool, 2017), pp. 149–74.

Breathnach, Ciara and Brian Gurrin, 'Maternal mortality, Dublin 1864–1905', *Social History of Medicine*, 31:1 (2018), pp. 79–105.

Breathnach, Ciara, 'Capital punishment in Irish prisons', *Health and History*, 22:1 (2020), pp. 104–25.

Breathnach, Ciara and Eunan O'Halpin, 'Sexual assault and fatal violence against women during the Irish War of Independence, 1919–1921: Kate Maher's murder in context', *Medical Humanities*, 48 (2022), pp. 94–103.

Breathnach, Ciara, 'Respiratory disease and death registration, Dublin 1900–1902', *Annales de Démographie Historique*, 142: 1 (2022), pp. 39–72.

Breathnach, Ciara and Ian Walsh (eds), *Original Inquest Papers of Dr Joseph E. Kenny, Dublin City Coroner, 1900* (forthcoming, Dublin, 2022).

Brugha, Traoloc and Dermot Walsh, 'Suicide past and present: the temporal constancy of under-reporting', *The British Journal of Psychiatry*, 132 (1978), pp. 177–9.

Buckley, Anthony D., '"On the club": Friendly Societies in Ireland', *Irish Economic and Social History*, 14 (1987), pp. 39–58.

Buckley, Sarah-Anne, *The Cruelty Man: Child Welfare, the NSPCC and the State in Ireland, 1899–1956* (Manchester, 2013).

Buckley, Sarah-Anne, 'Men, women and the family, 1730–1880', in James Kelly (ed.), *The Cambridge History of Ireland: Volume 3, 1730–1880* (Cambridge, 2017), pp. 231–54.

Burney, Ian, *Bodies of Evidence: Medicine and the Politics of the English Inquest, 1830–1926* (Baltimore, 2000).

Butler, Judith, 'Performative acts and gender constitution: an essay in phenomenology and feminist theory', *Theatre Journal*, 40:4 (1988), pp. 519–31.

Butler, Judith, 'Bodies in alliance and the politics of the street', http://eipcp.net/transversal/1011/butler/en (accessed 7 August 2018).

Cameron, Charles A., *How the Poor Live* (Dublin, 1904).

Campbell, Colm, *Emergency Law in Ireland, 1918–1925* (Oxford, 1994).

Cannadine, David, *History in our time* (New Haven, 1998).

Carroll, Patrick E., 'Medical police and the history of public health', *Medical History*, 46 (2002), pp. 461–94.

Carroll-Burke, Patrick, 'Material designs: engineering cultures and engineering states – Ireland 1650–1900', *Theory and Society*, 31:1 (2002), pp. 75–114.

Casey, Christine, *Dublin: The City within the Grand and Royal Canals and the Circular Road with the Phoenix Park* (New Haven, 2005).

Cherry, Richard E., 'The Eric Fines of ancient Irish law', *Journal of the Statistical and Social Inquiry Society of Ireland*, Vol. VIII, Part LXII (1884), pp. 544–51.

Clark, Gemma, 'Arson in modern Ireland: fire and protest before the Famine', in D.M. MacRaild and K. Hughes (eds), *Crime, Violence and the Irish in the Nineteenth Century* (Liverpool, 2017), pp. 211–26.

Clark, Michael J., 'General practice and coroner's practice: medico-legal work and the Irish medical profession, c.1830–c.1890', in Catherine Cox and Maria Luddy (eds), *Cultures of Care in Irish Medical History, 1750–1970* (Basingstoke, 2010), pp. 37–56.

Clarke, Amanda, '"Keepin' a home together": performing domestic security in Sean O'Casey's "The Plough and the Stars"', *The Canadian Journal of Irish Studies*, 38:1–2 (2014), pp. 208–27.

Coen, Mark and Niamh Howlin, 'The jury speaks: jury riders in the nineteenth and twentieth centuries', *American Journal of Legal History*, 58:4 (2018), pp. 505–34.

Conley, Carolyn, *Melancholy Accidents: The Meaning of Violence in Post-Famine Ireland* (New York, 1999).

Conley, Carolyn, 'The agreeable recreation of fighting', *Journal of Social History*, 33:1 (1999), pp. 57–72.

Conley, Carolyn, *Certain Other Countries: Homicide, Gender, and National Identity in Late Nineteenth-Century England, Ireland, Scotland, and Wales* (Columbus, 2007).

Connell, R.W., *Masculinities* (Cambridge, 2005, 2nd edn).

Connell, R.W. and James W. Messerschmidt, 'Hegemonic masculinity: rethinking the concept', *Gender & Society*, 19:6 (2005), pp. 829–59.

Corcoran, Michael, *Our Good Health: A History of Dublin's Water and Drainage* (Dublin, 2005).

Cox, Catherine, *Negotiating Insanity in the Southeast of Ireland, 1820–1900* (Manchester, 2012).

Crawford, E. Margaret, *Counting the People: A Survey of the Irish Censuses, 1813–1911* (Dublin, 2003).

Crossman, Virginia, *Poverty and the Poor Law in Ireland, 1850–1914* (Liverpool, 2013).

Cullen Rath, Richard, 'No corner for the devil to hide', in John Streane (ed.), *The Sound Studies Reader* (Abingdon, 2012).

Curran, Joseph, 'Charity, finance, and legitimacy: exploring stateless-capital status in early nineteenth-century Dublin and Edinburgh', *Journal of Urban History*, 47:4 (2021), pp. 753–70.

Curry, James and Ciarán Wallace, *Thomas Fitzpatrick and 'The Lepracaun Cartoon Monthly', 1905–1915* (Dublin, 2015).

Daly, Mary E., *Dublin, the Deposed Capital: A Social and Economic History, 1806–1914* (Cork, 1984).

Davin, Anna, *Growing Up Poor: Home, School and Street in London, 1870–1914* (London, 1996).

D'Cruze, Shani, *Crimes of Outrage: Sex, Violence and Victorian Working Women* (London, 1998).

de Nie, Michael, *The Eternal Paddy: Irish Identity and the British Press, 1798–1882* (Madison, 2004).

Dennison, S.R. and Oliver MacDonagh, *Guinness 1886–1939; from Incorporation to the Second World War* (Cork, 1998).

Dickson, David, 'In search of the old Irish Poor Law', in Rosalind Mitchison and Peter Roebuck (eds), *Economy and Society in Scotland and Ireland, 1500–1939* (Edinburgh, 1988), pp. 149–55.

Dickson, David, *Dublin: The Making of a Capital City* (Dublin, 2014).

Douglas, Mary, *Blame and Risk* (London, 1994).

Dukova, Anastasia, *A History of the Dublin Metropolitan Police and Its Colonial Legacy* (Basingstoke, 2016).

Dunbar, Holly, 'Women and alcohol during the First World War in Ireland', *Women's History Review*, 27:3 (2018), pp. 379–96.

Earner-Byrne, Lindsey, *Letters of the Catholic Poor: Poverty in Independent Ireland* (Cambridge, 2017).

Eleroy Curtis, William, *One Irish Summer* (New York, 1909).

Elliott, Marianne, *Wolfe Tone* (Liverpool, 2012).

Emmerichs, Mary Beth, 'Getting away with murder? Homicide and the coroners in 19th century London', *Social Science History*, 25:1 (2001), pp. 93–100.

Ewen, Shane, *Fighting Fires: Creating the British Fire Service, 1800–1978* (Basingstoke, 2010).

Ewen, Shane, *What Is Urban History?* (Cambridge, 2016).

Fallon, Las, *Dublin Fire Brigade and the Irish Revolution* (Dublin, 2012).

Farrell, Elaine, *Infanticide in the Irish Crown Files at Assizes, 1883–1900* (Dublin, 2012).

Farrell, Elaine, *'A Most "Diabolical Deed"': Infanticide and Irish Society, 1850–1900* (Manchester, 2013).

Farrell, Elaine, *Women, Crime and Punishment in Ireland: Life in the Nineteenth Century Convict Prison* (Cambridge, 2020).

Ferriter, Diarmaid, *A Nation of Extremes: The Pioneers in Twentieth-Century Ireland* (Dublin, 1999).

Ferriter, Diarmaid, 'Drink and society in twentieth-century Ireland', *Proceedings of the Royal Irish Academy: Archaeology, Culture, History, Literature, Vol. 115C, Food and Drink in Ireland* (2015), pp. 349–69.

Fitzpatrick, David M., *Oceans of Consolation: Personal Accounts of Irish Migration to Australia* (Cork, 1994).

Flanagan, Kieran, 'The Chief Secretary's Office, 1853–1914: a bureaucratic enigma', *Irish Historical Studies*, xxiv, no. 94 (1984), pp. 197–225.

Flanagan, Maureen A., *Constructing the Patriarchal City: Gender and the Built Environments of London, Dublin, Toronto, and Chicago, 1870s into the 1940s* (Philadelphia, 2018).

Foley, Michael, 'Colonialism and journalism in Ireland', *Journalism Studies*, 5:3 (2004), pp. 373–85.

Foley, Ronan, Healing Waters: Therapeutic Landscapes in Historic and Contemporary Ireland (Farnham, 2010).

Forbes, Thomas Rogers, 'Crowner's quest', *Transactions of the American Philosophical Society*, 68:1 (1978), pp. 1–52.

Forbes, T.R. *Surgeons at the Bailey: English Forensic Medicine to 1878* (London, 1985).

Foucault, Michel, *The History of Sexuality. Volume I: An Introduction*, translated from the French by Robert Hurley (New York, 1978).

Foucault, Michel, 'Technologies of the self', in L.H. Martin, H. Gutman, and P.H. Hutton (eds), *Technologies of the Self* (London, 1988).

Frost, Ginger, *Living in Sin: Cohabiting as Husband and Wife in Nineteenth-Century England* (Manchester, 2013).

Galavan, Susan, 'Building Victorian Dublin: Meade & Son and the expansion of the city', in Ciarán O'Neill (ed.), *Irish Elites in the Nineteenth Century* (Dublin, 2013), pp. 51–67.

Galavan, Susan, *Dublin's Bourgeois Homes: Building the Victorian Suburbs, 1850–1901* (London, 2017).

Garnham, Neal, *Association Football and Society in Pre-Partition Ireland* (Belfast, 2004).

Gates, Barbara T., *Victorian Suicide: Mad Crimes and Sad Histories* (Princeton, 1988).

Geary, Laurence M., 'The whole country was in motion: mendicancy and vagrancy in pre-Famine Ireland' in Jacqueline Hill and Colm Lennon (eds), *Luxury and Austerity: Historical Studies XXI* (Dublin, 1999), pp. 121–36.

Geary, Laurence M., 'The medical profession, health care and the Poor Law in nineteenth-century Ireland', in Virginia Crossman and Peter Gray (eds), *Poverty and Welfare in Ireland, 1838–1948* (Dublin, 2011).

Geary, Laurence M., '"The wages of sin is death": lock hospitals, venereal disease and gender in prefamine Ireland', in Margaret Preston and Margaret Ó hÓgartaigh (eds), *Gender and Medicine in Ireland, 1700–1951* (New York, 2012), pp. 165–73.

Geary, Laurence M., *The Land War in Ireland. Famine, Philanthropy, and Moonlighting* (Cork, forthcoming 2022).

Gentleman's and Citizen's Almanack (Dublin, 1842).

Geraghty, Hugh and Peter Rigney, 'The engineers' strike in Inchicore Railway Works, 1902', *Saothar*, 9 (1983), pp. 20–31.

Geraghty, Tom and Trevor Whitehead, *The Dublin Fire Brigade: A History of the Brigade, the Fires and the Emergencies* (Dublin, 2004).

Gethings, Caoimhe, 'Not so saved by the bell: the deodand in Irish and English law', *Irish Law Times*, 38:15 (2020), pp. 223–8.

Ginzburg, Carlo, John Tedeschi, and Anne C. Tedeschi, 'Microhistory: two or three things that I know about it', *Critical Inquiry*, 20 (1993), pp. 10–35.

Glaister, John, 'The law of infanticide: a plea for its revision', *The Edinburgh Medical Journal* (July 1895), pp. 1–18.

Goodbody, Rob, *Dublin, Part III, 1756–1847, Irish Historic Towns Atlas, No. 26* (Dublin, 2014).

Gray, Drew, *London's Shadows: The Dark Side of the Victorian City* (London, 2010).

Greer, Desmond and James W. Nicholson, *The Factory Acts in Ireland, 1802–1914* (Dublin, 2002).

Grey, Daniel, '"More ignorant and stupid than wilfully cruel": homicide trials and 'Baby-Farming' in England and Wales in the wake of the Children Act 1908', *Crimes and Misdemeanours*, 3:2 (2009), pp. 60–77.

Griffin, Ben, 'Hegemonic masculinity as a historical problem', *Gender & History*, 30 (2018), pp. 377–400.

Griffin, Brian, 'Cycling and gender in Victorian Ireland', *Éire-Ireland*, 41:1-2 (2006), pp. 213–41.

Griffin, Emma, 'The emotions of motherhood: love culture, and poverty in Victorian Britain', *The American Historical Review*, 123:1 (2018), pp. 60–85.

Griffin, Emma, *Bread Winner: An Intimate History of the Victorian Economy* (New Haven, 2020).

Hanna, Erika, *Modern Dublin: Urban Change and the Irish Past, 1957-1973* (Oxford, 2013).

Hession, Peter, 'Social authority and the urban environment in nineteenth-century Cork' (unpublished PhD thesis, University of Cambridge, 2018).

Hewitt, Martin, 'District visiting and the constitution of domestic space in the mid-nineteenth century', in Inga Bryden and Janet Floyd (eds), *Domestic Space: Reading the Nineteenth-Century Interior* (Manchester, 1999), pp. 120–41.

Hitchcock, Tim, 'A new history from below', *History Workshop Journal*, 57 (2004), pp. 294–8.

Holmes, Vicky, 'Absent fireguards and burnt children: coroners and the development of clause 15 of the Children Act 1908', *Law, Crime, and History* 2 (2012), pp. 21–58.

Holmes, Vicky, 'Death of an infant', *Home Cultures*, 11:3 (2014), pp. 305–31.

Holmes, Vicky, 'Penny death traps: the press, the poor, parliament, and the "Perilous" Penny Paraffin Lamp', *Victorian Review*, 40:2 (2014), pp. 125–42.

Holmes, Vicky, *In Bed with the Victorians: The Life-Cycle of Working-Class Marriage* (Basingstoke, 2017).

Hooper, Charlotte, *Manly States: Masculinities, International Relations, and Gender Politics* (New York, 2001).

Horrell, Sara and Jane Humphries, ' "The exploitation of little children": child labor and the family economy in the Industrial Revolution', *Explorations in Economic History*, 32:4 (1995), pp. 485–516.

Horrell, Sara, Jane Humphries, and Jacob Weisdorf, 'Family standards of living over the long run, England 1280-1850', *Past & Present*, 250:1 (2021), pp. 87–134.

Houston, R.A., 'Explanations for death by suicide in Northern Britain during the long eighteenth century', *History of Psychiatry*, 23:1 (2012), pp. 52–64.

Houston, R.A., *Peasant Petitions: Social Relations and Economic Life on Landed Estates, 1600-1850* (Basingstoke, 2014).

Houston, R.A., 'People, space, and law in late medieval and early modern Britain and Ireland', *Past & Present*, 230:1 (2016), pp. 47–89.

Howlin, Niamh, *Juries in Ireland: Laypersons and the Law in the Long Nineteenth Century* (Dublin, 2017).

Huband, William G., *A practical treatise on the law relating to the Grand Jury in criminal cases, the Coroner's Jury and the Petty Jury in Ireland* (London, 1896).

Hughes, Annmarie, 'The "non-criminal" class: wife-beating in Scotland (c.1800–1949)', *Crime, History and Societies*, 14:2 (2010), pp. 31–54.

Hurren, Elizabeth T., 'Remaking the medico-legal scene: a social history of the late-Victorian coroner in Oxford', *Journal of the History of Medicine and Allied Sciences*, 65:2 (2010), pp. 207–52.

Hurren, Elizabeth T. and Steven King 'Courtship at the coroner's court', *Social History* 40:2 (2015), pp. 185–207.

Ignatieff, Micheal, 'State, civil society, and total institutions: a critique of recent social histories of punishment', *Crime and Justice*, 3 (1981), pp. 153–92.

Inglis, Tom, 'Foucault, Bourdieu and the field of Irish sexuality', *Irish Journal of Sociology*, 7 (1997), pp. 5–28.

Inglis, Tom, 'Origins and legacies of Irish prudery: sexuality and social control in modern Ireland', *Éire-Ireland*, 30:3–4 (2005), pp. 9–37.

Jackson, Alvin, 'Ireland, the Union, and the Empire, 1800–1960', in Kevin Kenny (ed.), *Ireland and the British Empire* (Oxford, 2004), pp. 123–53.

Jackson, Mark, *New-Born Child Murder: Women, Illegitimacy and the Courts in Eighteenth-Century England* (Manchester, 1996).

Johnson, David, 'Trial by jury in Ireland, 1860–1914', *Journal of Legal History*, 8:3 (1996), pp. 270–93.

Johnston, J., 'Soda treatment of burns and scalds', *The British Medical Journal*, 2:922 (31 August 1878), p. 313.

Joyce, Patrick, *The Rule of Freedom: Liberalism and the Modern City* (London, 2003).

Joyce, James, 'A little cloud', in *Dubliners* (Dublin, 2012), pp. 81–96.

Joyce, Patrick, *The State of Freedom: A Social History of the British State since 1800* (Cambridge, 2013).

Kadel, Bradley, *Drink and culture in nineteenth-century Ireland: the alcohol trade and the politics of the Irish public house* (London, 2015).

Kaufman, Scott, ' "That Bantry jobber": William Martin Murphy and the critique of progress and productivity in "Ulysses" ', *European Joyce Studies*, 21:21 (2011), pp. 210–23.

Kearns, Kevin C., *Working Class Heroines: The Extraordinary Women of Dublin's Tenements* (Dublin, 2018).

Keats-Rohan, K.S.B., *Prosopography Approaches and Applications: A Handbook* (Oxford, 2007).

Kelleher, Margaret, *The Maamtrasna Murders: Language, Life and Death in Nineteenth-Century Ireland* (Dublin, 2018).

Kelly, Brendan D., *'He Lost Himself Completely': Shell Shock and Its Treatment at Dublin's Richmond War Hospital, 1916–19* (Dublin, 2014).

Kelly, Brendan D., *Hearing Voices: The History of Psychiatry in Ireland* (Dublin, 2016).

Kelly, Brendan D., 'Searching for the patient's voice in the Irish asylums', *Medical Humanities*, 42:2 (2016), pp. 87–91.

Kelly, James, 'Suicide in eighteenth-century Ireland', in James Kelly and Mary Ann Lyons (eds), *Death and Dying in Ireland, Britain and Europe* (Dublin, 2011), pp. 95–142.

Kelly, James, ' "An Unnatural Crime": infanticide in early nineteenth-century Ireland', *Irish Economic & Social History*, 46:1 (2019), pp. 66–110.

Kelly, Laura, *Irish Women in Medicine, c.1880s–1920s: Origins, Education and Careers* (Manchester, 2012).

Kelly, Laura, *Irish Medical Education and Student Culture, c.1850–1950* (Liverpool, 2017).

Kern, Leslie, *Feminist City: Claiming Space in a Man-Made World* (London, 2020).

King, Peter, *Crime and Law in England 1750–1850: Remaking Justice from the Margins* (Cambridge, 2006).

King, Steven, *Writing the Lives of the English Poor, 1750s–1830s* (Montreal, 2019).

Kleinberg, S.J., 'Women's employment in the public and private spheres, 1880–1920', *DQR Studies in Literature: Leiden*, 45 (2010), pp. 81–103.

Laite, Julia, *Common Prostitutes and Ordinary Citizens: Commercial Sex in London, 1885–1960* (London, 2011).

Langhamer, Claire, 'A public house is for all classes, men and women alike': women, leisure and drink in Second World War England', *Women's History Review*, 12:3 (2003), pp. 423–43.

Langhamer, Claire, *The English in Love: The Intimate Story of an Emotional Revolution* (Oxford, 2013).

Langhamer, Claire, ' "Who the hell are ordinary people?" Ordinariness as a category of historical analysis', *Transactions of the Royal Historical Society*, 28 (2018), pp. 175–95.

Laragy, Georgina, 'Suicide and insanity in post-Famine Ireland', in Catherine Cox and Maria Luddy (eds), *Cultures of Care in Irish Medical History, 1750–1970* (Basingstoke, 2010), pp. 79–91.

Laragy, Georgina, '"A peculiar species of felony": suicide, medicine, and the law in Victorian Britain and Ireland', *Journal of Social History*, 46:3 (2013), pp. 732–43.

Laragy, Georgina, 'Locating investigations into suicidal deaths in urban Ireland, 1901–1915', in Georgina Laragy, Olwen Purdue, and Jonathan Jeffery Wright (eds), *Urban Spaces in Nineteenth-Century Ireland* (Liverpool, 2018), pp. 144–61.

Leckey, Joseph J., 'The railway servants' strike in Co. Cork, 1898', *Saothar*, 2 (1976), pp. 39–45.

Lee, Joseph, 'On the accuracy of the pre-Famine Irish censuses', in J.M. Goldstrom and L.A. Clarkson (ed.), *Irish Population, Economy, and Society: Essays in Honour of the Late K.H. Connell* (Oxford, 1981), pp. 37–56.

Legg, Marie Louise, *Newspapers and Nationalism: The Irish Provincial Press, 1850–1892* (Dublin, 1999).

Lemire, Beverly, *The Business of Everyday Life: Gender, Practice and Social Politics in England, c.1600–1900* (Manchester, 2006).

Lomas, Janis, '"Delicate duties": issues of class and respectability in government policy towards the wives and widows of British soldiers in the era of the great war', *Women's History Review*, 9:1 (2000), pp. 123–47.

Loughnan, Arlie, '"Strange" case of the infanticide doctrine', *Oxford Journal of Legal Studies*, 32: 4 (2012), pp. 685–711.

Love, Christopher, *A Social History of Swimming in England, 1800–1918: Splashing in the Serpentine* (Abingdon, 2015).

Luckin, Bill, 'Drunk driving, drink driving: Britain, c.1800–1920', in Tom Crook and Mike Esbester (eds), *Governing Risks in Modern Britain: Danger, Safety and Accidents, c.1800–2000* (Basingstoke, 2016), pp. 171–94.

Luddy, Maria, *Prostitution and Irish society, 1800–1940* (Cambridge, 2007).

Lumsden, John, *An Investigation into the Income and Expenditure of Seventeen Brewery Families and a Study of their Diets* (Dublin, 1905).

Lynch, Patrick and John Vaisey, *Guinness's Brewery in the Irish Economy 1759–1876* (Cambridge, 2011).

Lyons, Martyn, *The Writing Culture of Ordinary People in Europe, c.1860–1920* (Cambridge, 2012).

McCabe, Ciarán, *Begging, Charity and Religion in Pre-Famine Ireland* (Liverpool, 2018).

McCabe, Ciarán, 'Humane society movement and the transnational exchange of medical knowledge', *Journal of the Royal College of Physicians of Edinburgh*, 49: 2 (2019), pp. 158–64.

McCarthy, P. Desmond and Dermot Walsh, 'Suicide in Dublin', *The British Medical Journal*, 1:5500 (4 June 1966), pp. 1393–6.

McCormick, Leanne, 'No sense of wrongdoing': abortion in Belfast 1917–1967', *Journal of Social History*, 49:1 (2015), pp. 125–48.

McDevitt, Patrick F., 'Muscular Catholicism: nationalism, masculinity and Gaelic team sports, 1884–1916', *Gender & History*, 9:2 (1997), pp. 262–84.

MacDonald, Ian, 'Picric acid in superficial burns', *The British Medical Journal*, 1:2002 (13 May 1899), p. 1152.

MacDonald, Michael, 'The secularization of suicide in England 1660–1800', *Past & Present*, 111 (1986), pp. 50–100.

McGarry, Fearghal, *The Rising: Ireland Easter 1916* (Oxford, 2017).

McHugh, Sarah, 'The institutional care of Ireland's elderly women, 1845–1908' (unpublished PhD thesis, Queen's University Belfast, 2021).

McIntosh, Gillian, 'Children, street trading and the representation of public space in Edwardian Ireland' in Maria Luddy and James Smith (eds), *Children, Childhood and Irish Society* (Dublin, 2014), pp. 46–64.

Mackenzie, Suzanne, 'Women in the city', in Richard Preet and Nigel Thrift (eds), *New Models in Geography: The Political-Economy Perspective* (London, 1989), pp. 109–26.

MacLeod, Christine and Alessandro Nuvolari, 'The pitfalls of prosopography: inventors in the "Dictionary of National Biography" ', *Technology and Culture*, 47:4 (2006), pp. 757–76.

McMahon, Richard, *Homicide in Pre-Famine and Famine Ireland* (Liverpool, 2013).

McMahon, Richard, Joachim Eibach, and Randolph Roth Source, 'Making sense of violence? Reflections on the history of interpersonal violence in Europe', *Crime, Histoire & Sociétés/Crime, History & Societies*, 17:2 (2013), pp. 5–26.

McManus, Ruth, 'Dublin's lodger phenomenon in the early twentieth century', *Irish Economic and Social History*, 45:1 (2018), pp. 23–46.

Magnússon, Gylfi Sigurður and István M. Szijártó, *What is Microhistory? Theory and Practice* (London, 2013).

Markwick, A., 'Treacle, a remedy for burns and scalds', *Provincial Medical & Surgical Journal (1844–1852)*, 11:26 (29 December 1847), p. 710.

Marsh, Patricia, *The Spanish Flu in Ireland: A Socio-Economic Shock to Ireland, 1918–1919* (London, 2021).

Mauger, Alice, ' "The Holy War Against Alcohol": alcoholism, medicine and psychiatry in Ireland, c.1890–1921', in Steven J. Taylor and Alice Brumby (eds), *Healthy Minds in the Twentieth Century: Mental Health in Historical Perspective* (Basingstoke, 2020), pp. 17–51.

Maume, Patrick, 'The Head Pacificator and Captain Rock: sedition, suicide and Honest Tom Steele', in Kyle Hughes and Donald MacRaild (eds), *Crime, Violence and the Irish in the Nineteenth Century* (Liverpool, 2017).

Miller, R. Shalders, Treatment of superficial burns and scalds, *The British Medical Journal*, 2:1868 (17 October 1896), p. 1168.

Milne, Ida, *Stacking the Coffins: The 1918–19 Flu Pandemic in Ireland* (Manchester, 2018).

Mokyr, Joel, *Why Ireland Starved: A Quantitative and Analytical History of the Irish* (London, 2005).

Mooney, Graham, *Intrusive Interventions: Public Health, Domestic Space, and Infectious Disease Surveillance in England 1840–1914* (Rochester, 2015).

Moss, Stella, 'Manly drinkers : masculinity and material culture in the interwar public house', in Jane Hamlett, Hannah Greig, and Leonie Hannan (eds), *Gender and Material Culture in Britain since 1600* (Basingstoke, 2015), pp. 138–52.

Mulholland, Marie, *The Politics and Relationships of Kathleen Lynn* (Dublin, 2002).

Munter, Robert, *The History of the Irish Newspaper, 1685–1760* (Cambridge, 1967).

Murphy, Francis J., 'Dublin trams 1872 1959', *Dublin Historical Record*, 33:1 (1979), pp. 2–9.

Murphy, James H., *The Politics of Dublin Corporation 1840–1900* (Dublin, 2020).

Murphy, John A. and Clíona Murphy, 'Burials and bigotry in early nineteenth-century Ireland', *Studia Hibernica*, 33 (2004/5), pp. 125–46.

Murphy, William, *Political Imprisonment and the Irish, 1912–1921* (Oxford, 2014).

Murray, Alexander, *Suicide in the Middle Ages: Volume 2: The Curse on Self-Murder* (Oxford, 2011).

Murray, Christopher, 'O'Casey and the city', in Nicolas Green and Chris Morash (eds), *The Oxford Handbook of Modern Irish Theatre* (Oxford, 2016), pp. 183–200.

NA, Proceedings of the Catholic Association in Dublin, 13 May 1823 to 11 February (London, 1825).

NA, *A Statistical Nosology, Comprising the Causes of Death, Classified and Alphabetically Arranged, with Notes and Observations* (Dublin, 1864).

NA, *Brennan v The Dublin United Tramways Company* [1901], 2 IR 241.

NA, *The Medical Directory The medical directory for [date] and general medical register, including The London and provincial medical directory, The medical directory for Scotland, The medical directory for Ireland, with a medical directory of the Army, Navy, and Mercantile Marine, a medical directory of registered practitioners resident abroad; also statistical and general information respecting the universities, colleges, schools, hospitals, dispensaries, societies, poor-law service, asylums for the insane, public services, &c., in the United Kingdom* (London, 1870–1910).

NA, *Thom's Irish Almanac and Official Directory of the United Kingdom of Great Britain and Ireland for the year, 1901, fifty eight annual publication* (Dublin, 1901).

NA, 'Docks as factories and the Workmen's Compensation Act – Hanlon v. North City Milling Company', *New Irish Jurist and Local Government Review*, 2 (1902), pp. 74–5.

NA, *Bulletin of the Bureau of Labor, Issues 50–55* (U.S. Government Printing Office, 1904).

NA, *Trial of Theobald Wolfe Tone for High Treason, before a Court Martial holden at Dublin on Saturday, November 10th, together with the Proceedings in the Court of King's Bench on Monday, November 12th*: 27 St Tr 613.

NA, The book of common-prayer, and administration of the sacraments, and other rites & ceremonies of the Church, according to the use of the Church of Ireland; together with the Psalter or Psalms of David, pointed as they are to be sung or said in churches. And the form and manner of making, ordaining, and consecrating of bishops, priests, & deacons Date: 1680 (TCD, http://gateway.proquest.com.proxy.lib.ul.ie/openurl?ctx_ver=Z39.88-2003& res_id=xri:eebo&rft_id=xri:eebo:image:31220:159).

Nash, David S., 'Towards an agenda for the wider study of shame: theorising from nine-teenth-century British evidence', in Judith Rowbotham, Marianna Muravyeva, and David Nash (eds), *Shame, Blame, and Culpability: Crime and Violence in the Modern State* (London, 2013), pp. 43–60.

Nash, David S. and Anne-Marie Kilday (eds), *Law, Crime and Deviance since 1700: Micro-Studies in the History of Crime* (London, 2016).

Naylor, I.L, B. Curtis, and J.J.R. Kirkpatrick, 'Treatment of bum scars and contractures in the early seventeenth century: Wilhelm Fabry's approach', *Medical History*, 40 (1996), pp. 472–86.

Nugent, Joseph, 'The sword and the prayerbook: ideals of authentic Irish manliness', *Victorian Studies*, 50:4 (2008), pp. 587–613.

Nugent, Joseph, 'The human snout: pigs, priests, and peasants in the parlor', *The Senses and Society*, 4:3 (2009), pp. 283–301.

Ó Gráda, Cormac, *Ireland Before and After the Famine: Explorations in Economic History, 1800–1925* (Manchester, 1993).

Ó Gráda, Cormac, *Jewish Ireland in the Age of Joyce: A Socioeconomic History* (Princeton, 2006).

Ó hÓgartaigh, Margaret, *Kathleen Lynn: Irishwoman, Patriot, Doctor* (Dublin, 2006).

O'Keeffe, Tadhg and Patrick Ryan, 'At the world's end: the lost landscape of Monto, Dublin's notorious red-light district', *Landscapes*, 10:1 (2009), pp. 21–38.

Ó Maonaigh, Aaron, '"Who were the Shoneens?": Irish militant nationalists and Association Football, 1913–1923', *Soccer & Society*, 18:5–6 (2017), pp. 631–47.

Osborough, W.N., 'Roman law in Ireland', *Irish Jurist*, 25/27 (1990/1992), pp. 212–68.

Paton, D. Noel, James C. Dunlop, and Maud Inglis, *Studies of the Diet of the Labouring Classes in Edinburgh: Carried Out Under the Auspices of the Town Council of the City of Edinburgh* (Edinburgh, 1901).

Perry, Reverend Joseph N., 'The right of ecclesiastical burial', *The Catholic Lawyer*, 28:4 (1983), 315–35.

Picker, John, 'The soundproof study', in John Streane (ed.), *The Sound Studies Reader* (Abingdon, 2012), pp. 141–51.

Pierce, Michael, 'The shadow of Seán: O'Casey, commitment and writing Dublin's working class', *Saothar*, 35 (2010), pp. 69–85.

Prunty, Jacinta, *Dublin's Slums 1800–1925: A Study in Urban Geography* (Dublin, 1998).

Purdue, Simon, 'Giving life and limb for empire: gender and occupational health in industrial Belfast, 1870–1914', *Irish Historical Studies*, 43:164 (2019), pp. 220–36.

Rabinow, Paul and Nikolas Rose, 'Biopower today', *BioSocieties*, 1 (2006), pp. 195–217.

Rains, Stephanie, *Commodity Culture and Social Class in Dublin 1850–1916* (Dublin, 2010).

Rattigan, Clíona, *What Else Could I Do? Single Mothers and Infanticide, Ireland 1900–1950* (Dublin, 2012).

Reay, Barry, *Microhistories: Demography, Society, and Culture in Rural England, 1800–1930* (Cambridge, 1996).

Reddy, William, *The Navigation of Feeling: A Framework for the History of Emotions* (Cambridge, 2001).

Reidy, Conor, *Criminal Irish Drunkards: The Inebriate Reformatory System 1900–1920* (Dublin, 2014).

Robinson, Michael, *Shell-Shocked British Army Veterans in Ireland, 1918–39: A Difficult Homecoming* (Manchester, 2018).

Rose, Gillian, 'Engendering the slum: photography in East London in the 1930s', *Gender, Place and Culture: A Journal of Feminist Geography*, 4:3 (1997), pp. 277–300.

Rose, Nikolas and Carlos Novas, 'Biological citizenship', in Aihwa Ong and Stephen J. Collier (eds), *Global Assemblages: Technology, Politics, and Ethics as Anthropological Problems* (Oxford, 2004).

Rouse, Paul, *The Hurlers: The First All-Ireland Championship and the Making of Modern Hurling* (Dublin, 2018).

Rowbotham, Judith, 'The shifting nature of blame', in Judith Rowbotham, Marianna Muravyeva, and David Nash (eds), *Shame, Blame, and Culpability: Crime and Violence in the Modern State* (London, 2013), pp. 64–79.

Rowley, Gwyn, 'British fire insurance plans: the Goad productions c.1885–c.1970', *Archives*, 17:74 (1985), pp. 67–78.

Rutherford, Vanessa, 'Muscles and morals: children's playground culture in Ireland, 1836–1918', in Leeann Lane and William Murphy (eds), *Leisure and the Irish in the Nineteenth Century* (Liverpool, 2016), pp. 61–79.

Rychner, Georgina, 'Defences to intimate partner homicide: historicising the relationship between provocation and temporary insanity in Victoria, Australia', *Law & History: Journal of the Australian and New Zealand Law and History Society*, 8:1 (2021), pp. 106–33.

Samuel, Raphael, *Theatres of Memory: Past and Present in Contemporary Culture* (London, 1996).

Schafer, R. Murray, *The Soundscape: Our Sonic Environment and the Tuning of the World* (New York, 1993).

Seebohm Rowntree, Benjamin, *A Study of Town Life* (London, 1901).

Sim, Joe and Tony Ward, 'The magistrate of the poor? Coroners and deaths in custody in nineteenth-century England', in Michael Clark and Catherine Crawford (eds), *Legal Medicine in History* (Cambridge, 1994), pp. 245–67.

Simmonds, Alecia, 'Legal records', in Katie Barclay, Sharon Crozier-De Rosa, and Peter N. Stearns (eds), *Sources for the History of Emotions: A Guide* (London, 2020), pp. 79–90.

Sokoll, Thomas, *Essex Pauper Letters, 1731–1837* (Oxford, 2001).

Steiner-Scott, Elizabeth, '"To bounce a boot off her now and then": domestic violence in post-Famine Ireland', in Maryann Valiulis and Mary O'Dowd (eds), *Women in Irish History: Essays in Honour of Margaret MacCurtain* (Dublin, 1997), pp. 125–43.

Stewart, D., 'Dublin City passenger transport services', *Journal of the Statistical and Social Inquiry Society of Ireland* (1955), p. 136.

Stone, Lawrence, 'Prosopography', *Daedalus, Historical Studies Today*, 100:1 (1971), pp. 46–79.

Szreter, Simon, 'Populations for studying the causes of Britain's fertility decline: communication communities', in P. Kreager, B. Winney, S. Uilaszek, and C. Capelli (eds), *Population in the Human Sciences: Concepts, Models, Evidence* (Oxford, 2015), pp. 172–95.

Tait, Clodagh, *Death, Burial and Commemoration in Ireland, 1550–1650* (Basingstoke, 2002).

Tarlow, Sarah and Emma Battell Lowman, *Harnessing the Power of the Criminal Corpse* (Basingstoke, 2018).

Tarr, Joel A. and Mark Tebeau, 'Housewives as home safety managers: the changing perception of the home as a place of hazard and risk, 1870–1940', in Roger Cooter and Bill Luckin (eds), *Accidents in History: Injuries, Fatalities and Social Relations* (Amsterdam, 1997), pp. 196–233.

Thomas, David, 'The Hackney Carriage in Cork: vehicle of a Victorian Irish city 1854–1902', *Irish Economic and Social History*, 45:1 (2018), pp. 136–54.

Thompson, E.P., *The Making of the English Working Class* (London, 1963).

Tosh, John, 'What should historians do with masculinity? Reflections on nineteenth-century Britain', *History Workshop Journal*, 38 (1994), pp. 179–202.

Turner, E.B., 'A report on cycling in health and disease: VIII. Training and racing', *The British Medical Journal*, 2:1854 (11 July 1896), pp. 98–9.

Turner, E.B., 'A report on cycling in health and disease: IX. Cycling accidents', *The British Medical Journal*, 2:1856 (25 July 1896), p. 203.

Urquhart, Diane, 'Irish divorce and domestic violence, 1857–1922', *Women's History Review*, 22:5 (2013), pp. 820–37.

Vaughan, William E., *Murder Trials in Ireland, 1836–1914* (Dublin, 2009).

Veblen, Thorstein, *The Theory of the Leisure Class: An Economic Study of Institutions* (New York, 1899).

Vickery, Amanda, 'Golden Age to Separate Spheres? A review of the categories and chronology of English women's history', *The Historical Journal*, 36:2 (1993), pp. 383–414.

Wallace, Ciarán, 'Civil society in search of a state: Dublin 1898–1922', *Urban History*, 45:3 (2018), pp. 426–52.

Walsh, Brendan, 'Life expectancy in Ireland since the 1870s', *The Economic and Social Review*, 48:2 (2017), pp. 127–43.

Walsh, Dermot, 'Suicide in Ireland in the 19th century', *Irish Journal of Psychological Medicine*, 34:3 (2017), pp. 177–81.

Walsh, Fionnuala, *Irish Women and the Great War* (Cambridge, 2020).

Walsh, Oonagh, 'Cure or custody: therapeutic philosophy at the Connaught District Lunatic Asylum', in Margaret Preston and Margaret Ó hÓgartaigh (eds), *Gender and Medicine in Ireland, 1700–1950* (Syracuse, 2012).

Weaver, John C., *Sadly Troubled History: The Meanings of Suicide in the Modern Age* (Montreal, 2009).

Wessling, Mary, 'Infanticide trials and forensic medicine: Wurttemberg', in Michael Clark and Catherine Crawford (eds), *Legal Medicine in History* (Cambridge, 1994), pp. 117–45.

Whitehead, Trevor, *Dublin Fire Fighters: A History of Fire Fighting, Rescue, and Ambulance work in the City of Dublin* (Dublin, 1970).

Wiener, Martin J., *Men of Blood: Violence, Manliness, and Criminal Justice in Victorian England* (Cambridge, 2012).

Wiggins, Deborah, 'The Burial Act of 1880, The Liberation Society and George Osborne Morgan', *Parliamentary History*, 15:2 (1996), pp. 173–89.

Wise, Sarah, *The Blackest Streets: The Life and Death of a Victorian Slum* (London, 2009).

Wolf, Nicholas, *An Irish-Speaking Island: State, Religion, Community, and the Linguistic Landscape in Ireland, 1770–1870* (Madison, 2014).

Wright, Charlotte, 'The English Canon Law relating to suicide victims', *Ecclesiastical Law Society*, 19 (2017), pp. 193–211.

Index